GLOBAL VIEW OF HIV INFECTION

Edited by **Vishwanath Venketaraman**

Global View of HIV Infection
Edited by Vishwanath Venketaraman

Published by InTech

Janeza Trdine 9, 51000 Rijeka, Croatia

Publishing Process Manager Alenka Urbancic

Technical Editor Teodora Smiljanic

Cover Designer InTech Design Team

Additional hard copies can be obtained from orders@intechopen.com

Global View of HIV Infection, Edited by Vishwanath Venketaraman
p. cm.
978-953-307-671-3

For EU product safety concerns:
IN TECH d.o.o., Prolaz Marije Krucifikse Kozulić 3, 51000 Rijeka, Croatia,
info@intechopen.com or visit our website at intechopen.com.

Meet the editor

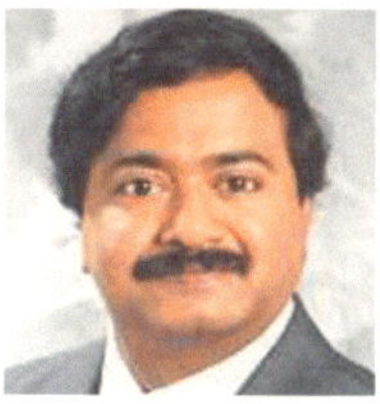

Upon completion of his doctorate in microbiology and immunology at the Tuberculosis Research Center in Chennai, India, Dr. Venketaraman was awarded a UNESCO fellowship to conduct post-doctoral research on tuberculosis at the University of Ferrara, Italy. Dr. Venketaraman continued his post-doctoral research at the University of Michigan Medical School and at the UMDNJ-New Jersey Medical School. Mycobacterial research has always fascinated Dr. Venketaraman, especially in characterization of the host immune defense mechanisms that are crucial for the control of Mycobacterium tuberculosis. Dr. Venketaraman has published more than 22 papers in peer-reviewed journals, and is currently an Assistant Professor at the College of Osteopathic Medicine of Pacific, Western University of Health Sciences, CA. His laboratory is actively trying to elucidate the role of glutathione in enhancing the host immune cell functions to control of Mycobacterium tuberculosis, a novel and previously undescribed phenomenon. More than eight publications were generated from this body of work. Most notably, the study on glutathione enhancing the functions of natural killer cells to control Mycobacterium tuberculosis infection, which was published in 2008 issue of "Journal of Interferon and cytokine research" and later cited in "Natural Immunology" as well as appeared on the cover page of the recent issue of "Journal of Interferon and Cytokine research" (March 2010). Dr. Venketaraman's long term goal is to discover immunomodulatory agents that can be given an adjunct to chemotherapy for controlling Mycobacterium tuberculosis infections in both non-HIV and HIV-infected individuals.

Contents

Preface

Both HIV-1 and HIV-2 cause AIDS, but HIV-1 is found worldwide, whereas HIV-2 is found primarily in West Africa.

It is estimated that approximately 40 million people worldwide are infected with HIV, and two-thirds of them live in the sub-Saharan Africa. Three regions, Africa, Asia, and Latin America, have the highest rates of new infections, and AIDS is the fourth leading cause of death worldwide. Since 1981, more than 980,000 cases of AIDS have been reported in the US alone, and according to CDC, more than 1,000,000 Americans may be infected with HIV.

HIV preferentially infects and kills CD4+ T lymphocytes, and by killing or damaging CD4+ T cells of the body's immune system, HIV progressively destroys the body's ability to fight infections. People diagnosed with AIDS often suffer from life-threatening diseases caused by opportunistic infections. HIV also infects other cells, such as macrophages, monocytes and dendritic cells.

This book provides a detailed overview on the HIV transmission, how HIV infection alters the host immune responses, and on the prevention and treatment of AIDS related diseases.

Vishwanath Venketaraman Ph.D.,
Assistant Professor
Microbiology/Immunology,
Department of Basic Medical Sciences,
College of Osteopathic Medicine of the Pacific,
Western University of Health Sciences
United States

Part 1

HIV and Altered Immune Responses

1

Infection for *Mycobacterium tuberculosis* and Nontuberculous Mycobacteria in the HIV/AIDS Patients

Lilian María Mederos Cuervo
National Reference Laboratory TB/Mycobacteria Collaborate Center PAHO / WHO
Tropical Medicine Institute Pedro Kourí (IPK)
Cuba

1. Introduction

Tuberculosis (TB) is a disease also know as consumption, wasting disease, and the white plague, it has affected humans for centuries. Until the mid-1800s, people thought that tuberculosis, or TB, was hereditary. They did not realize that it could be spread from person to person through the air. Also, until the 1940s and 1950s there was no cure for TB. For many people, a diagnosis of TB was a slow death sentence [1-4].

In 1865 a French surgeon, Jean-Antoine Villemin, proved that TB was contagious, and in 1882 a german scientist named Robert Koch discovered the bacteria causes TB, denominated as *Mycobacterium tuberculosis*. Yet half a century passed before drugs were discovered that could cure TB, until then, many people with TB were sent to sanatoriums, special rest homes where they followed a prescribed routine every day. A breakthrough came in 1943, an american scientist, Selman Waksman discovered a drug that could kill TB bacteria. Between 1943 and 1952, two more drugs were found, after these discoveries, many people with TB were cured and the death rate for TB in the United States dropped dramatically, and fewer and fewer people got TB [5].

A global health emergency [6, 7]:

- Someone in the world is newly infected with TB bacilli every second.
- Overall, one-third of the world's population is currently infected with the TB bacillus.
- 5-10 % of people who are infected with TB bacilli become sick or infectious at some time during their life.

TB program activities, reinforced by successful chemotherapy, resulted in a pronounced reduction of infection and death rates. The disease became greatly controlled but it never quite disappeared. Then, in around 1985, cases of TB began to rise again in industrialized countries. Several inter-related forces drove this resurgence, including increase in prison populations, homelessness, injection drug use, crowded housing and increased immigration from countries where TB continued to be endemic. Above all, the decline in TB control activities and the human immunodeficiency virus/acquired immunodeficiency syndrome (HIV/AIDS) epidemic were two major factors fuelling each other in the re-emergence of TB. People with HIV and TB infection are much more likely to develop TB. The HIV/AIDS epidemic has produced a devastating effect on TB control worldwide. While one out of ten immunocompetent people infected with *M. tuberculosis* will fall sick in their lifetimes, among those with HIV infection, one in ten per year will develop active TB. In developing countries, the impact of HIV infection on the TB situation, especially in the 20-35 age groups, is overwhelming. While wealthy industrialized countries with good public health care systems can be expected to keep TB under control, in much of the developing world a catastrophe awaits. In poorly developed countries, TB remains a significant threat to public health, as incidences remain high, even after the introduction of vaccination and drug treatment. The registered number of new cases of TB worldwide roughly correlates with economic conditions: highest incidences are seen in the countries of Africa, Asia, and Latin America with the lowest gross national products. Supervised treatment, including sometimes direct observation of therapy (DOT), was proposed as a means of helping patients to take their drugs regularly and complete treatment, thus achieving cure and preventing the development of drug resistance [5-7].

2. Transmission and pathogenesis

TB is spread from person through the air. When a person with pulmonary or laryngeal TB coughs, sneezes, speaks, or sings, droplet nuclei containing *Mycobacterium tuberculosis* are expelled into the air. Depending on the environment, these tiny particles (1-5 microns in diameter) can remain suspended in the air for several hours. If another person inhales air containing droplet nuclei, transmission may occur. The probability that TB will be transmitted depends on these factors [4, 5]:

- The infectiousness of the person with TB (the number of organisms expelled into the air).
- The environment in which exposure occurred.
- The duration of exposure and the virulence of the organism.

The best way to stop transmission is to isolate patients with infectious TB immediately and start effective TB therapy. Infectiousness declines rapidly after adequate therapy is started, as long as the patient adheres to the prescribed regimen. Persons at the highest risk of becoming infected with *Mycobacterium tuberculosis* are close contacts, the persons who had prolonged, frequent, or intense contact with a person with infectious TB. Close contacts may be family members, roommates, friends, coworkers, or others. Data collected by CDC since 1987 show that infection rates have been relatively stable, ranging form 21-23% for the contacts of infectious TB patients [6-9]. Some people with infection develop TB disease. This disease develops when the immune system cannot keep the tubercle bacilli under control and the bacilli begin to multiply rapidly. The risk that TB disease will develop is higher for some people than for others [3, 10-12]. Among contacts of persons with drug-resistant TB, infection rates seem to be similar. However, because they may have a poor response to treatment persons with drug-resistant disease are often infectious for longer periods and therefore have the potential to infect more contacts [10-13].

Extra pulmonary TB is rarely contagious; however, transmission from extrapulmonary sites has been reported during aerosol-producing procedures, such as autopsies and tissue irrigation [14-16].

3. Pathogenesis

The tubercle bacilli that alveoli are ingested by alveolar macrophages, the majority of these bacilli are destroyed or inhibited. A small number multiply intracellulary and are released when the macrophages die. These bacilli can spread through the lymphatic channels to regional lymph nodes and then through the bloodstream to more distant tissues and organs, including areas in which TB disease is most likely to develop: the apices of the lung, the kidneys, the brain, and bone. Extracellular bacilli attract macrophages form the bloodstream. The immune response kills most of the bacilli, leading to the formation of a granuloma. At this point the person has TB infection, which can be detected by using the tuberculin skin test. It may take 2-10 weeks for the infected person to develop a positive reaction to the tuberculin skin test. Immune responses soon develop to kill the bacilli. Within 2-10 weeks after infection, the immune system is usually able to halt the multiplication of the tubercle bacilli, preventing further spread [4, 17-19].

In persons infected with *Mycobacterium tuberculosis* but that don't have TB disease cannot spread the infection to other people. TB infection in persons who does not have TB disease is not considered a case of TB and referred to as ¨latent TB infection¨. In some persons, TB bacilli overcome the defenses or the immune system and begin to multiply, resulting in the progression from TB infection to TB disease. This process may occur soon after or many years after infection. Some study demonstrated that approximately 5% of person who have been infected with *Mycobacterium tuberculosis* will develop TB disease in the first year or two after infection and another 5% will develop disease some time later in life. Recent infection (with the past 2 years) with *Mycobacterium tuberculosis* is therefore an important risk factor for progression to TB disease and in approximately 10% of persons with normal immune system who are infected with *Mycobacterium tuberculosis* , TB disease will develop at some point [5-7].

Some medical conditions increase the risk that TB infection will progress to disease. Some studies suggest that the risk is mayor in inmmunosuppressed patients, for example persons with Diabetes mellitus, prolonged therapy with corticosteroids, immunosuppressive therapy, certain types of cancer, severe kidney disease, injection of illicit drugs, and infection with Human Immunodeficient Virus (HIV) [2,3,12].

TB disease most commomly affects the lung, 73% of TB cases are exclusively pulmonary, and however, TB is a systemic disease and may also commonly occur in the following ways; as pleural effusion in the central nervous, lymphatic, or genitourinary systems, as disseminated disease (military TB). Also the infection for *Mycobacterium tuberculosis* can occur in the other body sites; in the breast, skin, or peritoneum [16,20-23]. Extrapulmonary TB is more common in immunosuppressed persons and in young children; meningoencephalitis TB, lymphatic TB and military disease are particularly common in immunosuppressed persons, in some case the extrapulmonary TB is often accompanied by pulmonary TB [3, 8, 16-23].

4. Epidemiology of TB

TB infection is one of the most common infections in the world. It is estimated that 30-60% of adults in developing countries have TB infection. Annually about 8-10 million people develop TB disease and 2-3 million people die of the disease. TB disease is the leading cause of death due to infectious disease around the world [24, 25]. When the health department learns about a new case of TB, it should take steps to ensure that the person receives appropriate treatment. Is very important that the health authorities should also start a contact investigation, this means interviewing a person who has TB disease to determinate who may have been exposed to TB, this person are screened for TB infection and disease [8, 26-28].

In order to the decrease in the number of TB cases reported annually is very important to comply three factors [29]:

- To increase federal resources for TB control and other public health efforts.
- To improve prevention and TB control programs in state and local health department.
- To Increase attention to ensuring that patients complete drug therapy through directly observed therapy (DOT).

In the control of TB disease is also important to know the Groups at High Risk for TB [29, 30]:

People at Higher Risk for Exposure or Infection:

- Close contacts of people with infectious TB disease.
- People born in areas of the world where TB is common.
- Elderly people.
- Low-income groups with poor access to health care, including homeless people.
- People who inject illicit drugs.
- People who live or work in residential facilities (Example: nursing correctional facilities).
- Other people who may be exposed to TB on the job.
- People in other groups as identified by local public health officials.

People at Higher Risk for TB disease:

- People with other medical conditions that can increase the risk for TB.
- People recently infected with *Mycobacterium tuberculosis.*
- People with chest x-ray suggestive of previous TB disease.
- People who inject illicit drugs.
- People with HIV infection.

Infection with HIV makes people susceptible to rapidly progressive tuberculosis; over 10 millions peoples are infected with both HIV and *Mycobacterium tuberculosis* [8].

TB in Children:

The occurrence of TB infection and disease in children provide important information about the spread of TB in homes and communities. When a child has TB infection or disease is important to learn if [29-31]:

- Recent TB transmition.
- Other adults and children in the household or community have probably been exposed to TB; if they are infected, they may develop TB disease in the future.

4.1 Drug-resistant tuberculosis

Drug-resistant TB is transmitted in the same way as drug-susceptible TB. The earlier outbreaks of multidrugs-resistant (MDR) TB support the findings that drug-resistant TB is no less infectious than drug-susceptible TB, although prolonged periods of infectiousness that often occur in the patients with drug-resistant TB may facililate transmission. Drug resistance was divided in two types; primary resistance and secondary or acquired resistance. Primary resistance develops in persons who are initially infected, with resistant organisms. Second resistance, or acquired resistance develops during TB therapy, either because the patient was treated with an inadequate regimen or because the patient did not take the prescribed regimen appropriately [27, 29, 32]. The MDR-TB are resistant to rifampicin and isoniazid drugs. Recently drug-resistant tuberculosis (XDR-TB) is defined as tuberculosis caused by a *Mycobacterium tuberculosis* strain that is resistant to at least rifampicin and isoniazid among the first-line antitubercular drugs (MDR-TB) in addition to resistance to any fluroquinolones and at least one of three second-line drugs, namely amikacin, kanamycin and/or capreomycin. Current studies have described XDR-TB strains from all continents. Worldwide prevalence of XDR-TB is estimated in 6.6% in all the studied countries among MDR-TB strains. The emergence of XDR-TB strains is a reflection of poor tuberculosis management, and controlling its emergence constitutes an urgent global health reality and a challenge to tuberculosis control activities in all parts of the world, especially in developing countries and those lacking resources and as well as in countries with increasing prevalence of HIV/AIDS [32-34].

5. Diagnosis of tuberculosis

The systemic symptom of Tuberculosis include fever, chills, night sweats, appetite loss, weigh loss, and easy fatigability, the symptoms of pulmonary TB are productive and prolonged cough (>14-21 week) , chest pain and in some case the patient present hemoptysis. It is important to ask persons suspected of having tuberculosis about their history of TB exposure, infection, or disease. The clinicians may also contact the local health department for information about whether a patient has received tuberculosis treatment in the past, if the drug regimen was inadequate or if the patient may did not adhere to therapy, this disease may recur and may be drug resistant. Also is important to consider demographic factors; country of origin, age, ethnic or racial group and occupation, this factors may increase the patient's risk for exposure to TB or drug-resistant TB disease. Clinicians should determinate whether the patient has medical conditions, especially HIV infection, because this infection increases the risk for TB disease. All patients who do not know their current HIV status should be referred for HIV counseling and testing [26, 27].
The tuberculin skin test and the chest radiography, are two probes that help in the diagnostic for TB disease. Tuberculin skin testing useful for [29]:

- To examine a person who is not ill but may be infected with *Mycobacterium tuberculosis,* such as a person who has been exposed to someone who has TB. This test is the only way to diagnose tuberculosis infection before it has progressed to tuberculosis disease.
- To determine how many people in group are infected with *Mycobacterium tuberculosis.*
- To examine person who has symptoms of TB.

A negative reaction to the tuberculin skin test does not exclude the diagnosis of TB, especially for patients with severe TB illness or infection with HIV. Some persons may not react to the tuberculin skin test if they are tested too soon after being exposed to the infection. Generally it takes 2-10 week after infection for a person to develop an immune response to tuberculin. In children younger than 6 months of age may not react to the tuberculin skin test because their immune systems are not yet fully developed [32].

5.1 Chest radiography

The chest radiography is for:

- To detect abnormalities often seen in apical or posterior segments of upper lobe or superior segments of lower lobe.
- To detect atypical images in immunosuppressed persons an in HIV-positive persons.

In HIV-infected persons, pulmonary TB may appear in the chets radiograph. For example; TB disease may cause infiltrates without cavities in any lung zone, or it may cause mediastinal or hiliar lymphadenophaty with or without accompanying infiltrates and/or cavities. In HIV-positive persons, almost any abnormality on a chest radiographic may indicate TB. In fact, the radiograph of an HIV-positive person with TB disease may even appear entirely normal. Abnormalities on chest radiographs may be suggestive of, but are never diagnostic of TB. However, chest radiographic may be used to rule out the possibility of pulmonary TB in a person who has a positive reaction to the tuberculin skin test and no symptoms of disease [29, 31, 32, 34].

Summarizing the possibility of TB should be considered in persons who have these symptoms, person suspected of having this disease should be referred for a medical evaluation, which should include a medical history, a physical examination, a Mantoux tuberculin skin test or tuberculosis purified protein derivate (PPD) skin test, a chest radiograph. Also, it is very important any appropriate bacteriologic or histological examinations in this patients, principally in all inmmunosuppressed patients, of course including the HIV patients [29].

Person with symptoms of TB pulmonary disease should have at least three sputum specimens examined by smear and culture. The bets way would be to get serial specimens collected early in the morning on 3 consecutive days. A health care worked should be prepared and directly supervise at least during the first time sputum collection. This personal should give properly instructed in how to produce a good specimen, the patients should be informed that sputum is the material brought up form the lungs and that mucus from the nose or throat and saliva are not good specimens [35, 36].

Recommends for Specimen Collection:

- Get 3 sputum specimens for smear examination and culture.
- In persons unable to cough up sputum, induce sputum, bronchoscopy or gastric aspiration.
- Before chemotherapy and drug therapy is started.
- To use clean, sterile, one-use, plastic, disposable containers that have been washed with dichromate sulfuric acid and sterilized.
- To transport specimens to the laboratory as soon as possible.

5.2 Laboratory examination

Detection of acid-fast bacilli (AFB) in stained smears examined microscopically may provide the first bacteriologic of TB. The traditional method for to detect AFB is the Zielh-Neelsen coloration, it is a method more economic. There are other methods that increased sensitivity as fluorescent methods. Smear examination is an easy and quick procedure, because the results should be available within 24 hours of specimen collection. However, smear examination permits only the presumptive diagnosis of TB because many TB patients have negative AFB smears. The sensitivity of smear examination may be reduced if the directed inflammatory response and relative absence of cavitary lesions results in fewer organisms expectorated in sputum. There has been concern that the utility of sputum acid-fast smears may be reduced in HIV-infected populations [36, 37].

5.3 Extrapulmonary TB disease

This disease is not taking in account as causative agent of an extrapulmonary disease because the chest radiography is normal or tuberculin skin test is negative, or both. Mycobacteria may infect almost any organ in the body, the laboratory should expect to receive a variety of extrapulmonary specimens: aseptically collected body fluids, surgically excised tissue, aspirated or draining pus, and urine. Others ascetically collected specimens are the body fluids as spinal, pleural, pericardial, synovial, ascetic, blood, pus, and bone marrow are aseptically collected by the physician using aspiration techniques or surgical procedure. Acid-fast bacilli may be difficult to isolate from some of these specimens because they often are diluted by the large fluid volume [16-19, 37-39].

The identification of TB can be done by traditional culture materials include egg-based solid media, such as Löwenstein-Jensen medium, and synthetic solid media as Middlebrook 7H10 and 7H11 agars. The identification depends on the visualization of mycobacterial colonies and is limited by the slow growth rate of these organisms. A major advance in laboratory diagnosis of TB has been the development of systems based on detecting growth in liquid media with the use of radiometric methods as Bactec System. In this, the medium contains palmitic acid labeled with carbon-14. The metabolism of this fatty acid by growing mycobacteria liberates radioactive carbon dioxide, periodic sampling of the gasses in the culture-containing flask permits rapid detection of mycobacterial growth [40-41].

Species identification was accomplished with biochemical test that often involved additional diagnostic delays. Others techniques, currently being evaluated in a number of clinical settings include identification based on chromatography techniques for the studies of some specific lipids present in the wall of *Mycobacterium* [42, 43]. Also genetic probes are now availed for the identification of *Mycobacterium tuberculosis* and several other common mycobacterial species. These probes recognize species-specific sequences of ribosomal RNA. Theoretically, genetic probe as polymerase chain reaction (PCR), may permit diagnosis directly form patients specimens, eliminating the need for culture of organism. In practice, the utility of PCR has been limited by problems with the sensitivity and particularly, the specificity of results. In some laboratories, the sensitivity and specificity have been reported to exceed 85%. However, in several laboratories, false-positive rates ranged from 3% to 20%, and in one, 77% of positive results were false. In the last time the Genotype Mycobacteria Direct Assay (GTMD), a novel commercial assay based on nucleic acid sequence-based amplification technology, was evaluated for detection of *Mycobacterium tuberculosis* complex and some atypical mycobacterial species from clinical samples, and your sensitivity, specificity, positive predictive, and negative predictive were evaluated and these results were more better [44-46].

6. Nontuberculous mycobacteria in the environment

Environmental opportunistic mycobacteria are those that are recovered form natural and human influenced environments and can infect and cause disease in humans, animals, and birds. Other names for these mycobacteria are nontuberculous, however, they cause tuberculous lesions, also other name is atypical mycobacterial, it distinguish from "typical" *Mycobacterium tuberculosis,* and them nontuberculous mycobacteria (NTM). The environmental opportunistic mycobacteria are normal inhabitants of natural waters, drinking water, and soils. They can be isolated from biofilms, aerosol, and dusts. The distribution of NTM and the incidence of disease caused by them is perhaps are not fully understood in most parts of the world. NTM are widely distributed in nature and have been isolated from natural water, rap water, tap water, and water used in showers and surgical solutions [47-51].

It is common observation that environmental mycobacteria cause disease in individuals who offer some opportunity due to altered local or systemic immunity. Chronic obstructive pulmonary diseases, emphysema, pneumoconiosis, bronchiectasis, cystic fibrosis, thoracic scoliosis, aspiration due to esophageal disease, previous gastrectomy and chronic alcoholism are some of conditions which have been linked to disease due to NTM. While the reasons may be less clear in conditions like adenitis in children, such factors may be quite obvious in other conditions like bronchiectasis, surgical procedures, injections, break in skin surface due to wounds and generalized immune deficiency states like AIDS, use of immunosuppressive agents as used in transplant patients, etc [50, 51].

6.1 Pathogenesis

The mechanisms of pathogenesis of NTM are not very clear and have not been adequately investigated. Very low CD4 counts and defective cytokine response have been linked to severe infections in AIDS patients [50].

Nontuberculous mycobacteria have been reported to cause localized or disseminated disease depending on local predisposition and/or degree of immune deficit. In non-HIV patients, different NTM may cause localized pulmonary disease, adenitis, soft tissue infections, infections of joints and bones, bursae, skin ulcers and generalized disease in individuals like leukemia, transplant patients, etc. In AIDS patients the manifestations may range from localized to disseminated disease. Clinical features will include local organ specific signs and symptoms to persistent high grade fever, night sweats, anemia and weight loss in addition to nonspecific symptoms of malaise, anorexia, diarrhea, myalgia and occasional painful adenopathy [52-57].

7. Epidemiology of human infection with nontuberculous mycobacteria

The frequency of NTM pulmonary disease has been reported to be increasing on several continents. Changing patient populations, most notably from infection with HIV, have greatly increased the numbers of people at risk [57-60]. Studies addressing the epidemiology of NTM infection may be broadly divided into three types: cutaneous delayed-type hypersensitivity to NTM antigens has been used to study large samples of people in many countries. These studies have the strength of providing information regarding simple infection in large groups of people but suffer from the lack of information regarding the prevalence of disease. Another drawback of this study type reflects the relatively poor specificity of the skin test, as well as overlap in reactivity among various Mycobacterial species. The second useful type of epidemiologic study of NMT infection includes investigations reviewing consecutive isolates from a mycobacterial laboratory. In the presence of adequate laboratory protocols to avoid contamination with environmental organisms, these studies provide unequivocal evidence of infection but have the obvious shortcoming of a lack of clinical data, preventing the assessment regarding the presence or absence of disease. The final and most useful study type combines information from the mycobacterial laboratory and the clinician's assessment [55-62].

A true increase in rates of infection and disease could be related to the host, the pathogen, or some interaction between the two. Host changes leading to increased numbers of susceptibility could play an important role, with increased numbers of patients with inadequate defenses from diseases such as HIV infection, malignancy, or simply advanced age. Many investigations have observed decreasing rates of TB concomitant with the increases in NTM. Finally, an interaction between the host and pathogen could involve a major increase in pathogen exposure or potential inoculum size [63-67].

7.1 Clinical manifestations

Environmental opportunist or nontuberculous mycobacteria (NMT) include both slowly and rapidly growing. The range of infections caused by environmental opportunist mycobacteria is quite broad [8, 51].

7.2 Pulmonary infections

Mycobacterium avium-intracellulare complex (MAC) strains have been a major cause of pulmonary and other infections, principally in the HIV patients. MAC infections were commonly seen in chronic obstructive airway disease and in the in the geriatric patients too. *Mycobacterium kansasii and Mycobacterium scrofulaceum* have been considered an important cause of pulmonary infections. *Mycobacterium xenopi,* an unusual specie has been encountered as a pathogen in patients with other underlying lung diseases. Others species of slow grown as *Mycobacterium simiae* (*Mycobacterium 'habana'*), *Mycobacterium szulgai, Mycobacterium malmoense* and *Mycobacterium fortuitum* of rapid grown are other pathogens reported to be associated with pulmonary infections [51, 65-68].

7.3 Cutaneous infection

Mycobacterium szulgai, Mycobacterium marinum, Mycobacterium ulcerans and *Mycobacterium vaccae* have been reported to be a cause of skin infectious. *Mycobacterium marinum,* specie has been recognized as a causative organism of swimming pool granuloma or fish tank granuloma. It causes papular lesions in the extremities and may be confused with sporotricosis. *Mycobacterium ulcerans* is established cause of buruli ulcer, *Mycobacterium vaccae* has also been reported to be a cause of skin infections [51-56].

7.4 Wound infection bone, joints and bursae and sepsis

Mycobacterium fortuitum causes pyogenic lesions in the soft tissue, joints, bursae and injection abscesses, while *Mycobacterium chelonae abscessus* is a well known cause of wound infections, a new related species *Mycobacterum immunogenum* has been recently been recognized as a cause of sepsis. *Mycobacterium marinum* also causes infections of bones, joints, tendon sheaths especially in AIDS patients. *Mycobacterium smegmatis,* and more recently *Mycobacterium wolinskyi* and *Mycobacterium thermoresistible* have been reported to cause wound infection and also bacteraemia. *Mycobacterium terrae* complex (*Mycobacterium terrae, Mycobacterium nonchromogenicum* and *Mycobacterium triviale*) may be associated with mycobacterial disease. Also occasionally *Mycobacterium nonchromogenicum* and *Mycobacterium chelonae* have been identified as causes of acupuncture induced infections. *Mycobacterium septicum* a new rapidly growing species has been reported to be associated with catheter related bacteremia [49, 51, 57,58].

7.5 Lymphadenitis

Infection of the submaxillar, cervical, inguinal or preauricular lymph nodes is the most common presentation of NTM lymphadenitis. The involved lymph nodes are generally unilateral (95%) and not tender [54-57]. The nodes may enlarge rapidly, and even rupture, with formation of sinus tracts that result in prolonged local drainage. Other nodal groups outside of the head and neck may be involved occasionally. Distinguishing tuberculous from nontuberculous lymphadenitis is key because the former requires drug therapy and public health tracking, whereas the latter does not. A definitive diagnosis of NTM lymphadenitis is made by recovery of the causative organism form lymph node cultures. A simple diagnostic biopsy or incision and drainage of the involved lymph nodes should be avoided, since most of these procedures will be followed by fistulae formation with chronic drainage. However, even with excised nodes with compatible histopathology, only about 50% will yield positive cultures, because in some case these smear-positive, culture-negative cases may be due to fastidious species such as *Mycobacterium haemophilum* or *Mycobacterium genavence.* Approximately 80% of culture-proven cases of NTM lymphadenitis are due to *MAC*. It´s predominance is due to a change approximately from 20-30 years ago, when most geographic areas reported *Mycobacterium scrofulaceum* as the most common etiologic agent, only about 10% of the culture-proved mycobacterial cervical lymphadenitis in children is due to *Mycobacterium avium* complex and *Mycobacterium scrofulaceum.* Also *Mycobacterium haemophilum, Mycobacterium malmoense, Mycobacterium fortuitum* and others have been isolated from cases of lymphadenitis including HIV patients. In contrast, in adults more than 90% of the culture-proven mycobacterial lymphadenitis is due to *Mycobacterium tuberculosis* [8, 67, 70-76].

7.6 Disseminated disease in immunocompromized individuals

Disseminated disease due to NTM in AIDS patients usually occurs only in those with very advanced immunosuppressant, because these patients frequently have other complications, the diagnosis of mycobacterial infection may be confused or delayed. The diagnosis is exceedingly rare in person with >100 CD4 cells, and it should usually be suspected only in persons with <50 CD4 cells [53]. *MAC* have been found to be more commonly isolated from HIV-positive and HIV-negative patients, in their the portal of entry mainly through the gut [31 67,69]. Persistent high grade fever, night sweats, anemia and weight loss in addition to nonspecific symptoms of malaise, anorexia, diarrhoea, myalgia and occasional painfuladenopathy are common signs and symptoms associated with MAC disease in AIDS cases. Others pulmonary and extrapulmonary mycobacterial infections in AIDS patients are for *Mycobacterium kansasii , Mycobacterium scrofulaceum, Mycobacterium xenopi, Mycobacterium simiae, Mycobacterium fortuitum-Mycobacterium chelonei* complex, *Mycobacterium malmoense, Mycobacterium szulgai,* and more recently *Mycobacterium genavense, Mycobacterium haemophilum* and *Mycobacterium celatum* [74-82].

8. Identification of nontuberculous mycobacteria

Traditional identification of NTM, as well as *Mycobacterium tuberculosis,* has relied upon statistical probabilities of presenting a characteristic reaction pattern in battery biochemical test. The niacin test was the most useful for separating NTM and *Mycobacterium tuberculosis* because the former is usually negative, whereas isolates of *Mycobacterium tuberculosis* are positive. Runyon devised the first good scheme for grouping NTM based on growth rates and colony pigmentation. For the diagnostic of NTM is very important to know the growth rates and colony pigmentation, and biochemical test such as, niacin production, nitrate reduction, tween-80 hydrolysis, arylsulphatase, urease, tellurite reduction, catalase qualitative and quantitative, grown on MaConkey agar, sodium chloride tolerance, etc, are adequate to identify majority of clinically relevant mycobacteria. This strategy is very necessary and important for the diagnostic of NTM, however, some time consuming and is not conclusive for many isolates with variable characters. For this reason others alternative diagnostic techniques are recommended, for example, the analysis of the mycolic acids of mycobacteria by thin layer chromatography (TLC) and high performance liquid chromatography (HPLC), and more recently the identification and characterization of NTM by molecular methods, based on new knowledge about the gene sequences of mycobacteria many gene probes for the identification of isolates as well as amplification of specific gene fragments from the lesions and mycobacterial culture isolates have been developed; gene probes, polymerase chain reaction (PCR) techniques, DNA fingerprinting techniques, etc, [35-40, 43,44,48, 83, 84]

9. *Mycobacterium tuberculosis* and nontuberculous mycobacteria diseases in the HIV/AIDS patients

After years of worldwide decline of tuberculosis (TB), this disease has returned as a big problem in the Public Health. The resurgence of TB in the past decades is closely linked to acquired immunodeficiency syndrome (AIDS) pandemic. The high susceptibility of patients infected with the human immunodeficiency virus (HIV) to TB and others mycobacterial infections is unique, creating a lot of diagnostic and therapeutic challenges for clinicians [12,32,24]. Pulmonary tuberculosis is the most common manifestation of tuberculosis in adults infected with HIV [53,85,86].

HIV/TB co-infection occurs in various stages of HIV infection, with the clinical pattern correlating with the patient's immune status. In the early stages of HIV infection, when immunity is only partially compromised, the features are more typical of tuberculosis, commonly with upper lobe cavitations, and the disease resembles that seen in the pre-HIV era. HIV-infected patients present with atypical pulmonary disease due to immune deficiency advances, resembling primary tuberculosis or extra pulmonary and disseminated disease, commonly with hilar adenopathy and lower lobe infection [87].

9.1 Clinical symptoms in pulmonary tuberculosis

The clinical symptoms are severally similar in HIV-infected and HIV-negative patients. However, cough is reported less frequently by HIV-infected patients, probably because there is less cavitations, inflammation and endobronchial irritation as a result of a reduction in cell-mediated immunity. Similarly, haemoptysis, which results from caseous necrosis of the bronchial arteries, is less common in HIV-infected patients [87.88].

In general, the traits that characterize HIV-TB co-infection include the potential for rapid progression from primary infection to disseminated disease, atypical radiographic features of pulmonary disease, increased frequency of extrapulmonary disease and involvement of unusual sites of infection. All of these atypical features seem to occur more commonly with more advance stages of immunosuppression and the paradigm that emerges is one of typical TB early in the course of HIV infection and atypical manifestation with advanced HIV disease, in this case the atypical features included lower lobe alveolar opacities, multifocal alveolar opacities, interstitial infiltrates, mediastinal adenopathy and pleural effusions [24,30,67,69,89].

9.2 Clinical symptoms in extrapulmonary tuberculosis

The main manifestation of extrapulmonary tuberculosis in AIDS patients are lymphadenopathy, pleural effusion, meningitis, pericardial effusion and miliary tuberculosis. This diagnostic is often difficult because the patients with HIV are prone to all of the usual bacterial and viral infection that affect a non-HIV infected patients, so, the presentation of extrapulmonary tuberculosis in HIV-infected patients is generally no different [8, 69].

9.3 Nontuberculous mycobacterial infection in HIV/AIDS patients

The clinical relevant of NMT infection in HIV/AIDS patients are very frequent, this infection can be pulmonary and extrapulmonary and their symptoms are the same that *Mycobacterium tuberculosis* [51-54, 69]. Recently, the nontuberculous mycobacterial are also denominated as environmental opportunist mycobacterial. Normally, they live as environmental saprophytes and they cause opportunist disease in human. Many cases of NTM are associated with some form of immune deficiency in special HIV/AIDS patients. In this group of patients is frequently to find this mycobacterial species as etiological agent for this reason is very important their microbiology diagnostic which is different to *Mycobacterium tuberculosis* [90, 91].

Disseminate *Mycobacterium avium complex* (MAC) diseases was one of the first opportunist infections recognized in the syndrome of AIDS since 20 years ago. The interest of the diagnostic of disseminated MAC and others species of nontuberculous mycobacteria infection have been increased as a result of the HIV pandemic. The prevention and treatment in nontuberculous mycobacteria are life long because cure of them were not achievable in AIDS patients with profound immune suppression. The precise immune defect predisposing HIV/AIDS patients to disseminated diseases is unknown [92].

The main manifestation of pulmonary and extrapulmonary infections for *Mycobacterium tuberculosis* and nontuberculous mycobacterial are the same affecting lung, pleura, skin, lymphatic system and producing dissemination infection **(Figure 1, Figure 2), (Figure 3A-3B-3C, Figure 4A-4B)** [8, 63,69]. For this reason is very important the highly active antiretroviral therapy (HAART) for treatment of AIDS patients that has been associated with a market reduction in the incidence of most opportunistic infection [82,89,92].

So, is very important that the mycobacteriology laboratory should give a definitive diagnostic, because in immunosuppressed patients is important to find resistant alcohol acid bacillus in order to detect the co-infection with *Mycobacterium tuberculosis* which is the most frequently agent found. Nevertheless, others species of mycobacteria may be causing infection and should be search for.

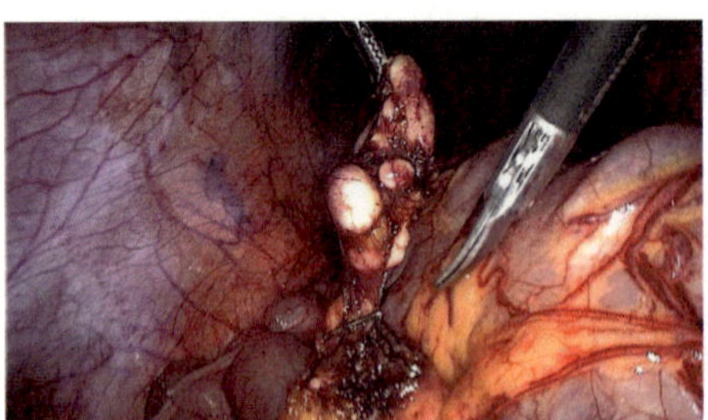

Fig. 1. Messenteric lymph nodes for *Mycobacterium tuberculosis* in AIDS patients.

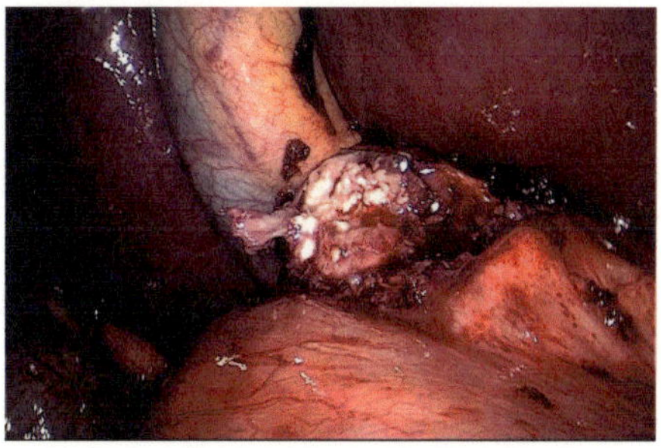

Fig. 2. Biopsy of liver pedicle lymph nodes for *Mycobacterium tuberculosis* in AIDS patients.

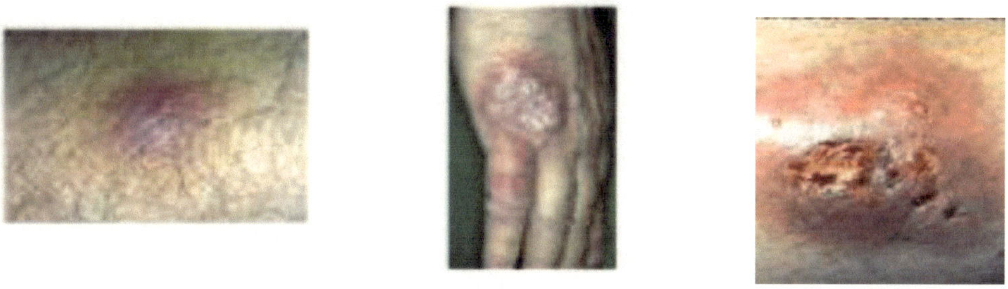

A B C

Fig. 3. AIDS patients with skin lesions from *Mycobacterium avium complex* (**Figure 3A, Figure 3B**) and *Mycobacterium fortuitum* (**Figure 3C**)

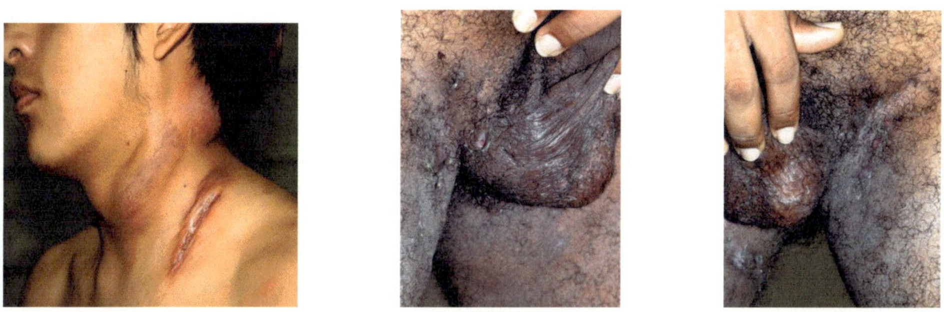

A B C

Fig. 4. Lymphadenitis cervical from *Mycobacterium tuberculosis* **(Figure 4A)**, inguinal-testes lesions from *Mycobacterium avium complex* in lymphatic system **(Figure 4B, Figure 4C)**.

10. References

[1] Center for Disease Control and Prevention. A strategic plan for the elimination of tuberculosis from the United States. MMWR 1989;38 (Suppl No. S-3).

[2] American Thoracic Society and Center for Disease Control and Prevention. Treatment of tuberculosis and tuberculosis infection in adults and children. Am J Respir Crit Care Med1994;149:1359-1374.

[3] Center for Disease Control and Prevention, National Center for HIV, STD, and TB Prevention Division of Tuberculosis Elimination. Trans mission and Pathogenesis of Tuberculosis. CDC 1995:8-19.
[4] Center for Disease Control and Prevention. Tuberculosis elimination revisited: obstacles, opportunities, and renewed commitment. MMWR 1999;48(No. RR-9).
[5] Benedek TG. The history of gold therapy for tuberculosis. J Hist Med Allied Sci 2004; 59: 50-89.
[6] Daniel TM. The history of tuberculosis. Respir Med 2006; 100: 1862-70.
[7] Hutton MD, Stead WW, Cauthen GM, Bloch AB, Ewing WM. Nosocomial transmission of tuberculosis associated with a draining abscess. J Infect Dis 1990;161:286-295.
[8] Kumar V, Abbas AK, Fausto N, Aster JC. Robbins and Cotran, Pathologic basis of disease. Professional Edition, Eigth Edition, Ed Saunders/Elsevier 2010;Chapter 8: 366-372.
[9] Cosma CL, Sherman DR, Ramakrishnan L. The secret lives of the pathogenic Mycobacteria. Annu Rev Microbiol 2003;57:641-671.
[10] Lundgren R, Norrman E, Asberg I. Tuberculosis infection transmitted at autopsy. Tubercle 1987;68:147-150.
[11] Tuberculosis and Human Immunodeficiency Virus Infection: Recommendations of the Advisory Committee for the Eliminations of Tuberculosis (ACET). MMWR Morb Mortal Wkly Rep 1989;23:250-4.
[12] Ussery XT, Bierman JA, Valway SE. Transmission of multidrug-resistant *Mycobacterium tuberculosis* among persons exposed in a medical examiner's office, New York. Infect Control Hosp Epidemiol 1995;16:160-165.
[13] Selwyn PA, Hartel D, Lewis VA. A prospective study of the risk of tuberculosis among intravenous drug users with human immunodeficiency virus infection. N Engl J Med 1989;320:545-550.
[14] Selwyn PA, Sckell BM, Alcabes P. High risk of active tuberculosis in HIV-infected drugs users with cutaneous anergy. JAMA 1992;268:504-509.
[15] Rieder HL, Snider DE Jr, Cauthen GM. Extrapulmonary tuberculosis lymphadenitis in the United States. Am Rev Respir Dis 1990;141:347-51.
[16] Shriner KA, Mathisen GE, Goetz MB. Comparison of mycobacterial lymphadenitis among persons infected with human immunodeficiency virus and seronegative controls. Clin Infect Dis 1992;15:601-5.
[17] Artesntein AW, Kim JH, Williams WJ, Chungg RC. Isolated peripheral tuberculous lymphadenitis in adults: current clinical and diagnostic issues. Clin Infect Dis 1995; 20:876-82.
[18] Rojas A, La Cruz H, Salinas P, Rangel D, Hernández M. Adenitis tuberculosa inguinal. Reporte de um caso. MedULA, 2006;15:37-9.
[19] Al Soub H, Al Alousi FS, Al-Khal AL. Tuberculoma of the cavernous sinus. *Sand J Infect Dis* 2001; 33: 868-70.
[20] Donald PR. Schoeman JF. Tuberculous Meningitis. *Tehe New England Journal of Medicine* 2004; 351:1719-1720.
[21] Karande S, Gupta V, Kulkarni M. Tuberculous Meningitis and HIV. *Indian Journal of Pediatric* 2005;72:7-9.

[22] Kaplan JB, Masur H, Holmes KK. Guidelines for preventing opportunistic infections among HIV infected persons. Recommendations of the US Public Health Service and the Infectious Diseases Society of America MMWR 2002;51(RR-8):1-52.
[23] Mederos LM, Banderas JF, Valdés L, Capó V, Fleites G, Martínez MR, Montoro EH. Meningitis y diseminación tuberculosa en paciente con el síndrome de inmunodeficiencia humana (sida). AVFT 2010;29:35-38.
[24] Rieder HL, Cauthen GM, Comstock GW, Snider DE. Epidemiology of tuberculosis in the Unites States. Epidemiol Rev 1989;11:79-98.
[25] Center for Disease Control and Prevention, National Center for HIV, STD, and TB Prevention Division of Tuberculosis Elimination. Epidemiology of Tuberculosis. CDC 1995:3-23.
[26] Center for Disease Control and Prevention. Tuberculosis morbility- United States, 1996. MMWR 1997;46:695-70.
[27] World Health Organization, Geneva. Toman´s Tuberculosis. Case detection, treatment, and monitoring: questions and answers. Ed. Frieden T, Second Edition, 2004.
[28] Department of Health and Human Services, Center for Disease Control and Prevention, Center for Disease Control and Prevention, National Center for HIV, STD, and TB Prevention Division of Tuberculosis Elimination. Core Curriculum on Tuberculosis. CDC, Fourth Edition, 2000: 15-21.
[29] World Health Organization. WHO Report. Global Tuberculosis Control. Surveillance, Planning, Financing, 2005.
[30] American Academic of Pediatrics. Tuberculosis. In: Peter G, ed. 1997 Red Book: Report of the Committee on Infectious Diseases. 24 th ed. Elk Grove Village, IL: American Academy of Pediatrics;1997:541-563.
[31] Center for Disease Control and Prevention. Prevention and treatment of tuberculosis among patients infected with human immunodeficiency virus: principles of therapy and revised recommendations. MMWR 1998;47(No. RR-20).
[32] Jain A, Mondal R. Extensively drug-resistant tuberculosis: current challenges and threats. FEMS Immunol Med Microbiol 2008;53:145-150.
[33] Jassal M, Bishai WR. Extensively drug-resistant tuberculosis. www.thelancet.com/infection Vol 9, January 2009.
[34] Cohen R, Muzaffar S, Capellan J, Azar H, Chinikamwala M. The validity of classic symptoms and chest radiographic configurations in predicting pulmonary tuberculosis. Chest 1996;109:420-23.
[35] Kent PT, Kubica GP. Public Health Mycobacteriology. A Guide for the Level III Laboratory. Department of Health and Human Services, Public Health Service, Centers for Disease Control, Atlanta, Georgia, 1985: 21-27.
[36] Tenover FC, Crawford JT, Huebner RE, Geiter LJ, Horsburgh LR, Good RC. The resource of tuberculosis: Is your laboratory ready?. J Clin Microbiol 1993:31:767-770.
[37] Crawford JT. New Technologies in the diagnosis. Semin Respir Infect 1994;9:62-70.
[38] Shinnick TN, Good RC. Diagnostic mycobacteriology laboratory practices. Clin Infect Dis 1995;21:291-9.
[39] Organización Panamericana de la Salud. Manual para el diagnostic bacteriológico de la Tuberculosis. Normas y Guía Técnicas. Parte II, Cultivo, 2008.

[40] Ruiz P, Zerolo FJ, Casal M. Comparison of susceptibility of *Mycobacterium tuberculisis* using the ESP Culture System II with that using the BACTEC Method. J Clin Microbiol 2000;38:4663-4664.

[41] Valero-Guillén PL, Martín-Luengo F, Larsson L, Jiménez J, Juhlin I, Portaels F. Fatty and mycolic acids of *Mycobactarium malmoense* . L Clin Microbiol 1988;26:153-154.

[42] Leite CQF, Souza CWO, Leite SRA. Identification of Mycobacteria by thin layer chromatographic analysis of mycolic acid and conventional biochemical method: Four years of experience. Mem Inst Oswaldo Cruz 1998;93:801-805.

[43] Mederos LM, Frantz JL, Perovani MA, Sardiñas M, Montoro EH. Identificación de Micobacterias no tuberculosas en pacientes VIH/SIDA por métodos convencionales y de fracciones de ácidos micólicos. Rev Soc Venezolana de Microbiología 2007;27:50-53.

[44] Forbes SA, Hicks KE. Direct detection of *Mycobacterium tuberculosis* in respiratory specimens in clinical laboratory by polymerase chain reaction. J Clin Microbiol 1993;31:1688.

[45] Noordhoek GT, Kolk AH, Bjune G et al. Sensitivity and specificity of PCR for detection of *Mycobacterium tuberculosis*: a blind comparison study among seven laboratories. J Clin Microbiol 1994;32:277.

[46] Franco-Alvarez F, Ruiz P, Gutierrez J, Casal M. Evaluation of the GenoType Mycobacteria Direct Assay for detection *Mycobacterium tuberculosis* complex and Four Atypical Mycobacterial Species in clinical samples. J of Clin Microbiol 2006;44:3025-3027.

[47] Wolinsky E. Nontuberculous mycobacteria and associated disease. Am Rev Respir Dis 1979;119:107-159.

[48] Wallace RJ Jr, O´Brein R, Glassroth J, Raleigh J, Dutta A. Diagnosis and treatment of disease caused by nontuberculous mycobacteria. Am Rev Respir Dis 1990;142:940-953.

[49] DeVita VT, Hellman S, Rosenberg SA. AIDS Etiology, Diagnosis, Treatment and Prevention. Fourth Edition, Chapter: Tuberculosis and Human Inmmunodeficiency Virus Infection 1997: 245-257, Lippincott-Raven Publishers, Philadelphia, New York.

[50] Murphy SM, Brook G, Birchall MA. HIV Infection and AIDS. Churchill Livinsgstone-ELSEVIER, Second Edition, Chapter: Tuberculosis 2000: 23-24, 63,71,119-120.

[51] Katoch VM. Infections due to non-tuberculous mycobacteria (NTM). Indian J Med Res 2004;120:290-304.

[52] García-Río I, Fernádez-Peñas P, Fernández-Herrera J, Gracía-Díez A. Infección cutánea por *Mycobacterium chelonae*. Revisión de seis casos. Clin Microbiol & Infection 2002;8:125-127.

[53] Guía Práctica Clínica de Dermatología Tropical. Colegio Ibero Latinoamericano de Dermatología (CILAD), Madrid, J´Editor Prof. Vilata JJ, Editora ¨adalia¨ , 2009; Capítulo ¨Micobacteriosis Atípica¨: 11-14.

[54] Saggese D, compadretti GC, Burnelli R. Nontuberculous mycobacterial adenitis in children: Diagnostic and therapeutic management. Am J Otolaryngol 2003; 24:79-84.

[55] Panesar J, Higgins K, Daya H, Forte V, Allen U. Nontuberculous mycobacterial cervical adenitis: a ten-year retrospective review. Laryngoscope 2003; 113:149-54.

[56] Barr KL, Lowe L, Su LD. *Mycobacterium marinum* infection simulating interstitial granuloma annulare: a report of two case. Am J Dermatopathol 2003;25:148-151.

[57] American Thoracic Society. Diagnosis and treatment of disease cause by nontuberculous mycobacteria. Am J Respir Crit Care Med 1997;156:S1-19.
[58] Moore JE, Kruijshaar ME, Ormerod LP, Drobniewski F, Abubakar I. Increasing reports of non-tuberculous mycobacteria in England, Wales and Norther Ireland, 1995-2006. BMC Public Health 2010;10:612, Article URL: http://www.biomedcentral.com/1471-2458/10/612.
[59] O´Brien RJ, Geiter LJ, Snider Jr. DE. The epidemiology of nontuberculous mycobacterial diseases in the United States. Results from a national survey. Am Rev Respir Dis 1987;135:1007-1014.
[60] Tsukamura, M, Kita N, Shimoide H, Arakawa H, Kuze A. Studies on the epidemiology of nontuberculous mycobacteriosis in Japan. Am Rev Respir Dis 1988;137:1280-1284.
[61] Frappier-Davignon L, Fortin R, Desy M. Sensitivity to "atypical" mycobacteria in high school children in two community health departments. Canadian J of Public Health 1989;80:335-338.
[62] Sackett DL. Bias in analytic research. J Chronic Dis 1979;32:51-63.
[63] de Armas Y, Capó V, González I, Mederos LM, Díaz R, de Waard JH, Rodríguez A, García Y, Cabanas R. Concomitant *Mycobacterium avium* infection and Hodgkin´s disease in lymph node from an HIV-negative child. Pathol Oncol Res 2011;17:139-140.
[64] Marras TK, Daley CL. Epidemiology of human pulmonary infection with nontuberculous mycobacteria. Clin Chest Med 2002;23:553-567.
[65] Chakrabarti A, Sharma M, Dubey ML. Isolation rates of different mycobacterial species from Chandinarh (north India). Indian J Res 1990;111-4.
[66] Levy-Frebaulth V, Pangon B, Bure A, Katima C, Marche C, David HL. *Mycobacterium simiae, Mycobacterium avium-intrecellulare* mixed infection in AIDS. J Clin Microbiol 1987;25:154-157.
[67] Wagner D, Young LS. Nontuberculous mycobacterial infections: a clinical review. Infection. 2004; 130: 257-70.
[68] Gupta AK, Nayar M, Chandra M. Critical appraisal cytology of fine needle aspiration cytology in tuberculosis lymphadenitis. Acta Cytol 1992;36:391-94.
[69] Ioachim HL, Medeiros LJ. Lymph Node Pathology. 2009;Chapter 21- Section III:130-135, and Chapter 23-Section III:137-143, Fourth Edition, Lippincott William & Wilkins, Wolters Kluwer Health.
[70] Mederos LM, González D, Pérez D, Paneque A, Montoro EH. Linfadenitis causada por *Mycobacterium malmoense* en paciente infectado con el virus de inmunodeficiencia humana. Rev Chil Infect 2004;21: 229-31.
[71] Mederos LM, González D, Montoro EH. Linfadenitis ulcerativa por *Mycobacterium fortuitum* en un paciente con sida. Enferm Infecc Microbiol Clin 2005;23:573-77.
[72] Mederos LM, Rodríguez ME, Mantecón B, Sardiñas M, Montoro EH. Adenitis submaxilar en niño causada por *Mycobacterium fortuitum* . Folia Dermatológica Cubana 2007;1:6-10.
[73] Nightingale SD, Byrd LT, Southern PM, Jockusch JD, Cal SX, Wynne BA. Incidence of *Mycobacterium avium-intracellulare*complex in humans immunodeficiency virus-positive patients. J Infetc Dis 1990;165:1082-1085.
[74] Horsburgh CR. *Mycobacterium avium* complex in deficiency syndrome infection in the acquired immuno. N Engla J Med 1991;324:1332-1338.

[75] Maloney JM, Gregg CM, Stephens DS, Manian FA, Rimland D. Infections caused by *Mycobacterium szulgai* in human. Rev Infect Dis 1987;9:1120-1126.

[76] Corti M, Palmero D. *Mycobacterium avium* complex infection in HIV/AIDS patients. Expert Rev Anti Infect Ther 2008;6:351-563.

[77] Mederos LM, Pomier O, Trujillo A, Fonseca C, Montoro EH. Micobacteriosis sistémica por *Mycobacterium avium* en paciente con SIDA. AVFT 2009;28:61-63.

[78] Lawn SD, Checkley A, Wansbrough MH. Acute bilateral parotiditis caused by *Mycobacterium scrofulaceum*: immune reconstruction disease in a patient with AIDS. Sex Trasm Infect 2005;5:361-73.

[79] Botteger EC, Teske A, Kirschner P, Bost S, Chang HR, Beer V. Disseminated *Mycobacterium genavense* infection in patients with AIDS. Lancet 1992;340:76-80.

[80] Dever LL, Martin JWm Seaworth B, Jorgense JH. Varied presentation and responses to treatment of infections caused by *Mycobacterium haemophilum* in patients with AIDS. Clin Infect Dis 1992;32:1195-2000.

[81] Jones D, Havlir DV. Nontuberculous mycobacteria in the HIV infected patient. Clin in Chest Med 2002;23: 312-24.

[82] Olalla J, Pombo M, Aguado JM, Rodríguez E, Palenque E, Costa JR, Riopérez. *Mycobacterium fortuitum* complex endocarditis-case report and literature review. Clin Microbiol & Infect 2002;8:197-201.

[83] Casal MM, Casal M. Las micobacterias atípicas como patógenos emergentes. Enf Emerg 2000;2:220-230.

[84] Zumla A, Grange J. Infection and disease caused by environmental mycobacteria. Curr Opin Pulm Med 2002;8:166-172.

[85] Lanjewar DN, Duggal RP. Pulmonary pathology in patients with AIDS: an autopsy study from Mumbai. HIV Med 2001; 2:266-271.

[86] Escombe AR, Moore DA, Gilman RH, Pan W, Navincova M, Ticona E, Martínez C, Caviedes L, Sheen P, Gonzalez A, Noakes CJ, Friedland JS, Evans CA. The Infectiousness of Tuberculosis Patients Coinfected with HIV. PLoS Med 2008;5: 188.

[87] Nunes EA, De Capitani EM, Coelho E, Panunto AC, Joaquim AO, Ramos Mde C. *Mycobacterium tuberculosis* and nontuberculous mycobacterial isolates among patients with recent HIV infection in Mozambique. J Bras Pneumol 2008;34:822-828.

[88] Buchacz K, Baker RK, Palella FJ, Chmiel JS, Lichtenstein KA, Novak RM, Wood KC, Brooks JT. AIDS-defining opportunistic illnesses in US patients, 1994-2007: a cohort study. AIDS 2010; 10:1549-1459.

[89] Browth-Elliot BA, Griffith DE, Wallace RJ. Diagnosis of nontuberculous mycobacterial infections. Clin Lab Med 2002;22:911-915.

[90] Catanzaro A. Diagnosis, differentiating colonization, infection, and disease. Clin Chest Med 2002;23:599-601.

[91] Horsburgh CJJr, Selik RM. Th epidemiology of disseminated nontuberculous mycobacterial infectio in the Acquired Immunodeficiency Syndrome (AIDS). Am Rev Respir Dis 1989;99:1-132.

[92] Dos Santos RP, Scheid K, Goldani LZ. Disseminated nontuberculous mycobacterial disease in patients with acquired immune deficiency syndrome in the south of Brazil. Trop Doct 2010;40:211-213.

2

Non-Tuberculous Mycobacteria in Uganda: A Problem or Not?

Adrian Muwonge[1], Ashemeire Patience[4], Clovice Kankya[2], Demelash Biffa[5], Eystein Skjerve[1] and James Oloya[3]

[1]*Department of Food Safety and Infection Biology, Norwegian School of Veterinary Science*
[2]*Department of Veterinary Public Health and Preventive Medicine, Faculty of Veterinary Medicine, Makerere University*
[3]*Department of Epidemiology and Biostatistics/ Population Health, college of Public health, 132 Coverdell centre, University of Georgia Athens,*
[4]*Faculty of Community Psychology, Makerere University,*
[5]*Schools of Veterinary Medicine, Hawassa University,*
[1]*Norway*
[2,4]*Uganda*
[3]*USA*
[5]*Ethiopia*

1. Introduction

1.1 HIV/AIDS

HIV/AIDS scourge has been and still is a devastating disease since its advent in the late 70's, claiming up to 25 million lives globally (WHO, 2010). The United Nations program on AIDS (UNAIDS) estimated that 39.5 million people were living with HIV/AIDS by the end of 2006, 63% of these were in Sub Saharan Africa. Furthermore, 4.3 million people were reported to be newly infected with HIV while 2.9 million had lost their lives to AIDS in 2006 alone (UNAIDS, 2010). It is also reported that young people of age 15 and above account for 40% of new infections (CWYF, 2007). Epidemiological models predict a growing trend of the disease most notably the alarming incidence of new infections in sub-Saharan Africa, Western Europe and Asia (UNAIDS, 2010).

1.2 HIV/AIDS in Uganda: Past and current situation

In many regards, Uganda is considered a global role model in awareness, prevention and control of HIV/AIDS (Aidsmap, 2006; Kaiser family foundation, 2005). The first cases of AIDS in Uganda were identified in Rakai district off the shores of Lake Victoria in 1982 (Serwadda et al 1985; MOH, 2006). AIDS was clinically characterized by wasting, this is why it is popularly known as 'slim disease' (Serwadda et al., 1985). Just as before, this disease is still characterized by opportunistic infections, notable are *Mycobacterium avium* complex infections which are usually the causes of fatality in victims (Serwadda et al., 1985; MOH, 2006). In the late 1980's a famous Ugandan Musician Philly Bongole Lutaaya paved the way for the awareness campaign by publically disclosing his sero-positive status at a time when the epidemic prevalence was up to 29% in peri-urban and urban areas of Uganda (Open Vision Club, 2004; Hooper, 1990; Hogle, 2002).

This campaign later evolved into the first ever control programme designed to educate the general population on measures of avoidance coined in the abbreviation ABC; 1) Abstinence, 2) being faithful to your partner and 3) the use of condoms (Hooper, 1990; Hogle, 2002). The success of this open campaign was characterized by a drastic fall in the incidence and prevalence of HIV/AIDS among young adults as well as pregnant women (Stoneburner, 2004; STI/AIDS, 2002). This prevalence has been kept at a record low in part due to this awareness, global funds and subsidies on anti-retroviral therapy in addition to a steady development in palliative treatment and counseling offered by nongovernmental organizations like 'The AIDS support organization' (TASO) (Hogle, 2002;UAC,2004;Ashemeire,2010). Unfortunately this effort together with the evolving life style trends today have bred an army of complacent and risk taking youth (Chinaview, 2008), therefore the resilience of this control strategy is yet to be fully tested. Early age at first sex is reported to be among the key risk factors for HIV infection. In this regard, records from the ministries of health and Gender Labour and Social Development estimates age at first sex being 16.7 and 18.8 for girls & boys respectively in 2005 (MGLSD,2004; MOH,2006). Furthermore, by age 17, half of young women are sexually active and 62.7% have already begun child bearing by the age of 19 (MOH, 2006). This explains the current prevalence estimated at 7% (UNAIDS, 2010) with the highest records of 17% and 18% in HIV/AIDS hot-spot districts of Mubende and Nakasongola, respectively (Anonymous, 2004 and Anonymous, 2008).

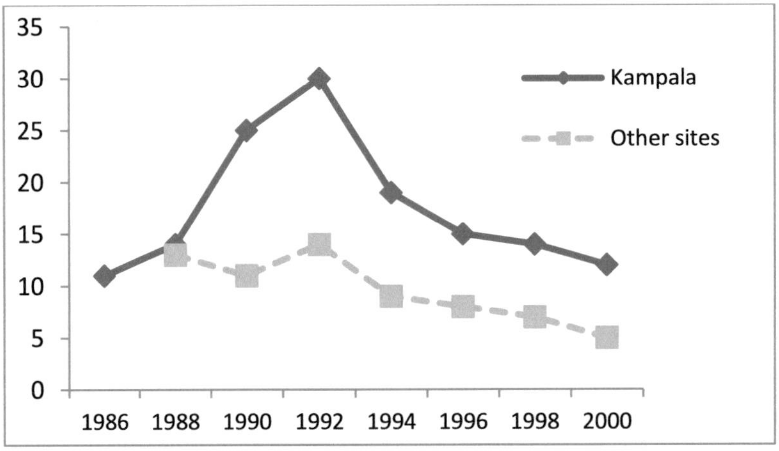

Fig. 1. Median HIV prevalence among pregnant women in Uganda (Hogle, 2002)

Likewise the Ministry of Health's indices in Uganda also indicate that to date this disease has affected approximately 7.4 % of the total national population and that 3.2% of the deaths that have occurred since its advent globally have been in Uganda (MOH,2006; UNAIDS, 2010). The socio-economic effects of AIDS on communities have recently been documented in a study conducted among public service officers with AIDS. It showed a significant increase in direct and indirect costs on HIV/AIDS related illness in addition to claiming the lives of family breadwinners. This has given rise to orphans who are left at the mercy of nongovernmental support groups (MOH report, 2010).

2. Mycobacterial infections in Uganda

Tuberculosis (TB) caused by *M. tuberculosis complex* group remains a major public health problem in Uganda. It is documented to be endemic in poor peri- urban and urban areas mainly due to; 1) congested living conditions (Banerjee, 1999; Tupasi, 2000; Asimwe et al., 2009), 2) high prevalence of HIV, malnutrition and use of immunesupressive therapy in use today (Cosivi, 1998; Asimwe, 2009). Uganda is ranked 16th among the countries with the highest burden of TB in Sub-Saharan Africa, with an estimated incidence rate of 559 cases per 100,000 per year (WHO, 2007). There are other pathogenic mycobacteria other than *M.tuberculosis* and *M.bovis* that have been documented in Uganda, and these include *M. ulcerans* and *M. leprae* (Giuseppe et al, 1997). *M. ulcerans,* the cause of Buruli Ulcer is a skin infection clinically characterized by a nodular skin lesion that busts open into a non healing ulcer (Giuseppe et al, 1997). In the 60's and 70's Buruli ulcer was reported in the Busoga District on the east side of the Victoria Nile, north of Lake Victoria (Barker, 1971). Although cases were known in the other parts of the country, it was unknown in the district before 1965. In this study Barker postulated that the outbreaks were related to the unprecedented flooding of the lakes of Uganda from 1962 to 1964 as a result of heavy rainfall (Barker, 1971). Leprosy in comparison to TB is an old disease documented in the Bible as affecting people even before Christ. It is caused by *M. leprae,* which damages the skin and the peripheral nervous system resulting in skin lesions and deformities, most often affecting the cooler places on the body for example, eyes, nose, earlobes, hands, feet, and testicles (Giuseppe et al, 1997). In Uganda, it was first documented in the South Eastern part in 1978 by a Christian based hospital (Kawuma, 1999). Currently, the prevalence of leprosy is 2.8 cases per 100,000 population, *with a case detection rate* of 2.5 per 100,000 (WHO, 2002&2004). In 2004, new cases were reported in Iganga, Hoima, Kabarole, Kyenjonjo, Rukungiri and Lira district. The latter had has as high as 86 new cases reported (Nation TB and Leprosy, 2004). Recent incidence reports on leprosy in Uganda showed a slight increase in the years 2004/05, but case detection rate continues to decline. It is therefore too early to envisage a Uganda free of leprosy.

At the beginning of the AIDS pandemic, Non-Tuberculous Mycobacteria (NTM) were reported as emerging pathogens responsible for opportunistic infections, found in almost half of HIV/AIDS infected patients, usually associated with CD4 cell counts B/100/ml and a survival of less than one year (Masur,1993). The species documented to cause opportunistic human infections are : *Mycobacterium avium, M. intracellulare, M. kansasii, M. paratuberculosis, M. scrofulaceum, M. simiae, M. habana, M. interjectum, M. xenopi, M. heckeshornense, M. szulgai, M. fortuitum, M. immunogenum, M.chelonae, M. marinum, M. genavense, M. haemophilum, M. celatum, M. conspicuum, M. malmoense, M. ulcerans, M. smegmatis, M. wolinskyi, M. goodii, M. thermoresistible, M. neoaurum, M. vaccae, M.palustre, M. elephantis, M. bohemicam and M. septicum* (Katoch, 2004). It has previously been estimated that up to one-quarter of all patients with AIDS will acquire this infection during their lifetime (Horsburgh, 1991). It is difficult to accurately describe the situation in Sub Saharan Africa since most of the data on which these inferences are made comes from northern Europe or North America (Horsburgh, 1989). Notably, these regions have experienced a gradual decline in the prevalence of TB and increase in mycobacterial infection caused by NTM's in the past several years (Claudio et al., 2008). It is still unclear if this trend is real or is the result of technologic developments in diagnostics (Claudio et al., 2008). Worse so, little has been done in developing countries especially in the sub Saharan Africa to capture this trend (Narang, 2008). Studies in 1990's in Kenya, Uganda, Tanzania, and the Ivory Coast (Gilks et al., 1995; Okello et al., 1990; Archibald et al., 1998; Lucas et al., 1993) concluded that disseminated NTM infections were relatively uncommon in Africa. On the contrary, recent studies in Zambia and South Africa using better diagnostic tools have actually reported a high prevalence of NTM infections in HIV/AIDS patients. These dismissed the previous notion and warned that the problem was bigger than previously documented (Clive, 2001; Buijtels, 2009).

3. Non tuberculous mycobacteria in the environment

The distribution of NTM and the incidence of NTM diseases is still an enigma in most parts of the world however; consistent reports show that NTM are widely distributed in nature. Therefore, the environment is regarded to the biggest reservoir and source of NTMs for animal and human hosts (Falkinham, 1996; Falkinham, 2009; Van ingen 2009). This is in resonance with earlier studies done in Ugandan environments, in which Stanford et al., in 1972 reported that areas around Kampala and Kyoga had 67%, 34% and 98%, 56% of NTM isolation from mud and grass respectively. Of the districts from which mud samples were taken, the isolation rate and the greatest variety of mycobacteria species recovered was from east Bunyoro (present day Kibaale District), southern Lango (present day Oyam, Apac and Dokolo districts) and northern Busoga (present day Kamuli district). Species isolated included *M. chelonae, M. fortuitum, M. avium* and others which were more prevalent in areas with surface water pH values between 5.5 and 5.7 (Barker et al., 1972). Subsequent studies showed that *Mycobacterium avium* complex (MAC) was the most prevalent in urban environments, these accounted for 43% of the recovered NTM from water and soil environments in Kampala, Uganda (Eaton et al., 1995).These were mostly recovered from water and soil with pH ranges (6.0, 6.0-6.9, and > 7.0) respectively. Meanwhile, the most recent studies in pastoral environments have shown that MAC accounted for 29% of NTM recovered in Mubende and Nakasongola (Kankya et al 2011). *M. gordonae, M. nonchromogenicum M. engbaekii, M. hiberniae, M. kubicae, M. simiae, M. arupense, M. terrae, M. parafortuitum* were some of the other NTM isolated from pastoral ecosystems of Uganda (Table 1). Water is considered to be the primary source of NTM infections in humans while domestic and wild animals may be reservoirs (Biet et al., 2005). In the highly mobile pastoral systems of Uganda, humans, livestock domestic and wildlife share open natural water sources. The sharing of these stagnant open water sources provides yet another NTM infection challenge at the human- environment-domestic/ wildlife interface (HELI) (Kankya et al 2010). Subsequent studies on these natural water sources and follow up of this water that was being used in households revealed a high prevalence of *Mycobacterium* species including those known to be pathogenic (Kankya et al., 2011). Host-environment interaction is a key element in colonization and maintenance of *Mycobacterium* in a niche (Falkinham 1996; Biet al , 2005). This is held true by the vast amounts of mycobacteria that were recently isolated from animal environments (Krizova et al., 2010; Ofukwu et al., 2010). Kankya et al 2011a also recovered a wide variety of NTMs from swine and cattle environments, which included *M. fortuitum peregrinum* complex, *M. avium* complex, *M. parafortuitum, M. hiberniae* and *M. engbaekii* (table 1).

Species	Host	Environmental source	Geographical location	Reported by
M. avium	Human, swine, cattle	Household & valley dam water, swine shelter, cattle kraal	Kampala, Karamoja, Mubende ,Kyoga,Toro and Nakasongola	Muwonge et al.,2011 under review, Kankya et al 2011;Oloya et al 2007; Eaton et al 1995; Stanford et al 1976
M. gordonae	Swine and human	Household & stream water	Mubende, Nakasongola,Kyoga, Toro and Kampala	Muwonge et al.,2011 under review, Kankya et al 2011; stanford et al 1976
M. avium subsp hominisuis	Swine and human		Karamoja and Mubende	Muwonge et al.,2011 under review;Oloya et al 2007a&b
M. intracellure	Swine, human, cattle	Household & valley dam water, swine shelter, cattle kraal	Mubende, Nakasongola and Karamoja	Muwonge et al.,2011 under review, Kankya et al 2011;Oloya et al 2007
M. fortuitum	Swine	Household & valley dam water, swine shelter, cattle kraal	Mubende and Nakasongola	Muwonge et al.,2011 under review, Kankya et al 2011;Oloya et al 2007
M. nonchromgenicum		Household, stream water	Mubende, Kampala, Kyoga and Toro	Kankya et al 2011; Stanford et al 1976
M. parafortuitum	Swine	Household water	Mubende and Nakasongola	Muwonge et al.,2011 under review, Kankya et al 2011
M. chubuense		Household water	Mubende and Nakasongola	Kankya et al 2011;
M. vanbaalenii		Household water	Mubende and Nakasongola	Kankya et al 2011;
M. engbaekii		cattle kraal	Mubende and Nakasongola	Kankya et al 2011;
M. kubicae		Household water	Mubende and Nakasongola	Kankya et al 2011;
M. simiae	Swine, human	Household water	Mubende, Nakasongola and Kampala	Kankya et al 2011; Muwonge et al.,2011 under review; Ssali, 1998
M. hiberniae		cattle kraal	Mubende and Nakasongola	Kankya et al 2011
M. terrae	Swine	Household water	Mubende and Nakasongola	Kankya et al 2011; Muwonge et al.,2011 under review
M. senuense	Swine	valley dam water	Mubende and Nakasongola	Kankya et al 2011; Muwonge et al.,2011 under review

Species	Host	Environmental source	Geographical location	Reported by
M. arupense		Household water	Mubende and Nakasongola	Kankya et al 2011
M. asiaticum	Swine		Mubende	Muwonge et al.,2011 under review
M. parascrofulaceum	Swine		Mubende	Muwonge et al.,2011 under review
M. bejali	Swine		Mubende and Nakasongola	Muwonge et al.,2011 under review
M. neoaurum	Swine, Human		Mubende,Kampala,Kyoga and Toro	Muwonge et al.,2011 under review; Stanford, 1976
M.duvalii	Swine, Human		Mubende, Toro, Kampala and Kyoga	Muwonge et al.,2011 under review; Stanford, 1976
M. smegmitis	Swine		Mubende	Muwonge et al.,2011 under review
M. salmonphilum	Swine		Mubende	Muwonge et al.,2011 under review
M. rhodesia	Swine		Mubende	Muwonge et al.,2011 under review
M. septicum	Swine		Mubende	Muwonge et al.,2011 under review
M. chelonae	Swine		Mubende Kampala,Kyoga	Muwonge et al.,2011 under review;Stanford, 1976
M. marinum	swine		Mubende	Muwonge et al.,2011 under review
M. komamatonse	Swine		Mubende	Muwonge et al.,2011 under review
Unidentified NTM	Cattle, human, swine	Valley dam water	Mubende, Karamoja and Kampala	Muwonge et al.,2011 under review; Oloya et al.,2007; Assimwe et al 2009

Table 1. Non-tuberculous mycobacteria isolated from Human, Animals and environments in Uganda

4. Non tuberculous mycobacteria in animals

The subject of NTM in humans and animals in the sub-Saharan Africa has received increasing attention in the recent past. Major concerns in the NTM transmission especially in immuno-compromised individuals has been associated with high levels of interactions occurring at the human-environment-livestock-wildlife interface.

4.1 Poultry

Avian tuberculosis is caused by *M. avium*, it is mostly known to occur in temperate zones and has been widely documented in North and South America and Australia (Barnes et al., 2003). In the United states Avian tuberculosis has been reported to be responsible the condemnation of 1870 per 100,000 birds slaughtered however the figures here were anticipated to be higher than this given that only visual inspection was used (Barnes et al., 2003). The incidence is reported to be low in South Africa while in Kenya it has only been documented in lesser flamingoes (Barnes et al., 2003). Uganda has 37 million chickens and about half a million turkey's. Unfortunately there has not been any studies done to document the prevalence of fowl tuberculosis despite the constant reports of clinical signs typical of this disease in poultry in the east and central region of Uganda (rural poultry farmers' personal communication).

4.2 Cattle

Bovine tuberculosis just like its human cousin *M. tuberculosis* has been given top priority in Uganda, simply because it is a well-documented zoonosis. Worldwide, the proportion of human cases caused by *Mycobacterium bovis* is estimated to be 3.1% of all forms of TB (Cosivi, 1998). In the most recent studies on the prevalence of bovine TB in pastoral areas of Uganda, tuberculin reactors were reported to be 6% of cattle in Mbarara district, an important dairy cattle area in the south west (Bernard et al., 2005), and a prevalence of 2·8% in nomadic cattle of Karamoja in the north east of the country (Oloya et al., 2006). Cattle herds in Uganda are concentrated along the cattle corridor that stretches from the south west to the north east through the central parts of the country. In another study done by Oloya (2007) in the same area gave the initial indication that Non tuberculous mycobacteria could be a public health force to reckon. This study found that NTMs were an integral part of bacteria isolated from disseminated tuberculous lesions and surprisingly these were almost equal in proportions (48.6:51.4) to *M.bovis* (Oloya et al 2007). Similarly a study done by Asimwe et al., 2009 on slaughtered cattle in Kampala revealed a similar pattern of isolation with *M.bovis* and NTMs accounting for 64.7% and 35.3% of the *mycobacterium* isolated from various tuberculous lymph node lesions respectively.

These finding further reaffirm the key role played by NTM in the tuberculosis pathogenesis. In two separate studies by Oloya et al., 2006 and Inangolet et al., 2007, shared water sources were identified as the responsible factor for a high prevalence of high avian reactors to the purified protein derivative (PPD) skin test.

The highest response to avian purified protein derivative (PPD) was observed in cattle 7-9 years old (figure 1) which was attributed to non specific immune response to environmental mycobacteria of the *Mycobacterium avium* complex prevalent in the natural water sources animals drink from. Therefore it is no longer disputable that NTMs are prevalent in cattle in Uganda but rather the effort should be on the role if any played by cattle in disseminating them to human populations.

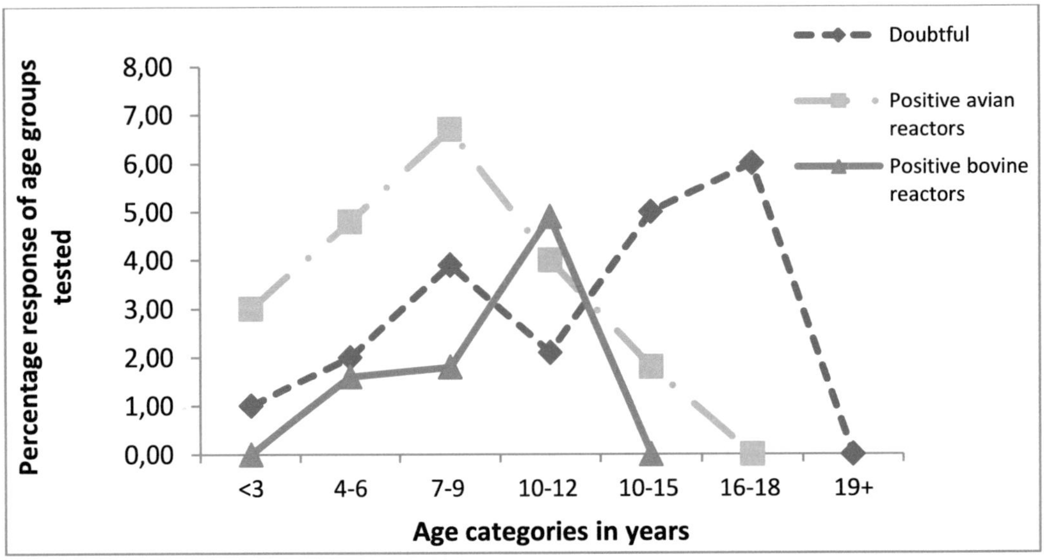

Fig. 2. Variation of skin reactions to comparative intradermal tuberculin test with age adapted from Oloya et al.,2006

4.3 Swine

Swine tuberculosis is a chronic infectious disease characterized by inflammatory reactions in various body parts but mostly in the digestive system. Calcification prone tubercles, inflamed lymph nodes and sarcoid-like granulomas are the most common features of this disease (Cvetnic, 2007; Coetzer, 2004; Ofukwu, 2010). The disease in swine is caused by *M. bohemicum, M. intracellulare, M. avium, M. hemophilum, M. malmose, M. szulgai, M. kansasii, M. scrofuleceum, M. tuberculosis, M.simiae, M. palustre, M. gordonae, M. terrae, M. xenopi and M. heckershornense* and other potentially pathogenic mycobacteria (PPM) (Jakko van Ingen, 2010, Cvetnic, 2007).

The only study in Uganda done on swine mycobacterial infection showed 9.3% and 3.1% prevalence based on necropsy examination and culture isolation, respectively (Muwonge et al 2010). A seasonal variation in prevalence of lesions typical of mycobacterial infections was also found in which lesions tended to increase after the rain season (figure 3).In a follow up molecular study on slaughter pigs in Mubende (Muwonge et al., 2011), *Mycobacterium avium* was the most prevalent *mycobacterium* specie accounting for 18% of the isolates from lymph nodes. Other species isolated included; *M. senuense, M. terrae, M. asiaticum, M. parascrofulaceum, M. bejali and M. neoaurum, M. simie, M. duvalii, M. smegmitis and M. parafortuitum,M.salmonphilum, M. rhodesia, M. septicum, M. chelonae, M. marinum,M. parafinicum, M. komamatonse and M. gordona* (Table 1).In general these findings are reflective of the NTMs load (infection/colonization) in swine reared in semi and free range systems, since the majority of the pigs in Uganda are reared in this system

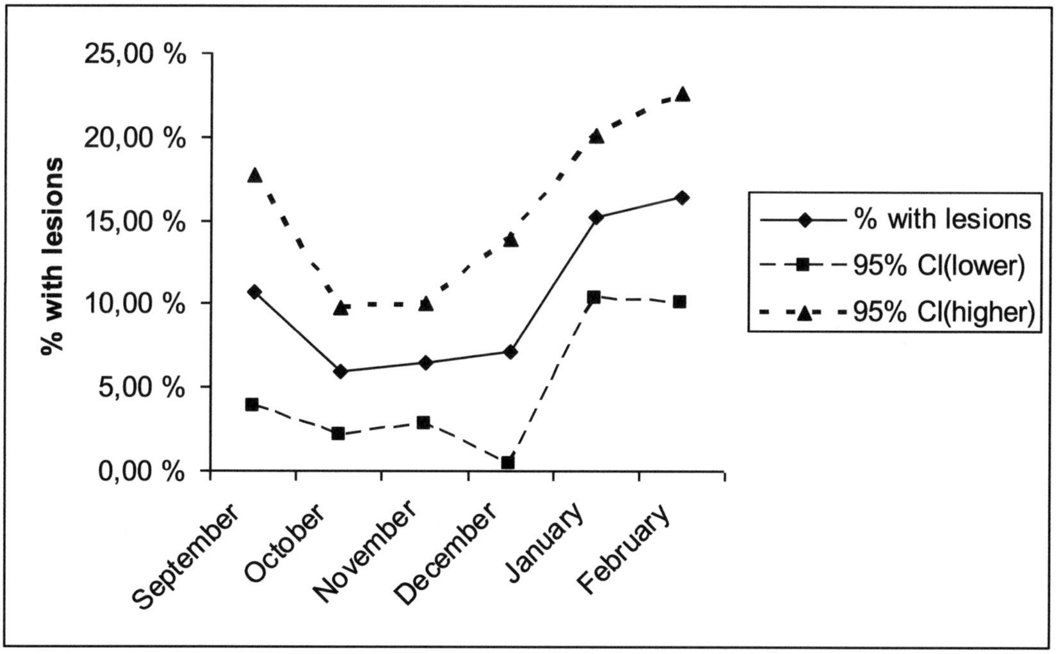

Fig. 3. Temperal occurrence of pathological lesions in slaughtered pigs in Mubende district (Muwonge et al., 2010)

5. Non-tuberculous mycobacteria in human

The absence of documented human to human transmission in the last 30 years has led to the conclusion that the environment is the source of NTM for human (Falkinham, 2009). In comparison to developed countries, NTM infections in humans are not well documented in Uganda. The few earlier studies did not show that disseminated *Mycobacterium avium* complex (MAC) infections was a problem in terminally sick AIDS patients unlike in the western world (Okello, 1990; Valadas, 2004; Chih-Cheng Lai, 2006). Subsequent studies further seem to support the absence of *M. avium* in HIV-infected Ugandans (Eaton et al., 1995). On the other hand Ugandan immigrants with AIDS in London had previously been diagnosed with symptomatic *mycobacterium avium* complex (MAC) infections (Nigel, 1993). These patients at the time of diagnosis had a CD4 count of $10X10^6/L$ and some had been receiving treatment for extra pulmonary tuberculosis (Nigel, 1993). This disparity in prevalence at the time was explained by the speculation that temperate areas were preferential niches for NTMs and the superiority in diagnostics. It is now known that it was the latter, Nambuya et al., (1988) documented the prevalence of tuberculous lymphadenitis (which today is known to be caused by MTCs and NTM) but surprisingly they were unable to culture specimen to prove the cause. In 1998 Ssali et al reported for the first time presence of disseminated MAC and *Mycobacterium simiae* infections in HIV/AIDS patients in Mulago hospital in Uganda. This study showed that mycobacteriamia among febrile HIV-infected Ugandan adults accounted for 13% (Ssali et al., 1998). *M. avium* is also known to be one of the leading causes of infant lymphadenitis worldwide (Coetzer, 2004; Johansen, 2007; Van Ingen et al., 2009). This is in agreement with a study done in Uganda on the cause of cervical lymphadenitis. In that study the prevalence was highest among infants below 7 years of age and *M. avium* was the most frequently isolated NTM in this group (Oloya et al 2007). It is a common observation that NTM cause disease in individuals whose immunity has been compromised (Wolinsky, 1979; Wallace et al.,1990; von Reyn et al 1994; Falkinham et al 2009). Pneumoconiosis, cystic fibrosis, bronchiestasis , smoking and chronic alcoholism are some of the predisposing factors to NTM infections. The current technological advancements in diagnostics seem to indicate a possible further identification of more NTM zoonoses. In Netherland, Komjin et al., (1999) showed a close genetic relatedness between *M. avium* subsp. *hominissuis* isolated from swine and humans. Since then many scholars have continued to document more evidence re affirming the role pigs play in the transmission of mycobacterial infections to immunecompromised and immunecompetent indivuals. In 2007, Oloya et al isolated *M. avium* subsp.*hominissuis* from tuberculous lesions in cattle and T.B patients with cervical lymphadenitis in pastoral areas of Karamoja in Uganda. The molecular findings showed a very high genetic relatedness between animal and human isolates (figure 4 and 5). Although the true source of human infection is still a matter of dispute, these findings tend to point us to zoonotic scenario, with shared environment, in this case water, playing an important role. The true picture of human non tuberculous infections in Uganda is yet to be unveiled, but studies done elsewhere in Africa have indicated that this problem is bigger than previously documented (Buitjel, 2009).

5.1 Diagnostics and therapeutics

The greatest mistake in disease treatment arises when a physician is not well armed with facts about the cause of visible clinical signs, in other words a good diagnosis precedes a better treatment. Given the ubiquitous presence of NTMs in the environment and animal hosts, establishing the true causal relationship is highly dependent on representative sampling and stringent laboratory practices as contamination can easily occur. Another important problem is the overlapping of clinical manifestation of the disease caused by *M.tuberculosis* which makes the specific diagnosis of NTM disease practically impossible in poor health care settings. In Uganda, definitive NTM diagnosis in clinical setting is rarely done therefore, at the time of treatment commencement the only diagnosis available is presence/absence of acid fast rod like bacteria. This diagnosis is arrived at with the use of Ziehl-Neelsen (ZN) staining (Nation leprosy and tuberculosis programme). Literature on ZN staining indicates that the specificity is compromised by bacteria like *Rodococcus* that have the same acid fast characteristics thus giving some false positives (Coetzer, 2004). Definitive diagnosis on the other hand requires that a physician knows exactly which type of *Mycobacterium* is causing the clinical signs. This can be achieved using fast clinical diagnostic methods like; gene probes, Ino-lipa and *Mycobacterium* growth indicator (MGIT).

Fig 4

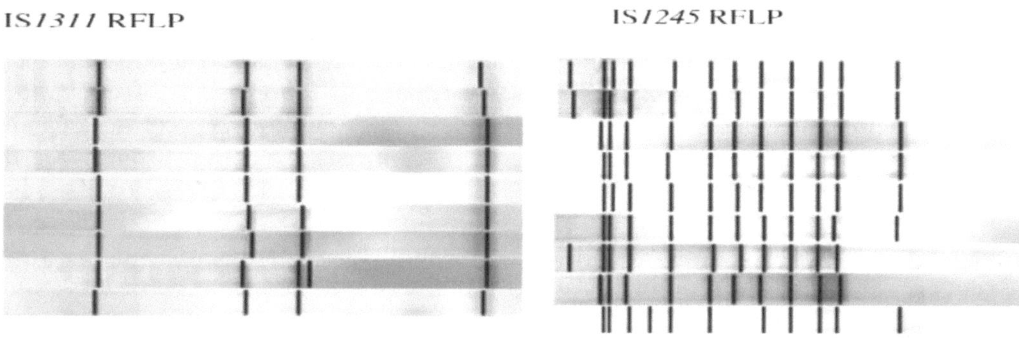

Fig 5

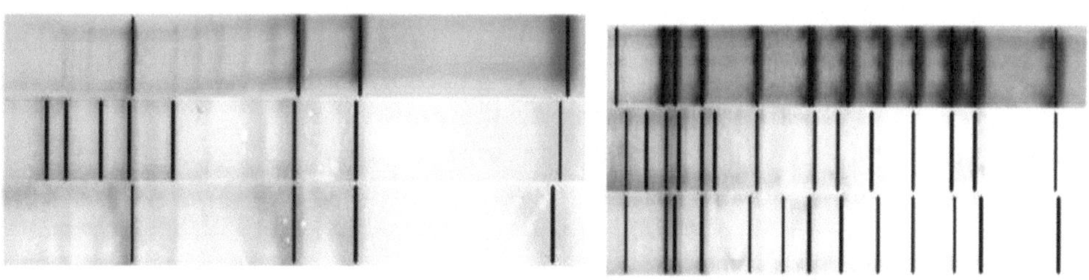

Fig. 4 & 5. Show the insertion sequences 1311 and 1245 of M. avium sub sp hominissuis isolated from humans with cervical lymphadenitis and cattle with disseminated tuberculosis respectively adapted from Oloya et al.,2007 a&b.

Most of these methods are available in Uganda however; they are mainly used for research and not routine clinical diagnostics. This is largely due to the fact that majority of people in Uganda cannot afford these extra costs to arrive at a definitive diagnosis. Fortunately, quick-cheaper, specific and sensitive diagnostic tools have been developed for example the ESAT-6 polymerase chain reaction primers which has been tailor-made to definitively diagnose *M. avium*, Serotyping methods using serotype specific sera for *Mycobacterium interacellulare scrofulaceum* (MAIS complex) and *M. avium* usually associated with AIDS patients can also be used in small and medium scale laboratories for definitive diagnosis (Kiehn et al., 1985; Singh et al., 2007; Wisselink et al 2010). NTM are generally resistant to the standard therapy Isoniazid, Rifampicin and Clarithromycin (Bum-Joon et al 2004). The reported resistance of *M. tuberculosis* (Asimwe et al., 2010) can be a contributing factor for the resistance in NTM due to constant exposure to these antibiotics as a result of lack of definitive diagnosis. There is optimism because of the consistent reported developments in medication which may improve on the treatment of NTMs for example dalfopristin, quinupristin and methoxy moieties of floroquinolones that are reported to have better effects (Lu et al., 2001; Braback, 2002; Singhai et al., 2010; Griffith et al., 2010). Their affectivity is however yet to be tested by the self prescriptive behavior common among Ugandans

5.2 Attitudes surrounding NTM

Uganda is blessed with a wide range of ethnic groups some with unique attitudes and perceptions with regard to prevention and control of infections (Nyanzi et al., 2005). Beliefs, myths, values, norms, taboos language, ritual and art are some of the cultural aspects that influence health of a given society. These cultural aspects describe the interaction between people, land and activities; they are also reported to influence the spread, control and prevention of diseases (Ntseane, 2004; Kyagaba, 2004). Tuberculosis, leprosy and Buruli ulcer are well documented simply because of the priority given to them by the Uganda health sector; this has negatively influenced the attitudes and perception of people towards the rest of NTMs that are regarded to be of less public health importance.

5.2.1 Socio-cultural attitudes in pastoral areas

In Uganda, studies done in rural areas have shown that there are many beliefs, attitudes and practices associated with NTM and other mycobacterial infections even when it is largely known that farming communities lack awareness with regards to mycobacterial infection, their epidemiology, and prevention and control strategies. Apart from mycobacterial infections due to zoonotic tuberculosis and classic tuberculosis; infections due to NTM have rarely been reported. Farming communities in Nakasongola and Mubende districts of Uganda lay their emphasis on the sharing of drinking water from open water sources with both domestic and wild animals as one of the major transmission route of NTM infection to humans and animals at the human-environment- livestock /wildlife interface (Kankya et al., 2010). Furthermore, attitude based studies have shown complacency in pastoral communities which is reflected in reports from service providers highlighted by statements like *"we teach community members that drinking un-boiled water is dangerous but they are stubborn as they continue to drink un-boiled water....many times they tell us that they have not died yet they have been drinking un-boiled water for decades"* commented; clinical officer Kiyuni Government Health Centre III, Mubende district Uganda (Kankya et al 2011 in press). Similarly in neighbouring sub county of Madudu residents said *"our grandparents and great grandparents used to drink un boiled water and milk and their cause of death was not as a result of drinking un boiled water and milk. We grew up drinking all these consumables raw, and that we have made it a cultural norm not to boil milk and water before consumption"* . Rural Africa is always punctuated with witchcraft, some communities have the belief that NTM infections can be caused by witchcraft (voodoo) and thus can be treated (Kankya et al 2011). Therefore families that have witches are believed to have the power to cause such diseases, and that this power can be inherited. Stigmatisation is probably one of the most important reason why these infections are under reported, rural communities are reported to say *"Some of us are sick and infected with mycobacterial infections such as tuberculosis, but we fear to disclose since these infections are associated with HIV/AIDS…"* (Kankya et al 2011). The affected individual would quickly be associated with HIV/AIDS. For the same reason, therefore affected individuals tend to shy away from seeking health services from the qualified health professionals. This aspect greatly impacts the health seeking behaviour (HSB) among the pastoral communities (Ashemeire, 2010).

5.3 Challenges and futures trends

The relative importance of mycobacterial diseases has been undergoing an evolution during the past few years, and further changes and modifications are expected to occur in the near future. The other concern especially in Africa has been the fact that non tuberculous mycobacteria diminishes the efficacy of the BCG (Brandt, 2002), the only available vaccine against tuberculosis. In a study done in Denmark it was shown in a mouse model that prior exposure to the Kalonga-Malawi environmental mycobacteria isolates resulted in reduction of efficacy or complete blockage of BCG activity (Brandt, 2002). This has however not yet been given its due attention in Uganda and therefore is anticipated to be a future challenge in the control of Tuberculosis especially in infants.

6. Conclusion

Non tuberculous mycobacterial infections have not been fully documented in Uganda because; 1) they are given less priority compared to TB regardless of the documented synergistic role they play in tuberculosis lesion development. 2) The dismissive attitude of communities, medical and veterinary fields as to their importance helps maintain their low priority status. With the wind of technological advancement in diagnostics and treatment blowing towards Africa, the increasing number of immune compromised individuals due to AIDS, it is anticipated that more infections due to NTM are likely to be discovered. Therefore the threat of NTM infections in Uganda is as real as the pandemic that precedes them.

7. Recommendations

1. NTMs are a force to reckon in the world today and therefore should be given priority by government, public, medical and veterinary fields.
2. The Ministry of Health and the available health marketing groups should put more emphasis on the campaigns geared towards a stigma free environment with regards to HIV/AIDS so as to improve the health reporting behavior among Ugandans

2a. The government should invest in disseminating free clean water sources like bore holes and piped spring water in rural areas to replace the valley dams which are reported to be the source of highly contaminated water.
2b. The government should improve the current waters sources for livestock and sensitize pastoral communities on the need to maintain them at reasonably high standards in a bid to reduce exposure to livestock.
3. The government should invest in research and innovation so that Ugandans develop tailor made diagnostic and therapeutic for Uganda and the great lakes region.

8. References

Aidsmap (2006). Is Uganda's HIV prevention success story 'unravelling' , Accessed march 2011, Retrieved from: http://www.aidsmap.com/page/1424728/

Anonymous.(2008). District State of Environment Report for Nakasongola District, pp(67) accessed December 2010, retrieved from: http://www.unpei.org/PDF/Uganda-NakasongolaDEP25may08.pdf

Anonymous. (2004). District State of Environment, Mubende District, pp21 accessed December 2010, retrieved from: http://www.nemaug.org/district_reports/mubende_2004_report.pdf

Archibald L, Dulk M, Pallangyo K, Reller B.(1998). Fatal *Mycobacterium tuberculosis* bloodstream infections in febrile hospitalized adults in Dar es Salaam, *Journal of Clinical Infectious Disease*, vol.26, pp(290–296)

Ashemeire P. (2010). Internship report: Palliative treatment at the AIDS support organization in Mbarara District, Department of community psychology Makerere University pp (22-23)

Asiimwe BB, Ghebremichae S, Kallenius G, Koivula T, Joloba ML.(2008). *Mycobacterium tuberculosis* spoligotypes and drug susceptibility pattern of isolates from tuberculosis patients in peri-urban Kampala, Uganda, *BMC Infectious Diseases*, vol.8, pp (101)

Asiimwe BB, Asiimwe J, Ghebremichae S, Kallenius G, Ashaba, Joloba FK, Koivula T.(2009).Molecular characterisation of *Mycobacterium bovis* isolates from cattle carcases at a city slaughterhouse in Uganda, *Veterinary Record. Vol.* 164, pp(655-658)

Banerjee A, Harries AD, Salaniponi FM.(1999). Differences in tuberculosis incidence rates in township and in rural populations in Ntcheu District, Malawi, *Transaction of the Royal Society of Tropica Medicine and Hygiene*, vol.93, No.4, pp(392-393)

Barker DJP.(1971). Buruli disease in a district of Uganda, *Journal of Tropical Medicine and Hygiene* vol. 74, pp (260-264)

Barker DJP, Clancey JK, Rao SK, 1972 *Mycobacterium* on vegetation in Uganda, *East African medical journal*,vol.49, pp(667-671)

Barnes HJ, Swayne DE, Glisson JR,Fadley AM,Macdougald LR. (1997). *Other bacterial dieases in Diseases of Poultry*, (11 edition), Willey Blackwell publishing company IOWA, page 838 Retrieved from <http://books.google.com/books?id=oBloqeMWktMC&pg=PA838&lpg=PA838&dq=m+avium+in+african+poultry&source=bl&ots=6DkwHUlYbw&sig=RQqwQY

uYkuL2z5jiW6kENfI8aqs&hl=en&ei=e4lrTZ3BGI2WswaR0tTdDA&sa=X&oi=book_result&ct=result&resnum=1&ved=0CB4Q6AEwAA#v=onepage&q=m%20avium%20in%20african%20poultry&f=false>

Biet F, Boschiroli ML, Thorel MF, Guilloteau LA.(2005). Zoonotic aspects of *Mycobacterium bovis* and *Mycobacterium avium-intracellulare* complex (MAC), *Journal of Veterinary Research*, vol.36, pp(411-436)

Braback M, Riesbeck K, Forsgren A.(2002).Susceptibilities of *Mycobacterium marinum* to gatifloxacin, gemifloxacin, levofloxacin, linezolid, moxifloxacin, telithromycin and quinupristin - dalfopristin (synercid) compared to its susceptibilities to reference macrolides and quinolones, *Journal of Antimicrobial Agents and Chemotherapy*, vol.46, pp (1114-1116)

Brandt L, Cunha JF, Weinreich A, Chilima B, Hirsch P, Appelberg R , Andersen P.(2002). Failure of the Mycobacterium bovis BCG vaccine: Some species of environmental mycobacteria block multiplication of BCG and induction of protective immunity to tuberculosis, *Journal of Infection and Immunity*, vol. 70, pp (672–678)

Buijtels CAMP, Marrianne AB, Graaf SDC, Parkinson S, Verbrugh AH, Petit LCP, Sooligen VD. (2009). Nontuberculous mycobacteria, Zambia, *Journal of EmergingInfectious Diseases*, vol.15, pp (242–248)

Bum-Joon K, Keun-Hwa L, Yeo-Jun Y, Eun-Mi P,Young-Gil P, Gil-Han B, Chang-Yong C, Yoon-Hoh K.(2004). Simultaneous identification of rifampin-resistant *Mycobacterium tuberculosis* and nontuberculous mycobacteria by polymerase chain reaction-single strand conformation polymorphism and sequence analysis of the RNA polymerase gene (rpoB), *Journal of Microbiological Methods* vol.58 pp (111 - 118)

Byarugaba F, Marcel CEE, Godreuil S, Grimaud P(2009).Pulmonary Tuberculosis and Mycobacterium bovis, Uganda, *Emerging Infectious Diseases* ,vol 15 accessed march 2011, retrieved from: www.cdc.gov/eid

Chinaview. (2008). 'Complacency, extramarital affairs pushing up Ugandan HIV infection rate', Acessed: march 2011 http://news.xinhuanet.com/english/2008-06/02/content_8302718.htm

Claudio P, Scarparo C.(2008). Review: Pulmonary infections associated with non-tuberculous mycobacteria in immunocompetent patients, *Lancet Infectious Disease*, vol.8, pp (323–334)

Clive AP, Alan SK, Mark H.(2001). Prevalence and Clinical Manifestations of Disseminated *Mycobacterium avium* Complex Infection in South Africans with Acquired Immunodeficiency Syndrome, *Journal of Clinical Infectious Diseases*, vol.33, pp (2068–2071)

Commonwealth youth forum (cwyf).(2007). Health,HIV/AIDS and development: A case for Uganda, accessed December 2010, retrieved from: http://www.aidsuganda.org/HIV%20PDf/comnwealth.pdf

Coetzer JAW, Tustin RC. (2004). *Infectious Diseases of livestock*, (3rd edition) Oxford University Press, New York, pp (1973-1987)

Cosivi O, Grange JM, Daborn CJ, Raviglione MC, Fujikura T, Cousins D.(1998). Zoonotic tuberculosis due to *Mycobacterium* bovis in developing countries, *Journal of Emerging Infectious Disease*, vol.4, pp (59–70).

Eaton T, Falkinham JO, III, Aisu TO, Daniel TM.(1995). Isolation and characteristics of *Mycobacterium avium* complex from water and soil samples in Uganda, *Journal of Tuberculosis and Lung Disease*, vol.76, pp(570-574)

Falkinham JO. (1996). Epidemiology of infection by nontuberculous mycobacteria, *Clinical Microbiology Review*, vol.9, pp (177-215)

Falkinham JO.(2009). Surrounded by mycobacteria: nontuberculous mycobacteria in the human environment, *Journal of Applied Microbiology*, vol.107, pp (356-367)

Gilks C, Brindle R, Mwachari C.(1995) Disseminated *Mycobacterium avium* infection among HIV-infected patients in Kenya. *Journal of Acquired Immune Deficiency Syndrom and Human Retrovirol*, vol.8, pp(195–198)

Giuseppe H, Katsambas A, Lotti T.(1997). Non-tuberculous mycobacterial skin infections, *Journal of the European Academy of Dermatology and Venereology*, vol. 9, pp (1-35)

Griffith DE, Wallace JR. (2010). Treatment of nontuberculous mycobacterial infections of the lung in HIV-negative patients, In: *Uptodate* March, 2011 Available from: September 2011 http://www.uptodate.com/contents/treatment-of-nontuberculous-mycobacterial-infections-of-the-lung-in-hiv-negative-patients

Hogle JA, Green E, Nantulya V,Stoneburner R, Stover J.(2002). What Happened inUganda? Declining HIV Prevalence, Behavior Change, and the National Response: PROJECT LESSONS LEARNED CASE STUDY,

U.S. *Agency for International Development* march, 2011 Available September 2002 http://www.usaid.gov/our_work/global_health/aids/Countries/africa/uganda_report.pdf

Hooper ED.(1990) 'AIDS epidemic moves south through Africa, *New Scientist* Acessed: march 2011 http://www.newscientist.com/article/mg12717241.400-aids-epidemic-moves-south-through-africa.html

Horsburgh CR, Selik RM.(1989). The epidemiology of disseminated non-tuberculous mycobacterial infection in the acquired immunodeficiency syndrome (AIDS), *American Review of Respiratory Disease*, vol.139, pp (4 -7)

Horsburgh CR.(1991). *Mycobacterium avium* complex infection in the acquired immunodeficiency syndrome. *New England Journal of Medicine*,vol 324 pp(1332–1338).

Johansen T, Olsen I, Jensen M, Dahle U, Holstad G, Djonne B. (2007). New probes used for IS1245 and IS1311 restriction fragment length polymorphism *of Mycobacterium avium* subsp. *avium* and *Mycobacterium avium* subsp. *hominissuis* isolates of human and animal origin in Norway, *BMC Microbiology*, vol. 7, pp (14)

Kaiser HJ Family Foundation (2005) Uganda's Decline in HIV/AIDS Prevalence Attributed to Increased Condom Use, Early Death From AIDS, *Study Says* Accessed February 2011, retrieved from: The body http://www.thebody.com/content/art9249.html

Kankya C, Muwonge A, Olet S, Munyeme M, Biffa D, Opuda-Asibo J, Skjerve E, Oloya J.(2010). Factors associated with pastoral community knowledge and occurrence of mycobacterial infections in Human-Animal Interface areas of Nakasongola and Mubende districts, Uganda, *BMC Public Health*, vol.10, pp 471.

Kankya C, Muwonge A, Djønne B, Munyeme M, Opuda-Asibo J, Skjerve E, Oloya J, Edvardsen V, Bjordal Johansen T.(2011a). Isolation of non-tuberculous mycobacteria from pastoral ecosystems of Uganda: Public Health significance, *BMC Public Health* BMC Public Health 11:320, http://www.biomedcentral.com/1471-2458/11/320

Kankya C, Mugisha A, Muwonge A, Skjerve E Kyomugisha E.(2011b). Myths, knowledge, attitudes, and perceptions linked to mycobacterial infection management among Ugandan pastoralists. *Journal of social behaviour and health sciences* in Press 2011

Katoc VM. (2004). Infections due to non-tuberculous mycobacteria (NTM), *Indian Journal of Medical Research*, vol. 120, pp (290-304)

Kawuma HJ, (1999) Early detection in leprosy' and 'The trends of leprosy control in Uganda, *International Leprosy Congress in Beijing* September 1999

Kiehn TE, Edwards FF, Brannon P, Tsang AY, Mary M, Jonathan WHG. (1985) Infections caused by MAC in immunocompromized patients ; diagnosis by blood culture and fecal examination, antimicrobial susceptability tests, and morphological and seroagglutination characterstics, *Journal of Clinical Microbiology*, vol. 21, pp (168-173).

Krizova K, Matlova L, Horvathova A, Moravkova M, Beran V, Boisselet T, Babak V, Slana I, Pavlik I.(2010).Mycobacteria in the environment of pig farms in the Czech Republic between 2003 and 2007. *Veterinarni Medicina*, vol.55, pp(55–69)

Liefoogh R, Baliddawa JB, Kipruto EM, Vermeire C, De Munynck AO. (1997). From their own perspective. A Kenyan community's perception of tuberculosis, *Tropical Medicine and International Health*, vol.2, pp(809-821)

Lu T, Zhao X, Li X, lic a -Wagner A , Wang J Y, Domagala J , et al.,(2001).Enhancement of fluroquinolones activity by C-8 halogen and methoxy moities: action against a gyrase resistant mutant of *Mycobacterium smegmatis* and a gyrase-topoisomerase IV double mutant of *Staphylococcus aureus*, *Journal of Antimicrobial Agents and Chemotherapy*, vol.45, pp (2703-2709)

Lucas S, Hounnou A, Peacock C, et al.(1993). The mortality and pathology of HIV infection in a West African city, *AIDS*, vol. 7, pp(1569–1579)

Masur H.(1993). Public Health Service Task Force on Prophylaxis and Therapy for *Mycobacterium avium* Complex: special report. Recommendations on prophylaxis and therapy for disseminated *Mycobacterium avium* complex disease in patients infected with the human immunodeficiency virus, *New England Journal of Medicine*, vol. 329, pp (898-904)

Ministry of Health Uganda (MOH). *(2006)*. 'Uganda: HIV/AIDS Sero-Behavioural Survey: 2004-05', accessed march 2011, retrieved from: http://www.measuredhs.com/pubs/pdf/AIS2/AIS2.pdf

Ministry of Health, Uganda(MOH) (2005). Final Draft - Health Sector Strategic Plan II 2005/06 - 2009/10, October 2005, accessed march 2011, retrieved from: http://www.who.int/rpc/evipnet/Health%20Sector%20Strategic%20Plan%20II%202009-2010.pdf

Ministry of Gender Labour and Social Development. (2004). National Strategic Programme Plan of Interventions for Orphans and Other Vulnerable Children Fiscal Year 2005/6-2009/10. Kampala:*Ministry of Gender Labour and Social Development,* accessed march 2011, retieved from:
http://www.aidsuganda.org/HIV%20PDf/comnwealth.pdf

Muwonge A, Kankya C, Godfroid J, Djonne B, Opuda-Asibo J, Biffa D, Skjerve E.(2010).Prevalence and associated risk factors of mycobacterial infections in slaughter pigs from Mubende district in Uganda, *Journal of Tropical Animal Health and Production,* vol.42, pp(905-913)

Muwonge A, Kankya C, Johansen TB, Djonne B, Godfroid J, Biffa D, Vigdis E, Skjerve E.(2011). Non-tuberculous mycobacteria isolated from slaughtered pigs in Mubende district, Uganda, *BMC Veterinary research (Under review)*

National Tuberculosis and Leprosy Program, Uganda. (2005). Status Report for Leprosy 2004, Accessed march 2011, retrieved from:
http://docs.google.com/viewer?a=v&q=cache:hdhWT8EccQIJ:www.kumihospital.org/reports/ZTLS%2520East%252005.doc+National+Tuberculosis+and+Leprosy+Program,+Uganda.+(2005).+Status+Report+for+Leprosy+2004,&hl=en&pid=bl&srcid=ADGEESgSuVljuLsCvaBic8bhpNBMX1NAgne886KXMrRL-BNSr-DV4FhX8nZq7-UnOjSxqcW5X1T4-UyZSYTeH-9ssQVwO5VM8m04ew89-E0ZobL13a4sL6Q606NFPppO5I2hHCZCXSsx&sig=AHIEtbSidkcnpZRCdO9em1yfPGESc7z11g

Nambuya A, Sewankambo N, Mugerwa J, Goodgame R, Lucas S.(1988). Tuberculous lymphadenitis associated with human immunodeficiency virus (HIV) in Uganda, *Journal of Clinical Pathology,* vol. 41, pp (93-96)

Narang P.(2008).Prevalence of non-tuberculous mycobacteria in India, *Indian Journal of Tuberculosis,* vol.55, pp (175-178)

Nkolo A ,Kalyesubula KS.(2006) Tour of the districts in the eastern zone of Uganda 12th to 23rd December 2005: Activity report *National tuberculosis and leprosy program* Retrieved from:
http://docs.google.com/viewer?a=v&q=cache:hdhWT8EccQIJ:www.kumihospital.org/reports/ZTLS%2520East%252005.doc+Nkolo+A+,Kalyesubula+KS.(2006)+TOUR+OF+THE+DISTRICTS+IN+THE+EASTERN+ZONE+OF+UGANDA+12th+to+23rd+DECEMBER+2005:+ACTIVITY+REPORT+NATIONAL+TUBERCULOSIS+ANDF+LEPROSY+PROGRAM&hl=en&pid=bl&srcid=ADGEESgSuVljuLsCvaBic8bhpNBMX1NAgne886KXMrRL-BNSr-DV4FhX8nZq7-UnOjSxqcW5X1T4-UyZSYTeH-9ssQVwO5VM8m04ew89E0ZobL13a4sL6Q606NFPppO5I2hHCZCXSsx&sig=AHIEtbQnCC5xETzpnbfIYaM14cI5oYcHAA

Ofukwo RA, lortyom BK, Akwuobu CA.(2010). Mycobacterium Avium and *Mycobacterium intracellulare* Infections in Slaughtered Pigs in Makurdi, North-Central Nigeria: An Emerging Zoonosis, *International Journal of Animal and Veterinary Advance,* vol.2,pp (43-46)

Okello D, Sewankambo N, Goodgame R.(1990). Absence of bacteremia with *Mycobacterium avium-intracellulare* in Ugandan patients with AIDS, *Journal of Infection and Disease,* vol. 162, pp(208–210)

Open vision youth club. (2004). My AIDS HERO,Accessed march 2011, retrieved from http://myhero.com/go/hero.asp?hero=PHILLY

Oloya J , Kazwala R, Lund A, Opuda-Asibo J,Biffa D, Skjerve E, Johansen TB, Djønne B,.(2007a). Characterisation of *mycobacteria* isolated from slaughter cattle in pastoral regions of Uganda, *BMC Microbiology*, vol. 7 95, doi: 10.1186/1471-2180-7-95

Oloya J, Muma JB, Opuda-Asibo J, Djønne B, Kazwala R, Skjerve E.(2007b). Risk factors for herd-level bovinetuberculosis seropositivity in transhumant cattle in Uganda, *Journal of Preventive Veterinary Medicine*, vol. 80, pp(318-329)

Serwadda D, Mugerwa RD, Sewankambo NK, Lwegaba A, Carswell JW, Kirya GB, Bayley AC, Downing RG, Tedder RS, Clayden SA. (1985) 'Slim Disease: A New Disease in Uganda and its Association with HTLV-III Infection' *Lancet* vol. 2, No.8460, pp(849-852)

Singh S, Gopinath K, Saba Shahbad MK, Singh B, Sharma P. (2007). Non tuberculous mycobacterial infections in Indian AIDS patients detected by a novel set of ESAT-6 polymerase chain reaction primers, *Japanese journal of infectious diseases*, vol.60, pp (14-18)

Singhal A, Gates C, Malhotra N, Irwin DA, Chansolme DH, Kohli V. (2010). Successful management of primary nontuberculous mycobacterial infection of hepatic allograft following orthotopic liver transplantation for hepatitis C, *Journal of Transplant and Infectious Disease,* Vol.13, No.1, pp (47–51)

Stanford JL, Paul RC.(1976). A preliminary study of the effects of contact with environmental mycobacteria on the patterns of sensitivity to a range of new tuberculins amongst Ugandan adults, *Journal of hygiene*, vol.76, pp (205)

Stoneburner RL, Low-Beer D. (2004). Population-level HIV declines and behavioral risk avoidance in Uganda, *Science*, vol. 30 No.304, pp (714-718)

Ssali FN, Kamya MR, Wabwire-Mangen F, Kasasa S, Joloba M, Williams D, Mugerwa RD, Ellner JJ, Johnson JL A.(1998). Prospective study of community-acquired bloodstream infections among febrile adults admitted to Mulago Hospital in Kampala, Uganda, Journal of Acquired Immune Deficiency Syndrom and Human Retrovirology. Vol.19, No.5,pp(484-489)

STD/AIDS Control Programme. (2002) Trends in HIV prevalence and sexual behavior, Accessed:March, 2011 http://gateway.nlm.nih.gov/MeetingAbstracts/ma?f=102253576.html

The Body. (2005).Uganda's Decline in HIV/AIDS Prevalence Attributed to Increased Condom Use, Early Death From AIDS, Study Says Accessed march 2011,retrieved from: http://www.thebody.com/content/art9249.html

Tupasi TE, Radhakrishna S, Quelapio MI, Villa ML, Pascual ML, RiveraAB, Sarmiento A, Co VM, Sarol JN, Beltran G, Legaspi JD, MangubatNV, Reyes AC, Solon M, Solon FS, Burton L, Mantala MJ.(2000). Tuberculosis in the urban poor settlements in the Philippines *International Journal of Tuberculosis and Lung Disease,* vol.4, No.1,pp(4-11).

UNAIDS (2010) 'UNAIDS report on the global AIDS epidemic, Accessed march 2011, retrieved from: http://www.unaids.org/globalreport/Global_report.htm

Uganda AIDS commission (UAC). (2004-a). The Revised National Strategic Framework for HIV/AIDS Activities in Uganda 2000/1 - 2005/6, A Guide for all HIV/AIDS Stakeholders, Uganda AIDS Commission, Kampala, Accessed march 2011 http://www.aidsuganda.org/HIV%20PDf/comnwealth.pdf

Van Ingen J, Boeree MJ, Dekhuijzen PN, Soolingen VD.(2009). Environmental sources of rapid growing nontuberculous mycobacteria causing disease in humans, Journal *of clinical Microbiology and Infection,* vol.15, pp(888-893)

Wisselink HJ, van Solt-Smits CB, Oorburg D, van Soolingen D, Overduin P, Maneschijn-Bonsing J, Stockhofe-Zurwieden N,Buys-Bergen H,Engel B Urlings BAP, Thole JER. (2010). Serodiagnosis of *Mycobacterium avium* infections in pigs, *Veterinary Microbiology,* vol.142, pp(401–40)

Wolinsky E. (1979). Non-tuberculous mycobacteria and associated disease, *American Review journal of Respiratory Diseases,* vol.119, pp (107-59)

Wolinsky E. (1995). Mycobacterial lymphadenitis in children: a prospective study of 105 nontuberculous cases with long-term follow-up, *Journal of Clinical Infectious Disease,* vol.20, pp(954–963)

WHO/UNAIDS/UNICEF (2010) 'Towards universal access: Scaling up priority HIV/AIDS interventions in the health sector, Accessed march 2011, retrieved from: http://www.who.int/hiv/pub/2010progressreport/en/index.html

WHO, Tropical Disease Research Website. Strategic direction for research in Leprosy, February 2002, 2004, accessed January 2011, retrieved from: http://www.who.int/tdrold/diseases/leprosy/direction.htm

World Health Organization (WHO). WHO Report (2007), global tuberculosis control, Uganda.WHO/HTM/TB/2007.376 Accessed 2008 march 2011, retrieved from: http://www.who.int/tb/publications/global_report/2007/pdf/uga.pdf

Part 2

HIV Transmission

3

Human Immunodeficiency Virus Transmission

Goselle Obed Nanjul[1,2]
[1]*School of Biological Sciences, Bangor University*
[2]*Applied Entomology and Parasitology Unit, Department of Zoology, University of Jos,*
[1]*UK*
[2]*Nigeria*

1. Introduction

Human Immunodeficiency Virus (HIV) is the causative organism of AIDS which has become one of the greatest public health challenges faced by mankind. AIDS was first identified in 1981 in Los Angeles, USA. Two types of HIV exist presently- HIV-1 and HIV-2 (Alizon et al., 2010; Adoga et al., 2010). HIV-1 was first isolated in the early 1980s (Barre-Sinoussi et al., 1983) and linked as causative agent of AIDS (Gallo et al., 1984). HIV-2 which is similar to HIV-1 was later identified in the developing world (Clavel, 1987, Clavel et al., 1986), but found to be less virulent and can differ in its response to antiretroviral agents. HIV-1 is classified into three groups [M, N and O] based on the genetic diversity. Group M (major) has 10 subtypes (A-J), and Group O (outlier) represents a number of highly divergent strains (Carr et al., 1998; Jassens et al., 1997 Chen et al., 2010). Francois Simon and his group reported a group N of HIV-1. Despite the phenotypic classification of HIV-1 into subtypes, the number of sequenced isolates remains limited (Sharp et al., 1994). Both strains are spread in the same way and have the same AIDS causing consequences. While HIV-1 has been reported to have a shorter incubation period of 7-10years, HIV-2 is considerably longer and often less severe (Barre-Sinoussi, 1996; WHO, 1989).

HIV infection is usually followed by a chronic progressive destruction of the immune and neurologic system (Price, 1996), which if not managed leads to the possible invasion and establishment of multiple opportunistic infections.(Lindo et al., 1998; Pozio et al., 1997) and malignancy (Schulz et al., 1996). Although on average, an infected individual spends several years without manifesting the disease, AIDS has always been certain. The time from infection to AIDS varies widely between individuals, from a few months to as many as 20 years with existing evidences accepting that 50% of individuals progress to AIDS in 7-10years and this has been accepted as the incubation period of the virus (Del Amo et al., 1998; WHO, 1994).

2. Portals of HIV transmission

The concentration of virus in a body fluid and the extent of exposure to body fluids determine to a great extent the transmission of a virus. Jaffe and McMahon-Pratt (1983) first indicated in their Epidemiological studies conducted in 1981 and 1982 that the major channel of transmission of AIDS were intimate sexual contact and contaminated blood. Gottlieb et al (1981); Masur et al (1981); Siegal et al (1981); Callazos et al (2010); van

Griensven and de Lin van Wijngaarden (2010) all described the syndrome in homosexual and bisexual men and, intravenous drug users, while Harris et al (1983); Padian et al (1991); Cameron et al (1989); Quinn et al (2000) and Decker et al (2010) recognised their mode of transmission through heterosexual activity. Evidences later showed that transmission recipients and haemophiliacs could contract the illness from blood or blood products (CDC, 1982; Peterson, 1992; CDC, 2010) and newborn infants get infected from their mothers' (Ammann et al., 1983; Scarlatti, 1996; Brookmeyer, 1991; Landesman, et al., 1996; Goedert et al., 1989; Mackelprang et al., 2010). Brookmeyer (1991); Stoneburner et al (1990) all agreed that the three principal means of transmission - blood, sexual contact and mother-to-child have not changed which could be attributed to a greater degree to the relative amount of the virus in various body fluids.

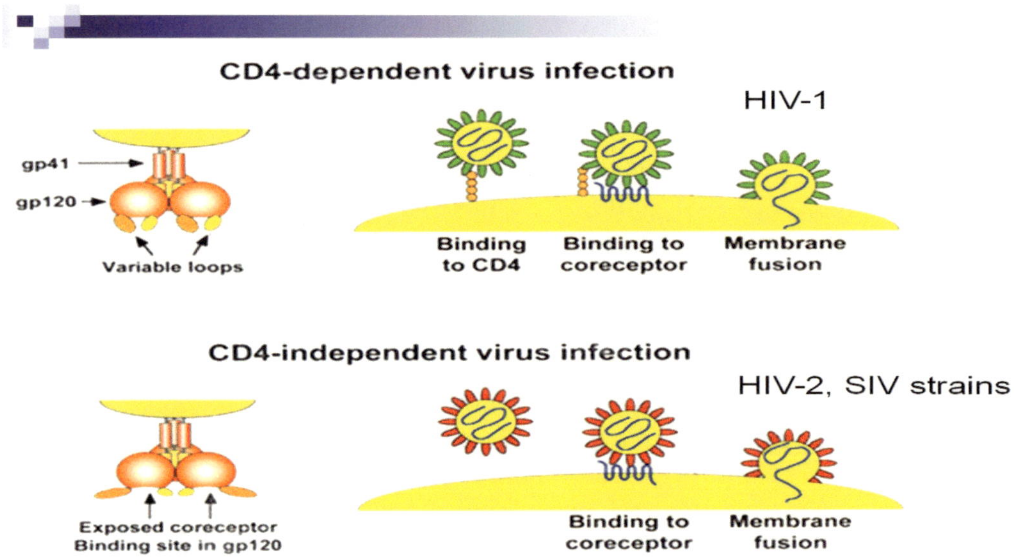

Fig. 1. Diagrammatic representation of HIV-1 and HIV-2 showing their dependent and independence on CD4+ [Courtesy-]

HIV is present in semen (including pre-seminal fluid), vaginal/cervical secretions and blood, breast milk expressed through feeding; organ donations; sharing infected objects (needles, tattoos and piercing) which are the main vehicles through which the virus is transmitted (Kim et al., 2010; Yu et al., 2010; Suligoi et al., 2010; Pruss et al., 2010 and Baggaley et al., 2010). The virus may also be present in saliva, tears, urine, cerebrospinal fluid and infected discharges, but these are not vehicles of which HIV is spread. Epidemiological survey do not support transmission through water or food, sharing eating utensils, coughing or sneezing, vomiting, toilets, swimming pools, insect bites, shaking of hands or other casual contacts, hence there is no public health reason for discrimination and or restrictions.

A study of French hospital patients by Grabar et al (2009) found that approximately 0.5% of HIV-1 infected individuals retain high levels of CD4+ T-cells and a low or clinically undetectable viral load without anti-retroviral treatment. These individuals are classified as HIV controllers or long-term non-progressors.

For conveniences, we will share the mode of infections into: Sexual and Non-sexual.

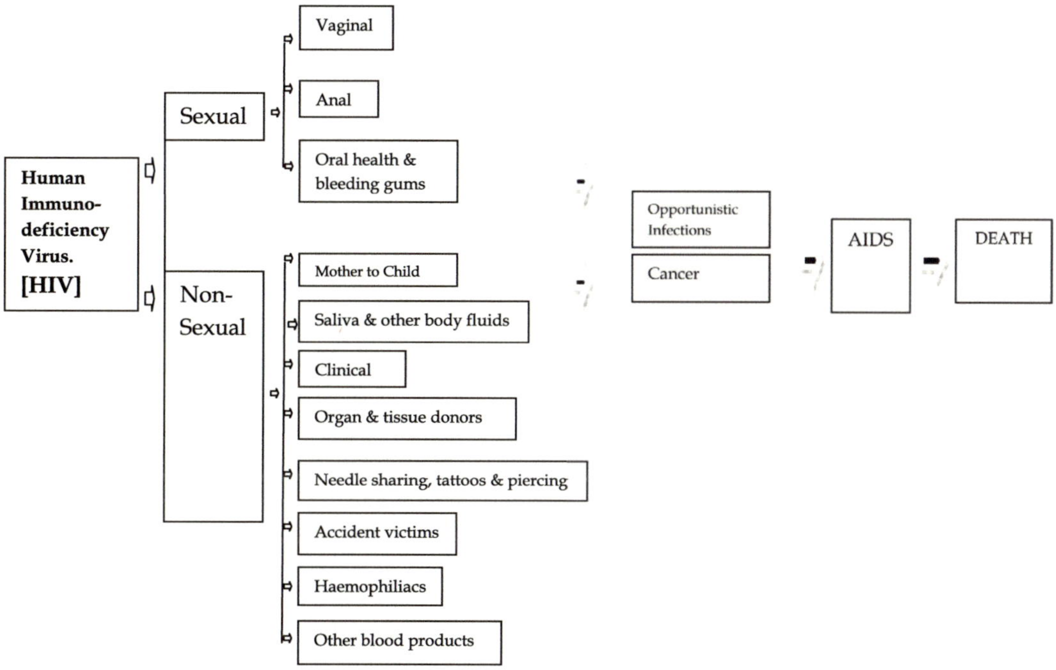

Fig. 2. Routes of Transmission of Human Immuno-deficiency Virus. [HIV]

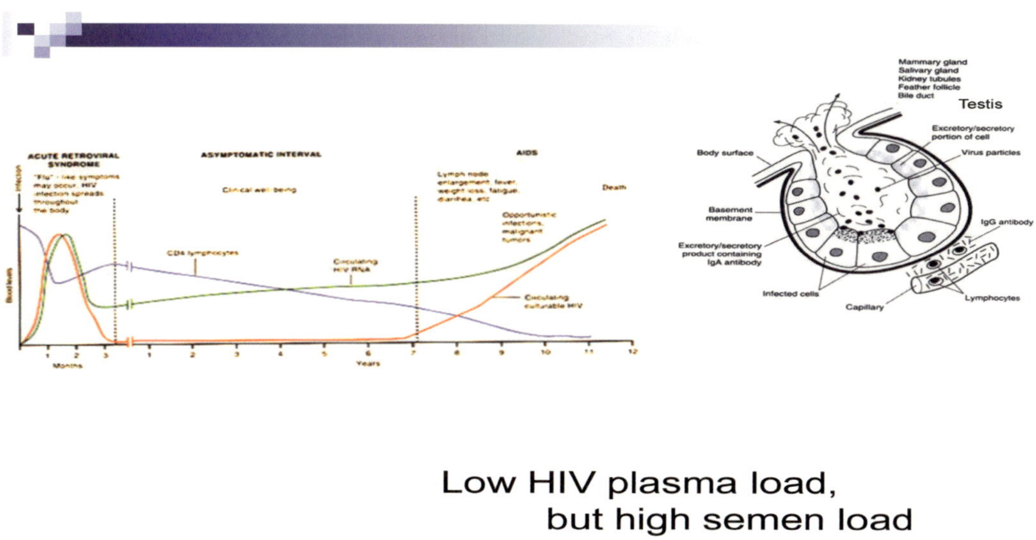

Fig. 3. Levels of HIV load in semen [Courtesy:...]

3. Vertical or Mother To Child Tranmission (MTCT)

The major source of paediatric infection of Human immunodeficiency virus one (HIV-1) is from mother to child. Since the first reported case of HIV-1 transmission in children in 1983, the global pandemic has had a serious impact on the health and survival of children. Transmission rates have been reported to be about 14% in industrialised countries and about 35-45% in developing countries especially in Africa (Bryson, 1996; Reinhardt et al., 1995).

It was estimated that MTCT accounts for over 1.5million HIV infection in children (Burton, 1996) with the WHO projecting between 5-10million child infections through MTCT during the next decade. HIV-2 though is related to HIV-1 is less readily transmitted from mother to child, this could be attributed to their differences which influences pathogenecity, natural history and therapy so that their susceptibility to antiretroviral therapy (ART) follows different mutation pathways to develop drug resistance (Mamata and Merchant, 2010).

According to Wollinsky et al (1992) as quoted by Pasquier et al (1998), the transmission of HIV-1 from mother to child occur *utero, intrapartum*, or postnatally by breastfeeding and a fourth dimension as reported by Pasquier et al (1998) which involves the transmission of multiple maternal variants to the infant and a rapid, fatal outcome in the child and the development of an HIV-based clinical disease in children seems to be correlated with the timing of the vertical transmission.

Infection in about two-thirds of children are thought to have occurred at the terminal end of pregnancy or at delivery with the disease progressing slowly; while in one-thirds, it is thought to progress rapidly to AIDS with increased indices of viral replication (De Rossi et al., 1998), these children appear to have been infected during pregnancy.

Infected children with slow progression to AIDS have a higher viral diversity than children who progress rapidly as evidenced in molecular variability studies (Halapi et al., 1996; Strunnikora et al., 1995) as reported in Adults (Delwart et al., 1997; Pasquier et al., 1998).

Although progress has been made in recent years in the curbing of MTCT, the mechanisms and timing of transmission remains uncertain and the relative contributions of each of the three modes of transmission is still not well defined. Bryson et al (1992) proposed that in most non-breastfeeding population; the lack of detection of virus in the child at birth might indicate that contamination took place at or shortly before delivery while detection of virus at birth indicates *utero* contamination. Evidences for both early and late utero transmission have been documented (Peckham and Gibb, 1995; Kuhn and Stein, 1995). Most prior estimates and hypothesis seem to agree that transmission usually occur during the *intrapartum* HIV exposure just as premature infants.

Perinatal or *Antepartum* HIV transmission has been documented as a route of infection estimated to occur in 13-30% of infants delivered to HIV-1 infected mothers (Andiman et al., 1990).

High proviral DNA/ or RNA concentration of virus is a risk factor for the transmission of HIV-1 from an untreated mother to infant. The reduction in such transmission after zidovudine is only partly explained by the reduction in plasma levels of viral RNA. To prevent HIV-1 transmission initiating maternal treatment with zidovudine is recommended regardless of the plasma level of HIV-1 RNA or the CD4+ Count (Sperling et al., 1996). Because of the different mutation pathways to develop drug resistance, pregnant women with detectable HIV-2 should be ideally managed using a Highly Active antiretroviral therapy (HAART) regimen to which the virus is sensitive. Non-nucleoside Reverse

Transcriptase Inhibitor (NNRTIs) and Fusion Inhibitor Enfuvirtide have no activity against HIV-2 and in the light of the current albeit limited data, zidovudine mono-therapy should not be used. These factors make it crucial that proper selection of and adherence to the first antiretroviral combination regimen is in place in order to achieve a successful treatment response. Though of recent, a combination of Combivir and nevarapine is given to mothers to prevent transmission of HIV to children. The Emergency Lower Segment Caesarian Section (ELSCS) could be planned at 38 weeks of gestation with regards to the mode of delivery if the viral load is undetectable or the mother is either symptomatic or has low CD4 cell count. HIV is present in breast milk and postnatal transmission via breastfeeding is an important component of MTCT in Sub-Saharan Africa (Kreiss, 1997). World-wide, an estimated one in three of vertical transmission may be due to breastfeeding with above 12months of age carrying higher risk (Bulterys et al., 1995). Kuhn and Stein (1997) demonstrated that under certain conditions prevailing in specific settings in developing countries, breast feeding for six months would be preferable to breast feeding beyond this age. Breastfeeding has been reported to account for 5-15% of infants becoming infected with HIV-1 after delivery (ECS 1991; Ryder et al., 1989; Mok et al., 1989). Although the placental entry of some infections is a critical aspect of these infections, the role of placental cells and the mechanism by which pathogens pass from the maternal to the foetal circulation varies. The placenta provides a barrier that prevents transmission of some viruses, but allows others to reach the foetal circulation. Mother to foetus placental transmission of some viruses occurs through transcytosis across placental cells. The placenta may also act as a reservoir in which virus replicates before reaching the foetus. Placental transmission of HIV-1 is a complex incompletely understood process which requires advanced studies (Al-husaini, 2009). The antiretroviral therapy, zidovudine (ZDV) is metabolized into its active form in the placenta (Qian et al., 1994). ZDV inhibits HIV replication within placental cells. To reach the foetal circulation, HIV-1 should cross the trophoblastic placental barrier (cytotrophoblasts and syncitiotrophoblasts). Blood borne maternal pathogens that arrive at the uteroplacental circulation and intervillous space may reach the foetus through the villous capillaries. HIV-1 has been detected on both the maternal and the foetal parts of the placenta. HIV-1 experiences replication in the placenta. The virus may cross the trophoblastic barrier by endocytosis, or by an injured villous surface. However, superficial breaks in syncytiotrophoblast cells do not radically affect the vertical transmission of viruses (Burton et al., 1996). The reverse transcriptase enzyme of HIV-1 is important in the life cycle of the virus by converting the single-stranded RNA genome into double-stranded DNA that integrates into the host chromosome. There is a lower degree of viral heterogeneity in transmitting mothers compared with nontransmitting mothers (Sundaravaradan et al., 2005).

Human chorionic gonadotropin (hCG) has been shown in vitro to inhibit reverse transcriptase and to block viral transmission between virus-carrying lymphocytes and placental trophoblasts (Bourinbaiar and Lee-Huang, 1995). However, role of hCG in protecting the foetus from vertical transmission HIV-1 needs to be studied. In summary, the restricted heterogeneity of HIV-1 in the infected mothers is more likely associated with lack of vertical transmission (Al-husaini, 2009).

As access to services for preventing the mother-to-child transmission of HIV has increased, the total number of children being born with HIV has also decreased. An estimated 370 000 [230 000–510 000] children were newly infected with HIV in 2009 (a drop of 24% from five years earlier)[UNAIDS, 2010].

4. Risk factors for vertical transmission of HIV

Documented evidence primarily based on PCR and virus culture studies or co-culture studies but short of serology which revealed maternal antibodies present in infants at birth showed that transmission of HIV from mother to child appears to occur in 11-60% of children delivered by HIV-positive mothers but reasons for the wide variations in virus transmission and sources of virus in newborn which could have provided approach to prevention are not known (Ades et. al., 1991; Courgnaud et. al., 1991; Lindgren et. al., 1991; Newell et. al., 1992; Scarlatti et. al., 1991; Tovo and Martino, 1988; Oxtoby, 1990; Rogers et. al., 1991).

Maternal, viral, obstetric, foetal, infant factors all affect transmission making it essentially multifactorial. Frequency of sexual activity, 'hard' drug ingestion during pregnancy, unprotected sexual intercourse, cigarette smoking during pregnancy, lack of adherence to drugs, HIV disease, degraded maternal immunocompetence or prolonged rupture of the amniotic membranes before delivery (Havens et al., 1997; Turner et al., 1996; Bryson, 1996; John and Kreiss, 1996; Lambert, 1996; Glenn and Dietrich, 1993).

The maternal factors involve transmission through the placenta to the unborn child, at the time of labour and delivery, or through breast-feeding. (CDC HIV/AIDS surveillance, October, 1989), seroconversion during pregnancy, advanced stage of the disease with high viral load and low immunity, concomitant malnutrition, micronutrient deficiencies, sexually transmitted diseases, no or suboptimal therapy; in the intranatal period, risk factors for increased transmission are mode of delivery, prolonged contact with maternal blood or cervicovaginal secretions, prolonged rupture of membranes, chorioamnionitis, invasive procedures like episiotomy, foetal scalp electrode, instrumental delivery; thin skin, susceptible mucous membranes, immature immune functions and low levels of maternal antibodies make prematurity a risk factor for increased transmission. In the postnatal period, risk factors are breast feeding, feeding with cracked nipples/mastitis, mixed feeding, new seroconversion of the mother, high viral load, low CD4 cell count; In the absence of any intervention, rates of MTCT of HIV-1 can vary from 15 to 30% in developed countries and increase to 30 to 45% in developing countries, the difference mainly attributable to infant feeding practices that comprise almost universally of breastfeeds for prolonged duration (De Cock et al., 2000 as quoted by Mamata and Merchant, 2001).

The foetus and mother circulatory systems though different, there still exists tiny mixing of blood that could serve as portal for the flow of infected maternal white blood cells or the AIDS virus in the maternal serum to be transmitted to the foetus with a confirmation found in the foetal tissues affirming such spread (CDC HIV/AIDS surveillance, October 1989; Glenn and Dietrich, 1993).

Bruising, abrasions and local swelling could occur to the baby and mother during labour owing to a great deal of trauma which produces visible and microscopic openings that could allow the virus to penetrate blood stream of infant. Another means of infection could be experienced or seen when the mother's perineum tears or if she receives an episiotomy which might lead to a large amounts of blood ingested by the baby or might get into the baby's mouth, eyes, rectum or vagina.

Glenn et al (1993) reported that breastfeeding is another means of risks exposure and it has been confirmed in the spread of hepatitis B from mother to infant and hepatitis B and AIDS as well which are thought to occur when the infant ingests the mothers blood through a cracked and bleeding nipples.

Other known correlates include high maternal plasma viremia, advanced clinical HIV disease, degraded maternal immunocompetence or prolonged rupture of the amniotic membranes before delivery. Others include vaginal delivery process and prematurity of low birth weight of the neonate (Bryson, 1996; John and Kreiss, 1996; Lambert, 1996).

High frequency of sexual activity and "hard" drug injection during pregnancy had previously been identified, along with unprotected sexual intercourse during pregnancy as certain behavioural risk factors for mother-to-child-transmission (Bulterys et al., 1997; Bulterys and Goedert, 1996). Firstly, unprotected intercourse might increase the concentration of strain diversity of HIV-1, particularly in the birth canal where ejaculated virus could be partially sequestered. Secondly, frequent intercourse might increase inflammation of the cervix or vagina either micro abrasion or if unprotected, by STDs. Third, frequent intercourse might increase the risk of chorioamnionitis or otherwise alter the integrity of the placenta (Bulterys and Goedert, 1996). Matheson et al (1997) found that continued drug users had significantly higher mother-to-child-transmission rates in maternal drug use during pregnancy. However, this was confounded by other variables such as premature delivery, prolonged membrane rupture, zidovudine non-use and unprotected sexual intercourse.

In the USA, cigarettes' smoking during pregnancy has been identified as independent risk factor for mother-to-child-transmission. The effect was greatest among women with critical evidence of more advanced HIV disease (Turner et al., 1996). Intensive nurse care management in supporting zidovudine use in women with HIV infection and their infants is a proven effective method in decreasing mother-to-child-transmission (Havens et al., 1997).

MTCT of HIV is influenced by multiple factors. Known correlates include high maternal plasma viremia, advanced clinical HIV disease, degraded maternal immunocompetence or prolonged rupture of the amniotic membranes before delivery. Others include vaginal delivery process and prematurity of low birth weight of the neonate (Bryson 1996; John and Kreiss, 1996; Lambert, 1996).

Results from zidovudine therapy to bridge MTCT have improved understanding of the pathophysiology of MTCT. First, the reduction in plasma viremia and MTCT (from 25.5% to 8.3%) by treating the mother and neonates suggests that relatively small changes in maternal viral load might have substantial effects on MTCT (Bulterys and Godert 1996; CDC, 1994). Secondly, cleaning of birth canal with chlorhexidine had no overall effect yet apparently did reduce MTCT for one subgroups of high-risk deliveries; those after 4hrs of membrane rupture (Scarlatti, 1996).

Maternal immunologic and virologic factors such as quantitative HIV-1 RNA (though insufficient) are strongly correlated with Mother-to-child-transmission. When stratified by the stage of HIV disease, the only group with significant association between viral load and mother-to-child-transmission were AIDS-free women with high $CD4^+$ Counts. The interactions of virus burden and maternal immune status has also demonstrated that $CD4^+$, $CD8^+$ cell subsets are percentages of $CD8^+$ cell subsets (e.g. activation markers CD8/CD38 and CD8/DR) were all associated with vertical transmission. Women in the highest $CD4^+$ cell percentage quartile or the lowest $CD8^+$ cell percentage quartile had only less than or equal to 4 percent of mother-to-child-transmission (Njoku, 2004).

5. Parental, saliva and other body fluids

Prior to Groopman and Greenspan (1996) report of oral manifestation of AIDS which increases the potentials of HIV transmission through several lesions which form exists for virus into the saliva, it was assumed that about 10% of both free virus and infected cells report in saliva were not very important in the spread of HIV (Groopman et al., 1984).
Dean et al (1988) and Mundy et al (1987) reported none or low level of pathogens in urine, sweat, breast milk, branchoalvolar lavage fluid, amniotic fluid, synovial fluid, faeces and tears which were not thought to be important source in virus transmission (Fujikawa et al., 1985), but this assumption has also changed with the report of Groopman and Greenspan (1996); Amory et al. (1992); Scarlatti (1996); van da Perre et al. (1991). Though not a natural source of HIV transmission, cerebrospinal fluid (CSF) in neurologic patients have been shown to contain large amount of virus when compared to other body fluids (Hollander and Levy, 1987; Ho et al., 1989).

6. Organs, blood, tissue donors and occupational health workers

Prior to 1985 (PPHS/MMWR, 1985; MMWR, 1985), when screening of blood, organ and tissue donors for HIV-1 antibody became available, several reports have documented the transmission of HIV-1 by transplantation of kidney (MMWR, 1987; Kumar et al., 1987; Erice et al., 1991; Schwartz et al., 1987; Prompt et al., 1985; L'age-Stehr et al., 1985; Neumayer et al., 1987; Quarto et al., 1989; Carbone et al., 1988), liver (MMWR, 1987; Kumar et al., 1987; Erice et al., 1991; Schwartz et al., 1987; Prompt et al., 1985; L'age-Stehr et al., 1985; Neumayer et al., 1987; Quarto et al., 1989; Carbone et al., 1988; Samuel et al., 1988), heart (Erice et al., 1991; Dummer et al., 1989), pancreas (Erice et al., 1991), bone (MMWR, 1988a) and possibly skin(Clarke, 1987) and In most cases involving donors whose serum had not been tested for HIV-1 antibody (MMWR, 1987; Kumar et al., 1987; Erice et al., 1991; Schwartz et al., 1987; Prompt et al., 1985; L'age-Stehr et al., 1985; Neumayer et al., 1987; Quarto et al., 1989; Carbone et al., 1988; Samuel et al., 1988; Dummer et al., 1989; MMWR, 1988a; Clarke, 1987).
As proposed by Simonds et al (1992), approaches to prevention could include: the screening of prospective donors and laboratory markers for HIV1 infection (MMWR, 1985); the inactivation of HIV-1 in allograft through processing techniques (Hilfenhaus et al., 1990; Kitchen et al., 1989; Wells et al., 1986) and the quarantining of tissues from living donors until repeated antibody testing more definitely excludes the possibility of subsequent seroconversion in the donor (MMWR, 1988a ; MMWR, 1988b).
The U.S. Centers for Disease Control and Prevention (2002) reported that in the health care industry there have been 57 confirmed cases and an additional 139 possible cases of health care workers in the U.S. who have become HIV positive from exposure to HIV in the work place. The Canadian HIV/AIDS Legal Network (2001) has also reported two of such cases in the laboratory workers and one health-care provider in Canada.

7. Horizontal (heterosexual) transmission

These could be through unprotected and protected sexual process. Ma et al (2010) reported that the probability of unprotected heterosexual transmission may vary with population and be influenced by many factors, these could include: the type of sex (Mastro et al., 1994: De Vincenzi, 1994; Varghese et al., 2002); bleeding during intercourse (Royce et al., 1997), semen viral load (Gupta et al., 1997; Tachet et al., 1999; Kalichman et al., 2008; Butler et al., 2008), stage of HIV infection (Mastro et al., 1994; Fauci et al., 1996; Wawer et al., 2005), co-morbid sexually transmitted diseases (Royce et al., 1997), vaginal or anal canal, co-occurring psychosocial risk factors (Safren et al., 2010).

Sexual forms of transmission are seen as a major portal of entry of HIV as 10-30% of seminal/vaginal fluids have transmissible virus (Royce et al., 1997; Henin et al., 1993).

In semen viral load, the males HIV-1 infected cells forms about 10^4 of the 10^6 leucocytes per ejaculation (Winkelstein et al., 1987), which confirms AIDS first association with sexual route, with the high prevalence in homosexual men. The virus subsequently became synonymous with heterosexual activity and is now attributed to the AIDS pandemic (UNAIDS 1986; Nkowane 1991; Stoneburner et al., 1990). Bouvier et al (1997) believes that vaginal pH neutralization by semen is a co-factor of HIV transmission.

The chances of transmission also depends on the type of sexually transmitted infections (STI), as co-infection with genital ulcers have been reported to increase the chances of transmission by increasing the susceptibility to HIV infection which also depends on HIV subtypes efficient (Gray et al., 2001; Mahiane et al., 2009; Limpakarnianarat et al., 1993; Wang, 2009; Xu, 2009).

Male circumcision have been documented to decrease the chances of HIV transmission (Mahiane et al., 2009; Lavreys et al., 1999; Gray et al., 2000; Reynolds et al., 2004; Gray et al., 2007; Donoval et al., 2006), but this also depends on the country (Ben et al., 2008; Sullivan et al., 2009; Ruan et al., 2009; Wawer et al., 2009).

The high level of heterosexual spread of HIV in Sub-Saharan Africa and developing countries where genital ulcers from existing venereal diseases (e.g. Chanchroid Chlamydia, Syphilis or Herpes virus infections) are aligned with increased HIV seroprevalence (UNAIDS, 1998, Hook et al., 1992; Plummer et al., 1991) could be tight to abrasions at the site of entry in the vagina or anal canal. Heise et al (1991) however reported that HIV could directly infect the bowel mucosa and perhaps cervical epithelium without the need for ulcerations which gave clue to the relatively low risk of the mucosal lining of the foreskin, urethral canal and oral genital contact (through minimal) to be implicated (Winkelstein et al., 1987).

Men having Sex with Men (MSM) have been reported as one of the first way of transmission of HIV. Various authors have showed evidence that the involvement of MSM could be traced to psychosocial behaviour (PB). These PB are said to be depression, violent victimisation, substance abuse, alcohol, psychiatric disorders, psychological distress, lower perceived social support (Berlan et al., 2010; King et al., 2008; Meyer , 2003; Cochran et al., 2003; Cochran and Mays, 2000; Gilman et al., 2001., Marshal et al., 2008; Mimiaga et al., 2009a; b; Safren and Heimberg, 1999; Stall et al., 2001; Chesney et al., 2003; The EXPLORE Study Team, 2004; Herbst et al., 2005). Although some studies have shown how substance use and high risk of HIV transmission are correlated (Stall et al., 2001; Hirshfield et al., 2004), most recent studies are now focussing on how *'syndemic'*- a situation where these diverse psychosocial issues could interact to enhance HIV risky behaviour among MSM (Mustanski et al., 2007; 2010; Stall et al., 2008; Centers for Disease Control and Prevention, 2010). However, varieties of cognitive behavioural interventions have been studied and validated for the treatment of mood and anxiety disorders (Barlow, 2008) behavioural activation therapy and HIV risk reduction counselling in MSM who abuse crystal methamphetamine (Mimiaga et al., 2010).

Addressing co-occurring psychosocial behaviour is a means to increase the effective size of current HIV prevention intervention and allow for more effective uptake by MSM, since they have been reported to be more than 44 times more likely to be newly diagnosed with HIV than other men (Purcell et al., 2010) and the focus on ameliorating disparities in HIV infection is essential for enhancing the health of MSM at the population level (Sanfren et al., 2010).

The Centers for Diseases Control and Prevention (CDC, 2007) reported the prevalence rate among heterosexual African American (AA) women and men with data indicating that more heterosexual AA women having a 74% HIV/AIDS prevalence as compared to the 27% in their male counterpart.

Myths and misperceptions of HIV/AIDS such as HIV being a genocide, suspicion of government information, belief that it is possible to identify risky partners by odour and appearance, belief that partners reported histories are accurate, misperceptions about the meaning of safe sex and the believe that specific classes of people (not one self) are at risk of HIV that resulted from sexual risk contributes to the risky behaviours of HIV transmission (Essien et al.,2002; Catania et al.,1994; Smith et al., 2000; Coleman et al., 2010; Coleman and Ball, 2007; Coleman, 2007).

The increase in the number of sexual partners also increases HIV transmission (Stranford, 1999; Coleman, 2007; Catania et al., 1994; Smith et al., 2000; Coleman et al., 2010; Coleman and Ball, 2007) with most under the influence of alcohol or drugs.

Unprotected oral and vaginal sex have been reported as a risk factor in the transmission of HIV especially where it is carried out in high risk settings, having sex more often under the influence of alcohol and/or drugs (Milam et al., 2006; Catania et al., 1994; Smith et al., 2000).

Even under protection for example the use of condoms, many cases has been reported where the barrier has failed especially where risky behaviours are undertaken. A case in study which made the People Living With HIV/AIDS (PLWHA) in Nigeria to sue the Federal Government of Nigeria to Court for promotion of condoms (Ogundele, 2010).

Though Tenofovir gel has been advocated for women to prevent HIV transmission (Karim et al., 2010).

The nature of HIV transmission from anecdotal records has not changed neither is a new means of transmission of the virus recorded. In view of this development, it is the earnest desire of this write up to bring to fore genealogical reports of the transmission of HIV and to also continue to write on the various modes of transmission as a way of curtailing the spread of the dreaded virus.

8. References

Adoga M .P., Nimzing, L., Mawak, J. D., Agwale, S. M. (2010). Human Immunodeficiency Virus Types 1 and 2: Sero-prevalence and Risk Factors Among a Nigerian Rural Population of Women of Child-bearing Age. *Shiraz E-Medical Journal* Vol. 11, No. 1: (29-33), Januar y, 2010. http://semj.sums.ac.ir/vol11/jan2010/87068.htm.

Ades, A.E., Newell, M.L., and Peckham, C.S., (1991). Children born to women with HIV-1 infection: natural history and risk of transmission. *Lancet*, 337: 253-260.

Andiman, W.A. et al. (1990). *American Journal of Diseases of Children*, 144:75.

Al-husaini, A.M. (2009). Role of placenta in the vertical transmission of HIV. *Journal of Perinatology*, 29:321-326.

Alizon, S., von Wyl, V., Stadler, T., Kouyos, D.R., Yerly, S., Hirschel, B., Boni, J., Shah, C., Klimkait, T., Furrer, H., Rauch, A., Vernazza, L. P., Bernasconi, E., Battegay, M., Burgisser, P., Telenti, A., Gunthard, F. H., Boenhoeffer, S., the Swiss HIV Cohort study (2010). Phylogenetic approach reveals that virus genotype largely determines HIV set-point viral load. *PLOS pathogens*, volume 6 issue 9, e1001123.

Ammann, A.J., Cowan, M.J., Wara, D.W., Weintrup, P., Dritz, S., Goldman, H. and Perkins, H.A. (1983). Acquired Immunodeficiency in an infant: possible transmission by means of blood products. *Lancet i:* 956-958.

Amory, J., Martin, N., Levy, J.A and Wara, W.W. (1992). The large molecular weight glycoprotein (MGI) a component of human saliva inhibits HIV-1 infectivity. *Clinical Research*, 40:51A (Abstract).

Andiman, W.A. et al. (1990). *American Journal of Diseases of Children*, 144:75.

Baggaley, R.F., White, R.G. and Boily, M. (2010). HIV transmission risk through anal intercourse: systematic review, meta-analysis and implifications for HIV prevention. *International Journal of Epidemiology*, 39: 1048-1063.

Barlow DH, ed. Clinical Handbook of Psychological Disorders: A Step-by-Step Treatment Manual. 4th ed. New York, NY: Guilford Press; 2008.

Barre-Sinoussi, F., Cherman, J.C., Rey, F., Nugeyre, M.T., Chamaret, S., Gruest, J., Dauguet, C., Axler-Blin, C., Vezinet-Brun, F., Rouzioux, W., Rozenbaum, W. and Montagnier, L. (1983). Isolation of a T-lymphotrophic retrovirus from a patient at risk for AIDS. *Science*, 220:868-871.

Barre-Sinoussi, F. (1996). HIV as the cause of AIDS. *Lancet*, 348:31-35.

Ben, K., Xu, J., Lu, L., Yao, J.P., Min, X.D., Li, W.Y., Tao, *J.*, Wang, *J.*, Li, J.J., Cao, X.M. (2008). Promoting male circumcision in China for preventing HIV infection and improving reproductive health. *National Journal of Andrology* 14(4), 291-297. (In Chinese-English version read).

Berlan, E.D., Corliss, H.L., Field, A.E., Goodman, E., Bryn Austin, S. (2010). Sexual orientation and bullying among adolescents in the Growing up Today Study. *Journal of Adolescence Health*; 46:366–371.

Brookmeyer, R. (1991). Reconstruction and future trends of the AIDS epidemic in the United States. *Science*, 253:37-42.

Bourinbaiar, A.S., Lee-Huang, S.(1995). Anti-HIV effect of beta subunit of human chorionic gonadotropin (beta hCG) in vitro. *Immunology Letters*; 44(1): 13–18.

Bouvier, P., Rougemont, A., Breslow, N., Doumbo, O., Delley, V., Dicko, A., Diakite, M.., Mauris, A., Robert, C. (1997). Seasonality and malaria in a West African village: does high parasite density predict fever incidence? *American Journal of Epidemiology*, 145:850-857.

Brabin, B.J. (1983). An analysis of malaria in pregnancy in Africa. *Bulletine of World Health Organisation*, 61:1005-1016.

Bryson, Y. J. (1996). Perinatal HIV-1 transmission: recent advances and therapeutic interventions. *AIDS*, 10:S33–S42.

Bryson, Y. J., Luzuriaga, K., Sullivan, J.L. and Wara, D.W. (1992). Proposed definitions for in utero versus intrapartum transmission of HIV-1. *New England Journal of Medicine*, 327:1246–1247.

Bulterys, M.., Chao, A., Dushimimana, A. and Saah, A. (1995). HIV-1 seroconversion after 20months of age in a cohort of breastfed children born to HIV-1 infected women in Rwanda (letter). *AIDS*, 9:93-94.

Bulterys, M. and Goedert, J.M. (1996). From biology to sexual behaviour-towards the prevention of mother to child transmission of HIV/AIDS. *AIDS*, 10:1287-1289.

Bulterys, M.., Landesman, S., Burns, D.N., Rubin-Stein, A. and Goedert, J.J. (1997). Sexual behaviour and injection drug use during pregnancy and vertical transmission of HIV-1. *Journal of Acquired Immunodeficiency Syndrome and Human Retrovirology*, 15:76-82.

Butler, D. M., Smith, D. M., Cachay E. R., Edward, R., Hightower, G. K., Nugent, C. T., Richman, D. D., Little, S. J. (2008). Herpes simplex virus 2 serostatus and viral loads of HIV-1 in blood and semen as risk factors for HIV transmission among men who have sex with men. *AIDS*, 22(13), 1667-1671.

Burton, G.J., O'Shea, S., Rostron, T., Mullen, J.E., Aiyer, S., Skepper, J.N., Smith, R. and Banatvala, J.E. (1996). Significance of placental damage in vertical transmission of human immunodeficiency virus. Journal of Medical Virology, 50: 237–243.

Catania, J. A., Coates, T. J., Golden, E., Dolcini, M. M., Peterson, J., Kegeles, S., Siegel, D., Fullilove, M.T. (1994). Correlates of condom use among Black, Hispanic, and White heterosexuals in San Francisco: The AMEN longitudinal survey. *AIDS Education and Prevention*, 6(1), 12–26.

Canadian HIV/AIDS Legal Network. (2001). Testing of persons believed to be the source of an accidental occupational exposure to HBV, HCV, or HIV: A backgrounder (Health Canada, Canadian Strategy on HIV/AIDS Information Sheet). Retrieved September 1, 2007, from http://www.aidslaw.ca/maincontent/issues/testing.htm.

Cameron, D.W., D'Costa, L.J., Maitha, G. M., Cheang, Piot, P., M., Simonsen, J.N., Ronald, A.R., Gakinya, M.N., Ndinya-Achola, J.L., Brunham, R.C. and Plummer, F.A. (1989). Female to male transmission of human immunodeficiency virus type 1: risk factors for seroconversion in men. *Lancet,* volume 334, issue 8660: 403-407.

Carr, J.K., Suleiman, M.O., Albert, J., Sanders-Buell, E., Gotte, D., Bird, D.L. and McCutchan, F.E. (1998). Full genome sequences of HIV-1 subtypes G and A/G heterotype recombinants. *Journal of Virology*, 247:22-31.

Carbone, L.G., Cohen, D.J., Hardy, M.A., Benvenisty, A.I., Scully, B.E., Appel, G.B. (1988). Determination of AIDS after renal transplantation. *American Journal of Kidney Diseases*, 11:387-92.

Centers for Disease Control (1982). *Pneumocystis carini* pneumonia among persons with haemophilia. *Morbidity and Mortality Weekly Report,* 31:365-367.

Centers for Disease Control, "HIV/AIDS Surveillance", October 1989.

Centres for Disease Control and Prevention (1994). Zidovudine for the prevention of HIV transmission from mother to infant. *Morbidity and Mortality Weekly Report*, 43:285-287.

Centers for Disease Control and Prevention (CDC) HIV/AIDS Surveillance Report. (2007). Atlanta: US Department of Health and Human Services, (17), 1–54. Coleman, C. L. (2007). Health beliefs and high risk sexual behaviour among

HIV infected African American men. *Applied Nursing Research*, 20, 110–115.

Centers for Disease Control and Prevention (2010). HIV transmission through transfusion-Missouri and Colorado, (2008). *Morbidity and Mortality Weekly Report*, 59 (41): 1335-9.

Chen, J.H., Wong, k., Chen, Z., Chan, K., Lam, H., To, S. W., Cheng, C., Yuen, K., Yam, W. (2010). Increased genetic diversity of HIV-1 circulating in Hong Kong. *PLOS one*, volume 5, issue 8, e12198.

Chesney, M.A., Koblin, B.A., Barresi, P.J., Husnik, M.J., Celum, L.C., Colfax, G., Mayer, K., McKirnan, D., Judson, N.F., Huang, Y., Coates, J.T.(2003). An individually tailored intervention for HIV prevention: baseline data from the EXPLORE study. *American Journal of Public Health*, 93:933–938.

Clavel, F., Guetard, D., Brun-Vezinet, F., Chamaret, S., Rey, M.A., Santos-Ferreira, M.O., Laurent, A.G., Danduet, C., Klatzmann, D., Champalimand, and Montagnier, (1986). Isolation of a new human retrovirus from West African patients with AIDS. *Science*, 233: 343-346.

Clavel, F. (1987). The West African AIDS virus. *AIDS*, 1:135-140.

Clarke, J.A. (1987). HIV transmission and skin grafts. *Lancet*, 1:983.

Collazos, J., Asensi, V., Carton, J.A. (2010). Association of HIV transmission categories with sociodemographic, viroimmunological and clinical parameters of HIV- infected patients. *Epidemiology and Infection*, 138(7): 1016-1024.

Cochran, S.D., Mays, V.M. (2000). Lifetime prevalence of suicide symptoms and affective disorders among men reporting same-sex sexual partners: Results from NHANES III. *American Journal of Public Health*, 2000; 90:573–578.

Cochran, S.D., Sullivan, J.G., Mays, V.M. (2003). Prevalence of mental disorders, psychological distress, and mental services use among lesbian, gay, and bisexual adults in the United States. Journal of Consulting and Clinical Psychology,. 2003; 71: 53–61.

Coleman, C. L. (2007). Health beliefs and high risk sexual behaviour among HIV infected African American men. *Applied Nursing Research*, 20, 110–115.

Coleman, C. L. and Ball, K. (2007). Determinants of perceived barriers to use condoms among HIV infected African American men middle-aged and older. *Journal of Advanced Nursing*, (60), 368–376.

Coleman, C.L. and Ball, K. (2010). Sexual diversity and HIV risk among older heterosexual African American males who are seropositive. *Applied Nursing Research*, 23: 122-129.

Contag, C. H., Ehrnst, A., Duda, J., Bohlin, A.B., Lindgren, S., Learn, G.H. and Mullins, J.I. (1997). Mother-to-infant transmission of human immunodeficiency virus type 1 involving five envelope sequence subtypes. *Journal of Virology*, 71:1292–1300.

Courgnard, V., Laure, F., Brossard, A., Goudeau, A., Barin, F., and Brechot, C. (1991). Frequent and early *in utero* HIV-1 infection. *AIDS Research on Human Retroviruses*, 7:337-341.

Dean, N.C., Golden, J.A., Evans, L., Wornock, M.L., Addison, T.E., Hopewell, P.C. and Levy, J.A. (1998). HIV recovery from bronchoalveolar lavage fluid in patients with AIDS. *Chest*, 93:1173-1176.

Decker, M.R., McCauley, H.L., Phuengsamram, D., Janyam, S., Seage, G. R. and Silverman, J.G. (2010). Violence victimisation, sexual risk and sexually transmitted infection symptoms among female sex workers in Thailand. *Sexually Transmitted Infections*, 86(3): 236-240.

De Cock, K.M., Fowler, M.G., Mercier, E., de Vincenzi, I., Saba, J., Hoff, E., Alnwick, J.D., Rogers, M., Shaffer, N. (2000). Prevention of mother-to-child HIV transmission in resource-poor countries: translating research into policy and practice. Journal of American Medical Association, 283(9):1175–82.

Del Amo, J., Petruckevitch, A., Philips, A., Johnson, A.M., Stephenson, J., Desmond, N., Hanscheid. T., Low, N., Newell, A., Obasi, A., Paine, K., Pym, A., Theodore, C.M. and De Cock, K.M. (1998). Disease progression and survival in HIV-1 infected Africans in London. *AIDS*, 12 (10): 1203-1209.

Delwart, E. L., Pan, H., Sheppard, H.W., Wolpert, D., Neumann, A.U., Korber, B. and Mullins. J.I. (1997). Slower evolution of human immunodeficiency virus type 1 quasispecies during progression to AIDS. *Journal of Virology*, 71: 7498–7508.

De Vincenzi , I. (1994). A longitudinal study of human immunodeficiency virus transmission by heterosexual partners. *New England Journal of Medicine*, 331(6), 341-346.

De Rossi, A., Masiero, S., Giaquinto, C., Ruga, E., Comar, M., Giacca, M. and Chieco-Bianchi, L. (1996). Dynamics of viral replication in infants with vertically acquired human immunodeficiency virus type 1 infection. *Journal of Clinical Infections*. 2:323–330.

Donoval, B. A., Landay, A. L., Moses, S., Agot, K., Ndinya-Achola, J.O., Nyagaya, E.A., MacLean, I., Bailey, R.C. (2006). HIV-1 target cells in foreskins of African men with varying histories of sexually transmitted infections. *American Journal of Clinical Pathology* 125(3), 386-391.

Dummer, J.S., Erb, S., Breinig, M.K., Ho, M., Rinaldo, C.R. Jr., Gupta, P., Ragni, M.V., Tzakis, A., Makowka, L., Van Thiel D. (1989). Infection with HIV in the Pittsburg transplant population: a study of 583 donors and 1043 recipients, 1981-1986. *Transplantation*, 47: 134-40.

Essien, E. J., Meshack, A. F., & Ross, M. W. (2002). Misperceptions about HIV transmission among heterosexual African-American and Latino men and women. *Journal of the National Medical Association*, 94(5), 304–312.

Erice, A., Rhame, F.S., Heussner, R.C., Dunn, D.L., Balfour, H.H. Jr. (1991). HIV infection in patients with solid organ transplants: report of five cases and review. *Rev Infectious Diseases*, 13:537-47.

European Collaborative Study (1991). *Lancet*, 337:253.

Fauci A S, Pantaleo G, Stanley S., Weissman, D. (1996). Immunopathogenic mechanisms of HIV infection. *Annals of Internal Medicine* 124(7), 654-663.

Fujikawa, L.S., Salahuddin, S.Z., Palestine, A.G., Nussenblatt, R.B., and Gallo, R.C. (1985). Isolation of human T-lymphotropic virus type III from the tears of a patient with acquired immunodeficiency syndrome. *Lancet*, ii: 529-530.

Gallo, R.C., Salahuddin, Z., Popovic, M., Shearer, G.M., Kaplan, M., Haynes, B.F., Palker, T.J., Redfield, R., Oleske, J. and Satai, B. (1984). Frequent detection and isolation of cytopathic retroviruses HTLV-III) from patients with HIV and at risk for AIDS. *Science*, 224:500-503.

Glenn, W.G. and Dietrich, E. John.(1993). *The AIDS Epidemic, Balancing Comparison and Justice.* Multnomah, Oregon, U.S.A. *Multnomah* Press, 1990. .... 1990 Inter-Varsity

Christian Fellowship of the *U.S.*, PO Box 7985, Madison, WI, 53707-7895. 800-828-2100

Gilman, S.E., Cochran, S.D., Mays, V.M., Hughes, M., Ostrow, D., and Kessler, R.C.(2001). Risk of psychiatric disorders among individuals reporting same-sex sexual partners in the National Comorbidity Survey. *American Journal of Public Health*, 2001;91:933–939.

Goedert, J.J., Drummond, E.J., Minkoff, L.H., Stevens, R., Blattner, A.W., Mendez, H., Robert-Guroff, M., Holman, S., Rubinstein, A., Willoughby, A. and Landesman, H.S. (1989). Mother-to-infant transmission of HIV-1: association with prematurity or low anti-gp120. *Lancet*, vol. 3342, issue 8679: 1351-4.

Gottlieb, M.S. Shcroff, R., Schanker, H., Weisman, J.D., Fan, P.T., Wolf, R.A., and Saxon, A. (1981). *Pneumocystis carinii* pneumonia and mucosal candidiasis in previously healthy homosexual men. *New England Journal of Medicine*, 305:1425-1430.

Grabar, S., Selinger-Leneman, H., Abgrak, S., Pialoux, G., Weiss, L. and Costagliola, D. (2009). Prevalence and comparative characteristics of long-term non-progressors and HIV controller patients in French hospital database on HIV. *AIDS*, 23(9):1163-1169. Doi.10.1097/QAD.obo13e32832644c8PMD19444075.

Gray, R H, Kiwanuka N, Quinn T C, *et al.* (2000). Male circumcision and HIV acquisition and transmission: cohort studies in Rakai, Uganda. *AIDS*, 14(15), 2371-2381.

Gray R H, Wawer M J, Brookmeyer R, *et al.* (2001). Probability of HIV-1 transmission per coital act in monogamous, heterosexual, HIV-1-discordant couples in Rakai, Uganda. *The Lancet*, 357(9263), 1149-1153.

Gray, R. H., Kigozi, G., Serwadda, D., Makumbi, F., Watya, S., Nalugoda, F., Kiwanuka, N., Moulton , H.L., Chaudhary, A.M.., Chen, M.Z., Sewankambo, N.K., Wabwire-Mangen , F., Bacon, M.C., Williams, F.MC., Opendi, P., Reynolds, S.J., Laeyendecker, O., Quinn , T.C., Wawer, M.J. (2007). Male circumcision for HIV prevention in men in Rakai, Uganda: a randomised trial. *The Lancet*, 369(9562), 657-666.

Groopman, D. and Greenspan, J.S. (1996). HIV-related oral disease. *Lancet*, 348: 729-733.

Groopman, J.E., Salahuddin, S.Z., Sarngadharan, M.G., Markham, D., Gonda, M., Sliski, A. and Gallo, R.C. (1984). HTLV-III in saliva of people with AIDS. Sexual men at risk for AIDS. *Science*, 226:447-449.

Gupta, P., Mellors, J., Kingsley, L., Riddler, S., Singh, M.K., Schreiber, S., Cronin, M. and Rinaldo, C.R. (1997). High viral load in semen of human immunodeficiency virus type 1-infected men at all stages of disease and its reduction by therapy with protease and nonnucleoside reverse transcriptase inhibitors. *Journal of Virology*, 71(8), 6271-6275.

Halapi, E., Gigliotti, D., Hodara, V., Scarlatti, G., Tovo, P.A., DeMaria, A., Wigezll, H. and Rossi, P. (1996). Detection of CD8 T-cell expansions with restricted T-cell receptor V usage in infants vertically infected by HIV-1. *AIDS*, 10: 1621–1626.

Harris, C., Small, C.B., Klein, R.S., Friedland, G.H., Moll, B., Emeson, E.E., Spigland, I. and Steigbigel, N.H. (1983). Immunodeficiency in female sexual partners of men with the AIDS. *New England Journal of Medicine*, 308:1181-1184.

Havens, P.L., Cuene, B.E., Hand, J.R., Gern, J.E., Sullivan, B.W. and Chusid, M.J. (1997). The puzzle of HIV-1 subtypes in Africa. *AIDS*, 11:705-712.

Heise, C., Dandekar, S., Kumar, P., Duplantie, R., Donovan, R.M. and Halsted, C.H. (1991). HIV infection of enterocytes and monuclear cells in human jejuna mucosa. *Gastroenterology*, 100:1521-1527.

Henin, Y., Mandelbrot, L., Henrion, R., Pradinaud, R., Couland, J. and Montagnier, L. (1993). Virus excretion in the cervicovaginal secretions of pregnant and non-pregnant HIV-infected women. *Journal of Acquired Immunodeficiency Syndrome*, 6: 72-75.

Herbst, J.H., Sherba, R.T., Crepaz, N., DeLuca J.B., Zohrabyan L, Stall, R.D., Lyles, C.M. (2005). HIV/AIDS Prevention Research Synthesis Team A meta-analytic review of HIV behavioral interventions for reducing sexual risk behaviour of men who have sex with men. *Journal of Acquired Immune Deficiency Syndrome*, 2005; 39:228–241.

Hilfenhaus, J.W., Gregersen, J.P., Mehdi, S., Volk, R. (1990). Inactivation of HIV-1 and HIV-2 by various manufacturing procedures for human plasma proteins. *Cancer Detection and Prevention Journal*, 14:369-75.

Hirshfield, S., Remien, R., Humberstone, M., Walavalkar, I., Chiasson, M. (2004). Substance use and high-risk sex among men who have sex with men: A national online study in the USA. AIDS Care 2004; 16:1036–1047.

Hollander, H. and Levy, J.A. (1987). Neurologic abnormalities and recovery of HIV from cerebrospinal fluid. *Annals of Internal Medicine*, 106: 692-695.

Ho, D.D., Rota, T.R., Schooley, R.T., Kaplan, J.C., Allan, J.D., Groopman, J.E., Resnick, L., Felsenstein, D., Andrews, C.A. and Hirsch, M.S. (1995). Isolation of HTLV-III from cerebrospinal fluid and neural tissues of patients with neurologic syndromes related to the AIDS. *New England Journal of Medicine*, 313:1493-1497.

Hook, E.W., Cannon, R.O., Nahmias, A.J., Lee, F.F., Campbell, C.H., Glasser, D. and Quian, T.C. (1992). Herpes simplex virus infection as a risk factor for the HIV infection in heterosexuals. *Journal of Infectious Diseases*, 165:251-255.

Human immunodeficiency virus infection transmitted from an organ donor screened for HIV antibody-North Carolina. *MMWR* 1987; 36:306-8.

Jaffe, C.L. and McMahon-Pratt, D. (1983). Monoclonal antibodies specific for *Leishmania tropica*: characterization of antigens associated with stage and species-specific determinants. *Journal of Immunology*, 131:1987-1993.

Jassens, W., Bure, A., Nkengasong, J.N. (1997). The puzzle of HIV-1 subtypes in Africa. *AIDS*, 11: 705-712.

John, G.C. and Kreiss, J. (1996). Mother-to-child transmission of HIV type 1. *Epidemiological Reviews*, 18:149-157.

Landesman, H.S., Kalish, A.L., Burns, N.D., Minkoff, H., Fox, E.H., Zorrilla, C., Garcia, P., Fowler, G.H., Mofenson, L. and Toumala, R. (1996). Obstetrical factors and the transmission of HIV-1 from mother to child. *New England Journal of Medicine*, 334; 1617-23.

Karim, Q.A., Karim, S.S.A., Frohlich, J.A., Grobler, C.A., Baxter, C., Mansoor, E.L., Kharsany, A.B.M., Sibeko, S., Mlisana, P.K., Omar, Z., Gengiah, N.T., Maarschalk, S., Arulappan, N., Mlotshwa, M., Morris, L., Taylor, D. (2010). Effectiveness and safety of Tenofovir gel and antiretroviral microbicide, for the prevention of HIV infection in women. CAPRISA 004 Trial Group. Science, 3rd Sept vol. 329:1168-1174.

Kalichman, S. C., Berto, G. D. and Eaton L (2008). Human immunodeficiency virus viral load in blood plasma and semen: review and implications of empirical findings. *SexuallyTransmitted Diseases* 35(1), 55-60.

Kitchen, A.D., Mann, G.F., Harrison, J.F., Zuckerman, A.J. (1989). Effect of gamma irradiation on the HIV and human coagulation proteins. *Vox Sang*, 56: 2323-9.

Kim, K.A., Yolamanova, M., Zirafi, O., Roan, N.R., Staendker, L., Forssmann, W.G., Burgener, A., Dejucq-Rainsford, N., Hahn, B.H., Shaw, G.M., Greene, W.C., Kirchhoff, F., Munch, J. (2010). Semen-mediated enhancement of HIV infection is donor-dependent and correlates with the levels of SEVI *Retrovirology*, 7: Article 55. doi: 10.1186/1742-4690-7-55

King M, Semlyen J, Tai SS, et al. (2008).A systematic review of mental disorder, suicide, and deliberate self harm in lesbian, gay, and bisexual people. *BMC Psychiatry*, 2008; 18:70. doi: 10.1186/1471-244X-8-70.

Kuhn, L. and Stein, Z.A. (1995). Mother-to-infant HIV transmission: timing risk factors and prevention. *Paediatric Perinatal Epidemiology*, 9:1-29.

Kumar, P., Pearson, J.E., Martin, D.H., Leech, S.H., Buisseret, P.D. , Bezbak, H.C., Gonzalez, F.M., Royer, J.R., Streicher, H.Z., Saxinger, W.C. (1987). Transmission of HIV by transplantation of a renal allograft, with development of the acquired immunodeficiency syndrome. *Annals of Internal Medicine*, 1987; 106:244-5.

Kresis, J. (1997). Breastfeeding and vertical transmission of HIV-1. *Acta Paediatrica*, 421 (Suppl.):113-117 (1985). HTLV-III infection in kidney transplant recipients. Lancet, 2:1361-2.

Lambert, J.S. (1996). Paediatric HIV infection. *Current Opinion in Paediatrics*, 8:606-614.

Lavreys L, Rakwar J P, Thompson M L, *et al.* (1999). Effect of circumcision on incidence of human immunodeficiency virus type 1 and other sexually transmitted diseases: a prospective cohort study of trucking company employees in Kenya. *The Journal of Infectious Diseases*, 180, 330-336.

Limpakarnianarat, K., Mastro, T. D., Yindeeyoungyeon, W., *et al.* (1993). STDS in female prostitutes in northern Thailand. *International Conference of AIDS*, 9, 687 (abstract no. PO-C10-2820).

Lindo, J.F., Dubon, J.M., Ager, A.L., De Gwurville, E.M., Gabriele, S.H., Karkalla, W.F., Baum, K.M. and Palmer, C.J. (1998). Intestinal parasitic infections in HIV-positive and HIV-negative individuals in San Pedrosula, Honduras. *American Journal of Tropical Medicine and Hygiene*, 58(4):431-435.

Lindgren, S., Anzen, B., Bohlin, A., Lidman, K. (1991). HIV and child-bearing: clinical outcome and aspects of mother-to-infant transmission. *AIDS*, 5:1111-6.

Ma, W. J., Wang, J.J., Reilly, K.H., Bi, A.M., Kumismith, W.G., and Wang, N. (2010). Estimation of Probability of Unprotected Heterosexual Vaginal Transmission of HIV-1 from Clients to Female Sex Workers in Kaiyuan, Yunnan Province, China. *Biomedical and Environmental Sciences*, 23: 287-292 (2010)

Mackelprang, R.D., Carrington, M., John-Stewart, G., Lohman-Payne, B., Richardson, B. A., Wamalwa, D., Gao, X., Majiwa, M., Mbori-Ngacha, D., Farquhar, C. (2010).

Maternal human leucocyte antigen A* 2301 is associated with increased mother-to-child HIV-1 transmission. *Journal of Infectious Diseases*, 202(8): 1273-7.

Mahiane, S. G., Legeai, C., Taljaard, D., Latouche, A., Puren, A., Peillon, A., Bretagnolle, J., Lissouba, P., Nguema, E.P., Gassiat, E., Auvert, B.(2009). Transmission probabilities of HIV and herpes simplex virus type 2, effect of male circumcision and interaction: a longitudinal study in a township of South Africa. *AIDS* 23 (3), 377-383.

Mamatha, M.L. and Merchant, H.R. (2010). Vertical Transmission of HIV–An Update. *Indian Journal of Pediatrics* (2010) 77:1270–1276 DOI 10.1007/s12098-010-0184-0

Marshal, M.P., Friedman, M.S., Stall, R., King, K.M., Jonathan Miles, J., Gold, M.A., Oscar G. Bukstein, G.O., Jennifer Q. Morse, J.Q. (2008). Sexual orientation and adolescent substance use: a meta-analysis and methodological review. *Addiction*. 2008; 103:546–556.

Mastro, T., Satten, G., Nopkesorn, T., Sangkharomya, S., Longini, I. (1994). Probability of female-to-male transmission of HIV-1 in Thailand. *Lancet*, 1994; 343: 204-207.

Masur, H., Michelis, M.A. and Greene, J.B. (1981). An outbreak of community-acquired *Pneumocystis carinii* pneumonia. *New England Journal of Medicine*, 305: 1431-1438.

Meyer, I.H. (2003). Prejudice, social stress, and mental health in lesbian, gay, and bisexual populations: conceptual issues and research evidence. *Psychological Bulletin*, 2003; 129:674–697.

Mimiaga, M.J., Case, P., Johnson, C.V., Safren, S.A., Mayer, K.H. (2009). Preexposure antiretroviral prophylaxis attitudes in high-risk Boston area men who report having sex with men: limited knowledge and experience but potential for increased utilization after education. *Journal of Acquired Immune Deficiency Syndrome*, 2009; 50(1):77–83.

Mimiaga, M.J., Noonan, E., Donnell, D., Safren, S.A., Koenen, K. C., Gortmaker, S., O'Cleirigh, C., Chesney, M. A., Coates, T. J., Koblin, B. A., Mayer, K. H.(2009). Childhood sexual abuse is highly associated with HIV risk taking behaviour and infection among MSM in the EXPLORE Study. *Journal Acquired Immune Deficiency Syndrome*. 2009; 51: 340–348.

Mimiaga, M.J., Reisner, S.L., Pantalone, DW, et al. An open phase pilot of behavioral activation therapy and risk reduction counseling for MSM with crystal methamphetamine abuse at risk for HIV infection. Paper Session 2.

Presented at: Society of Behavioral Medicine 2010 Annual Meeting; April 7–10, 2010; Seattle, Washington. PowerPoint available at: http://www.sbm.org/meeting/2010/presentations/Thursday/Paper%20Sessions/Paper%20Session%2002/An%20open%20phase%20pilot%20of%20behavioral%20activation%20therapy.pdf. Accessed August 10, 2010.

Milam, J., Richardson, J. L., Espinoza, L., & Stoyanoff, S. (2006). Correlates of unprotected sex among adult heterosexual men living with HIV. *Journal of Urban Health*, 83(4), 669–681.

Mok, J.Y.Q. et al (1989). *Archives of Disease in Children*, 64:1140.

Mundy, D.C., Schinazi, R.F., Ressell-Gerber, A., Nahmias, A.J. and Randal, H.W. (1987). HIV virus isolated from amniotic fluid. *Lancet*, II: 459-460.

Mustanski, B., Garofalo, R., Herrick, A., Donenberg, G. (2007). Psychosocial health problems increase risk for HIV among urban young men who have sex with men: preliminary evidence of a syndemic in need of attention. *Annals Behavioural Medicine*, 2007; 34:37–45.

Newell, M.L., Dunn, D., Peckham, C.S., Ades, A.E., Pardi, G. and Semprini, A.E., (1992). Risk factors for mother-to-child transmission of HIV-1. *Lancet*, 339:1007-1012.

Newell, M.L., Peckham, C., Dunn, D. and Ades, A. (1994). Natural transmission of vertically acquired HIV type infection. *Paediatrics*, 94:815-819.

Neumayer, H.H., Fassbinder, W., Kresse, S., Wagner, K. (1985). HTLV-III antibody screening in kidney transplant recipients and patients receiving maintenance haemodialysis. *Transplantation Proceedings*, 19:2169-71.

Njoku, M.O (2004). Studies on the prevalence, seroepidemiology of Cryptosporidiosis and some cofactors in the immune responses and pathogenesis of HIV infection in North Central Nigeria. PhD thesis page 65.

Nkowane, B.M. (1991). Prevalence and incidence of HIV infection in Africa: a review of data published in 1990. *AIDS*, 5:S7-S16.

Ogundele, B. (2010). HIV/AIDS patients want court to stop promotion of condoms. Nigerian Tribune, Wednesday nov, 03, 2010. http://tribune.com.ng/index.php/news/13032-hivaids-patients-want-court-to-stop-pro.accessed 03/11/2010.

Oxtoby, M.J. (1990). Perinatally acquired HIV infection. *Pediatrics Infectious Disease Journal*, 9:609-19.

Padian, N. S., Shiboski, S. C. and Jewell, N. P. (1991). Female-to-male transmission of human immunodeficiency virus. *JAMA*, 266(12), 1664-1667.

Pasquier, C., Cayrou, C., Blancher, A., Tourne-Petheil, C., Berrebi, A., Tricoire, J., Puel, J. and Izopet, J. (1998). Molecular evidence for mother-to-child transmission of multiple variants by analysis of RNA and DNA sequences of human immunodeficiency virus type 1. *Journal of Virology*, 1998; 72: 8,493-8,501.

Peckham, C., and D. Gibb. (1995). Mother-to-child transmission of the human immunodeficiency virus. *New England Journal Medicine*, 333:298–302.

Peterson, C. (1992). Cryptosporidiosis in patients infected with the Human Immunodeficiency Virus. *Clinical Infectious Diseases*, 15: 903-909.

Plummer, F.A., Simonsen, J.N., Cameron, J.O., Ndinya-Achola, J.O., Kresis, J.K., Gakinya, M.N., Waiyaki, P., Cheang, M., Piot, P., Ronald, A.R. and Ngugi, E.N. (1991). Co-factors in male-female sexual transmission of HIV type 1. *Journal of Infectious Diseases*, 163: 233-239.

Pozio, E., Rezza, G., Boschini, A., Pezzotti, P., Tamburini, A., Rossi, P., Difine, M., Smacchia, A.C., Schiesari, A., Gattei, E, E., Zuccani, R. and Ballarini, P. (1997). Clinical Cryptosporidiosis and HIV-induced immunosuppression: findings from a longitudinal study of HIV-positive and HIV-negative former injection drug users. *Journal of Infectious Diseases*, 176: 969-975.

Price, R.W. (1996). Neurological complications of HIV infection. *Lancet*, 348:445-452.

Prompt, C.A., Reiss, M.M., Grillo, F.M., Kopstein, J., Kraemer, E., Manfro, R.C., Maia, M.H., Comiran, J.B. (1985). Transmission of AIDS virus at renal transplantation. *Lancet*, 2:672.

Provisional Public Health Service inter-agency recommendations for screening donated blood and plasma for antibody to the virus causing AIDS. *MMWR*, 1985; 34:1-5.

Pruss, A., Caspari, G., Kruger, D.H., Blumel, J., Nubling, C.M., Gurtler, L., Gerlich, W. H. (2010). Tissue donation and virus safety: more nucleic acid amplification testing is needed. *Transplant Infectious Disease*, 12 (5): 375-386.

Purcell, D.W., Johnson, C., Lansky, A., Prejean, J., Stein, R., Denning, P., Gaul, Z., Weinstock, H., Su, J., & Crepaz, N. (2010). Calculating HIV and syphilis rates for risk groups: estimating the national population size of men who have sex with men. Abstract #22896. Presented at: 2010 National STD Prevention Conference; March 10, 2010; Atlanta, GA. Available at: http:// www.cdc.gov/hiv/topics/msm/resources/research/msm.htm. Accessed June 1, 2010.

Quarto, M.., Germinario, C., Fontana, A., Bartuni, S. (1989). HIV transmission through kidney transplantation from a living related donor. *New England Journey Medicine*, 320:1754.

Qian, M., Bui, T., Ho, R.J., Unadkat, J.D. (1994) Metabolism of 30-azido-30-deoxythymidine (AZT) in human placental trophoblasts and Hofbauer cells. *Biochemical Pharmacology*, 48(2): 383–389.

Quinn, C.T., Wawer, J.M., Sewankambo, N., Serwadda, D., Li, C., Wabwire-mangen, F., Meehan, M.O., Lutalo, T. and Gray, H.R. (2000). Viral load and heterosexual transmission of HIV-1. *New England Journal of Medicine*, 342:921-9.

Reinhardt, P. P., Reinhardt, B., Lathey, J.L. and Spector, S.A. (1995). Human cord blood mononuclear cells are preferentially infected by non-syncytiuminducing, macrophage-tropic human immunodeficiency virus type 1 isolates. *Journal of Clinical Microbiology*, 33:292–297.

Reynolds, S. J., Shepherd, M. E., Risbud, A. R., Gangakhedkar, R.R., Brookmeyer, R.S. (2004). Male circumcision and risk of HIV-1 and other sexually transmitted infections in India. *The Lancet*, 363(9414), 1039-1040.

Rogers, M.F., Ou, C-Y., Kilbourne, B., and Schochetman, G. (1991). Advances and problems in the diagnosis of human immunodeficiency virus infection in infants. *Pediatrics Infectious Disease Journal*, 10:523-531.

Royce, R.A., Sena, A., Cates Jr., W. and Cohen, M.S. (1997). Sexual transmission of HIV. *New England Journal of Medicine*, 336 (15): 1072-1078.

Ruan, Y. H., Qian, H. Z., Li, D. L., Shi, W., *Li*, Q.C., Liang, H.Y., Yang, Y., Luo, F.J., Vermund, S.H., Shao, Y.M. (2009). Willingness to Be Circumcised for Preventing HIV among Chinese Men Who Have Sex with Men. *AIDS Patient Care and STDs*, 23(5), 315-321.

Ryder, R.W., Nsa, W., Hassig, S.E., Behets, F., Rayfield, M., Ekungola, B., Nelson, M.A., Mulenda, U., Francis, H., Mwandagalirwa, K., Davachi, F., Rogers, M., Nzilambi, N., Greenberg, A., Mann, J., Quinn, T.C., Piot, P. and James W. Curran, J.W. (1989). Perinatal Transmission of the human immunodeficiency virus type 1 to infants of seropositive women in Zaire. *New England Journal of Medicine,* 320, 1637-1642.

Safren, S.A. and Heimberg, R.G. (1999). Depression, hopelessness, suicidality, and related factors in sexual minority and heterosexual adolescents. *Journal of Consulting and Clinical Psychology,* 1999; 67:859–866.

Safren, S.A., Sari, L., Reisner, A. H., Mimiaga, M.J. and Stall, R.D. (2010). Mental Health and HIV Risk in Men Who Have Sex With Men. *Journal of Acquired Immune Deficiency Syndrome,* 2010; 55:S74–S77.

Safren, S.A., Traeger, L., Skeer, M.R., O'Cleirigh, C., Meade, C.S., Covahey, C., Mayer, K.H. (2010). Testing a social-cognitive model of HIV transmission risk behaviours in HIV-infected MSM with and without depression. *Journal of Health Psychology,* 2010; 29:215–221.

Samuel, D., Castaing, D., Adam, R., Saliba, F., Chamaret, S., Misset, J.L., Montagnier, L., Bismuth, H. (1988). Fatal acute HIV infection with aplastic anaemia, transmitted by liver graft. *Lancet,* 1:1221-2.

Scarlatti, G., Lombardi, V., Plebanic, N., Vegni, C., Ferraris, G., Bucceri, A., Fenyo, E.M., Wigzell, H., Rossi, P. and Albert, J. (1991) Polymerase chain reaction, virus isolation and antigen assay in HIV-1-antibody-positive mothers and their children., *AIDS,* 5:1173-1178.

Semen banking, organ and tissue transplantation, and HIV antibody testing. *MMWR* 1988; 37:57-8, 63.

Schulz, T.F., Boshoff, C.H. and Weiss, R.A. (1996). HIV infection and neoplasia. *Lancet,* 587-591.

Scarlatti, G. (1996). Paediatric HIV infection. *Lancet,* 348: 863-868.

Schwarz, A., Hoffmann, F., L'age-Stehr, J., Tegzess, A.M., Offermann, G. (1987). HIV transmission by organ donation: outcome in cornea and kidney recipients. *Transplantation,* 44:21-4.

Sharp, P.M., Robertson, D.L., Gao, F. and Hahn, B.H. (1994). Origins and diversity of HIV. *AIDS,* 8 (Suppl. 1): S27-S42.

Siegal, F.P., Lopez, C. and Hammer, G.S. (1981). Severe AIDS in male homosexuals, manifested by chronic perianal ulcerative herpes simplex lesions. *New England Journal of Medicine,* 305: 1439-1444.

Simonds, R.J., Holmberg, S.D., Hurwitz, L.R., Coleman, T.R., Bottenfield, S., Conley, L.J., Kohlenberg, H.S., Castro, G.K., Dahan, A.B., Schable, A.C., Rayfield, A.M. and Rogers, M.F. (1992). Transmission of HIV-1 from a seronegative organ and tissue donor. The New England Journal of Medicine, March, 329:726-32.

Smith, D.K., Gwinn, M., Selik, R.M., Miller, K.S., Dean-Gaitor, H., Thompson, P.I., De Cock, K.M., Gayle, H.D. (2000). HIV/AIDS among African Americans: progress or progression? *AIDS;* 2000; 14(9):1237-1248.

Sperling, S.R., Shapiro, E.D., Coombs, W.R., Todd, A.J., Herman, A.S., McSherry, D.G., et al. (1996). Maternal viral load, zidovudine treatment, and the risk of transmission of human immunodeficiency virus type 1 from mother to infant. Paediatric AIDS Clinical Trials Group Protocol 076 Study Group. *New England Journal of Medicine,* 1996; 335:1621–9.

Stall, R., Paul, J.P., *Greenwood, G.,* Pollack, L.M., Bein, E., Crosby, G.M., Mills, T.C., Binson, D., Coates, T.J., Catania, J.A. (2001). Alcohol use, drug use, and alcohol related problems among men who have sex with men: The Urban Men's Health Study. *Addiction,* 2001; 96:1589–1601.

Stall, R., Friedman, M., Catania, J.(2008) Interacting epidemics and gay men's health: a theory of syndemic production among urban gay men. In: Wolitski RJ, Stall R, Valdiserri RO, eds. Unequal Opportunity: Health Disparities Affecting Gay and Bisexual Men in the United States. New York, NY: Oxford University Press; 2008:251.

Stoneburner, R.C., Chiasson, M., Weisfuse, I.B. and Thomas, P.A. (1990). The epidemic of AIDS and HIV-1 infection among homosexuals in New York City. *AIDS,* 4: 99-106.

Strunnikova, N., Ray, S.C., Livingston, R.A., Rubalcaba, E. and Viscidi, R.P. (1995). Convergent evolution within the V3 loop domain of human immunodeficiency virus type 1 in association with disease progression. *Journal of Virology,* 69:7548–7558.

Suligoi, B., Raimondo, M., Regine, V., Salfa, M.C., Camoni, L.(2010). Epidemiology of HIV infection in blood donations in Europe and Italy. *Blood Transfusion,* 8(3): 178-85.

Sullivan, S. G., Ma, W., Duan, S. D., *et al.* (2009). Attitudes towards circumcision among Chinese men. *JAIDS Journal of Acquired Immune Deficiency Syndromes* 50(2), 238-240.

Sundaravaradan, V., Hahn, T. and Ahmad, N. (2005). Conservation of functional domains and limited heterogeneity of HIV-1 reverse transcriptase gene following vertical transmission. *Retrovirology,* 2005; 2: 36.

Tachet, A., Dulioust, E., Salmon, D, *et al.* (1999). Detection and quantification of HIV-1 in semen: identification of a

subpopulation of men at high potential risk of viral sexual transmission. *AIDS,* 13(7), 823-831.

Testing donors of organs, tissues, and semen for antibody to HLTV-III/lymphadenopathy-associated virus. *MMWR* 1985; 34:294.

The EXPLORE Study Team. Effects of a behavioural intervention to reduce acquisition of HIV infection among men who have sex with men: the EXPLORE randomised controlled study. *Lancet,* 2004; 364:41–50.

Tovo, P.A. and de Martino, M. (1988). Epidemiology, Clinical features, and prognostic factors of paediatric HIV infection. *Lancet,* ii: 1043-1045.

Transmission of HIV through bone transplantation: case report and public health recommendations. *MMWR,* 1988; 37:597-9.

Turner, B.J., Hauck, W.W., Fanning, T.R. and Markson, L.E. (1996). Cigarette smoking and maternal-child HIV transmission. *Journal of AIDS and Human Retrovirology,* 14: 327-337.

UNAIDS (2010). Global Report. UNAIDS Report on the global AIDS epidemic. Copyright © 2010 Joint United Nations Programme on HIV/AIDS (UNAIDS).

U.S. Centers for Disease Control and Prevention. (2002). Surveillance of health care personnel with HIV/AIDS. Retrieved May 15, 2008, from http://www.cdc.gov/ncidod/dhqp/bp_hiv_hp_with.html.

Van Griensven, F. and de Lin van Wijngaarden, J.W. (2010). A review of the epidemiology of HIV infection and prevention responses among MSM in Asia. *AIDS*, 24 Suppl. 3: S30-40.

Van de Perre, P., Simon, A., Msellati, P., Hitimana, D.G., Vaira, D., Bazubagira, A., Van Goethem, C., Stevens, A.M., Karita, E., Sondag-Thull, D., Dabis, F. and Lepage, P. (1991). Postnatal transmission of HIV type 1 from mother to infant. *New England Journal of Medicine*, 325: 593-598.

Varghese, B., Maher, J.E., Peterman, T. A., Branson, B. M. and Steketee, R. W. (2002). Reducing the risk of sexual HIV transmission: quantifying the per-act risk for HIV on the basis of choice of partner, sex act, and condom use. *Sexually Transmitted Diseases*, 29(1), 38-43.

Wang, L.D. (2009). *AIDS*. 1st ed. Beijing: Beijing Publishing House.

Wang L, Wang N, Wang L Y, *et al*. (2009). The 2007 estimates for people at risk for and living with HIV in China: progress and challenges. *Journal of Acquired Immune Deficiency Syndromes*, 50(4): 414-418.

Ward, J.W., Holberg, S.D., Allen, J.R., et al. (1988). Transmission of HIV by blood transfusions screened as negative for HIV antibody. New Eng J Med, 318:473-8.

Wawer, M. J., Gray, R. H., Sewankambo, N. K., *et al*. (2005). Rates of HIV-1 transmission per coital act, by stage of HIV-1infection, in Rakai, Uganda. *Journal of Infectious Diseases*, 191(9): 1403-1409.

Wawer, M.J, Makumbi F, Kigozi G, *et al*. (2009). Circumcision in HIV-infected men and its effect on HIV transmission to female partners in Rakai, Uganda: a randomised controlled trial. *The Lancet* 374(9685), 229-237.

Wells, M.A., Wittek, A.E., Epstein, J.S. et al., (1986). Inactivation and partition of human T-cell lymphotrophic virus, type III, during ethanol fractionation of plasma. *Transfusion*, 26:210-3.

Winkelstein, W. Jr., Lyman, D.M., Padian, N., Grant, R., Samuel, M., Wiley, J.A., Anderson, R.E., Lang, W., Riggs, J. and Levy, J.A. (1987). Sexual practices and risk of infection by the Human Immunodeficiency Virus: The San Francisco Men's Health Study. *Journal of American Medical Association*, 257: 321-325.

Wolinsky, S. M., Wike, C.M., Korber, B.T.M., Hutto, C., Parks, W.P., Rosenblum, L.L., Kunstman, K.J., Furtado, M.R. and J. L. Munoz. (1992). Selective transmission of human immunodeficiency virus type-1 variants from mothers to infants. *Science*, 255:1134–1137.

World Health Organisaztion (1989). HIV-2 working Group: Criteria for HIV-2 serodiagnosis, Marseille, France.

World Health Organization and Global programme on AIDS, WHO/GPA (1994). The HIV/AIDS pandemic: Overview. WHO/GPA/TCO/SEF/94.4.

Xu, J. (2009). Prospective cohort study to the incidence of HIV/STIs among FSWs in Kaiyuan City. PhD [dissertation].Beijing, China: China Center for Disease Control and Prevention.

Yu, M. and Vajdy, M. (2010). Mucosal HIV transmission and vaccination strategies through oral compared with vaginal and rectal routes. *Expert Opinion on Biological Therapy*, 10(8): 1181-1195.

4

HIV/AIDS Transmission Dynamics in Male Prisons

C.P. Bhunu*and S. Mushayabasa
Department of Applied Mathematics, Modelling Biomedical Systems Research Group
National University of Science and Technology, Bulawayo
Zimbabwe

1. Introduction

The imprisonment of large numbers of drug addicts has the potential to create environments within which social networks that enhances the transmission of infectious diseases form (7–11; 14). About 668,000 men and women are incarcerated in sub-Saharan Africa with South Africa having the highest prison population with 157,402 people behind bars in the region and 335 prisoners per 100,000 of the national population; it has the ninth largest prison population in the world (21). International data show that HIV prevalence among prisoners is between six to fifty times higher than that of the general adult population. For example, in the USA the ratio is 6:1, in France it is 10:1; in Switzerland 27:1 and in Mauritius 50:1 (17). On a global scale, the prison population is growing rapidly, with high incarceration rates leading to overcrowding, which largely stems from national law and criminal justice policies. In most countries, overcrowding and poor physical conditions prevail (20). This phenomenon poses significant health concerns with regard to control of infectious diseases-and HIV prevention and care most of all (21). Prisons are high risk settings for HIV transmission. However, HIV prevention, treatment are not adequately developed and implemented to respond to HIV in prisons (13). There is evidence to show that health programmes for the particular needs of imprisoned drug users are not enough in USA and Canada (15; 22). In Russia, a study of intravenous drug users demonstrated the critical role of prisons in the transmission of HIV through high levels of needle (syringes) sharing among the imprisoned (23).

Prison populations are predominantly male and most prisons are male-only institutions, including the prison staff. In such a gender exclusive environment, male-to-male sexual activity (prisoner-to-prisoner and guard-to-prisoner) is frequent (18). While much of the sex among men in prisons is consensual, rape and sexual abuse are often used to exercise dominance in the culture of violence that is typical of prison life (19). Inmate rape, including male rape, is considered one of the most ignored crimes. Sexual and physical abuse in custody remains a tremendous human rights problem (1). Intravenous drug use, tattooing and the following aspects of man-to-man sexual activity in prison make it a high risk for HIV transmission: anal intercourse, rape and the presence of sexually transmitted infections (STIs). Related problems in prisons across Southern Africa include overcrowding, shortages, corruption, and the presence of juveniles alongside adult prisoners. The potential for the spread of HIV is also increased by a lack of information and education, and a lack of proper medical care. STIs, if left untreated, can greatly increase a person's vulnerability to HIV

*Visiting Fellow, Clare Hall College, University of Cambridge

through sexual contact, UNAIDS noted (26). Men get tattooed in prison (12). In the absence of proper precautions and access to safe equipment tattooing can be a high-risk activity for the transmission of HIV (24; 25).
The literature and development of mathematical epidemiology is well documented (2; 3; 6). This paper seeks to use mathematical models to gain insights on transimission of HIV among male prisoners while in prison in the context of homosexuality and intravenous drug use. The rest of this paper is organized as follows. In the next section, the model and its basic properties are presented. In Section 3, we determine stability analysis of the equilibria states. Numerical simualtions are presented in Section 4 and finally the last section concludes the paper.

2. Model description

The model sub-divides the total male prisoner population into the following sub-populations of susceptible intravenous drug users $S_d(t)$, susceptible non-drug users $S_n(t)$, intravenous drug using HIV-only infected people not yet showing AIDS symptoms $I_n(t)$, non-drug using HIV-only infected people not yet showing AIDS symptoms $I_d(t)$, intravenous drug using AIDS cases $A_d(t)$ and non-drug using AIDS cases $A_d(t)$. There is sexual interaction between intravenous drug users and non-drug users making HIV transmission across different these two distinct distinct groups possible. The population is patterns is heterogeneous mixing with regard to sexual behaviour. The total population is given by;

$$N(t) = N_d(t) + N_n(t),\ N_d(t) = S_d(t) + I_d(t) + A_d(t),\ N_n(t) = S_n(t) + I_n(t) + A_n(t), \quad (1)$$

with $N_n(t)$ and $N_d(t)$ being the total number of non-drug using and intravenous drug using male prisoners (intravenous drug users-IDU), respectively. The group j members make c_j, $j = (d, n)$ sexual contacts per unit time, and that a fraction of the contacts made by a member of group j is with a member of group i is p_{j_i}, $i = (d, n)$. Then $p_{n_n} + p_{n_d} = p_{d_d} + p_{d_n} = 1$. The total number of sexual contacts per unit time by members of group 'n' (non-drug users) with members of group 'd' (intravenous drug users) is $c_n p_{n_d} N_n$ and because this must be equal to the number of contacts made by members of group 'd' with members of group 'n', we have a balance relation

$$\frac{p_{n_d} c_n}{N_d} = \frac{p_{d_n} c_d}{N_n}. \quad (2)$$

In this case the sexual contact rates (partner acquistion rates) c_d and c_n are saturating terms for the total population and the mixing proportions may change with time. It is worth mentioning here that intravenous drug users are more likely to have more sexual partners than the general population. Therefore, $c_d = \mathcal{B} c_n$, $\mathcal{B} \geq 1$. We assume that male prisoners in AIDS stage of the disease are nolonger sexually active as they are nolonger capable of attracting sexual mates among prisoners. Also drug using AIDS patients nolonger share their needles with others as other prisoners do not like sharing needles with someone whose AIDS symptoms are visible. The forces of HIV infection for intravenous drug users and non-drug users in the male prison are:

$$\lambda_{d_h} = \frac{p_{d_d} c_d \beta_d I_d}{N_d} + \frac{p_{d_n} c_d \beta_n I_n}{N_n} + \frac{c_{d_2} \beta_{d_2} I_d}{N_d},$$
$$\text{and } \lambda_{n_h} = \frac{p_{n_n} c_n \beta_n I_n}{N_n} + \frac{p_{n_d} c_n \beta_d I_d}{N_d}, \text{ respectively} \quad (3)$$

with β_i, $i = (n,d)$ is probabbility on individual being infected with HIV by an individual from the n- or d-class per sexual contact; c_j, $j = (n,d)$ are the number of sexual partners an individual acquires per year (partner acquistion rates); β_{d_2} is the probability an intravenous drug user getting HIV infection through sharing non-sterile needles during drug injections and c_{d_2} are the number drug sharing partners an individual acquires.
It is assumed people are recruited into prison at rate Λ through committing various crimes and the following proportions π_1, π_2, π_3 and π_4 recruited enter the classes $S_n(t)$, $S_d(t)$, $I_n(t)$ and $I_d(t)$, respectively. We further assume that AIDS cases are too sick to commit a crime, so there are no recruitment of prisoners already in the AIDS stage of disease. Furthermore, it is assumed that intravenous drug using prisoners showing AIDS symptoms are nolonger able to exert peer pressure strong enough to make one become a drug user. Individuals in $S_n(t)$ and $I_n(t)$ acquire drug misusing habits at rate $\lambda_d(t)$ due to peer pressure and move into $S_d(t)$ and $I_d(t$, respectively with

$$\lambda_{d_d} = \frac{\beta_{d_1} c_{d_1} (S_d + I_d)}{N_d}, \tag{4}$$

where β_{d_1} is the probability of becoming an intravenous drug user (IDU) following contact with an IDU and c_{d_1} are the number of contacts necessary for one to become an IDU (partner acquistion rate). Individuals in $S_n(t)$ class acquire HIV infection at a rate $\lambda_{n_h}(t)$ to move into $I_n(t)$. Individuals in $S_d(t)$ class acquire HIV infection at a rate $\lambda_{d_h}(t)$ to move $I_d(t)$ class. Individuals infected with HIV-only not yet displaying symptoms $(I_n(t), I_d(t))$ progress to the AIDS stage $((A_n(t), A_d(t))$ at a rate γ. Individuals in $A_d(t)$ leave the intravenous drug using habits at a rate α to get into $A_n(t)$ class. Individuals in all classes experience natural death at a rate μ and those in AIDS stage of the disease experience an additional disease induced death at a rate ν. Individuals in all classes leave the prison at rate ω upon completion of their sentences. Individuals in the AIDS stage of the disease (final terminal stages) are further released from prison due to sickness at rate ϕ. The model flow diagram is shown in Figure 1. Based on these assumptions the following system of differential equations describe the model.

$$\begin{aligned}
S_n'(t) &= \pi_1 \Lambda - (\lambda_d + \lambda_{n_h}) S_n - (\mu + \omega) S_n, \\
I_n'(t) &= \pi_3 \Lambda + \lambda_{n_h} S_n - \lambda_d I_n - (\mu + \omega + \gamma) I_n, \\
A_n'(t) &= \gamma I_n + \alpha A_d - (\mu + \omega + \phi + \nu) A_n, \\
S_d'(t) &= \pi_2 \Lambda + \lambda_d S_n - \lambda_{d_h} S_d - (\mu + \omega) S_d, \\
I_d'(t) &= \pi_4 \Lambda + \lambda_{d_h} S_d + \lambda_d I_n - (\mu + \omega + \gamma) I_d, \\
A_d'(t) &= \gamma I_d - (\mu + \alpha + \omega + \phi + \nu) A_n.
\end{aligned} \tag{5}$$

2.1 Model basic properties

In this section, we study the basic results of solutions of model system (5), which are essential in the proofs of stability results.

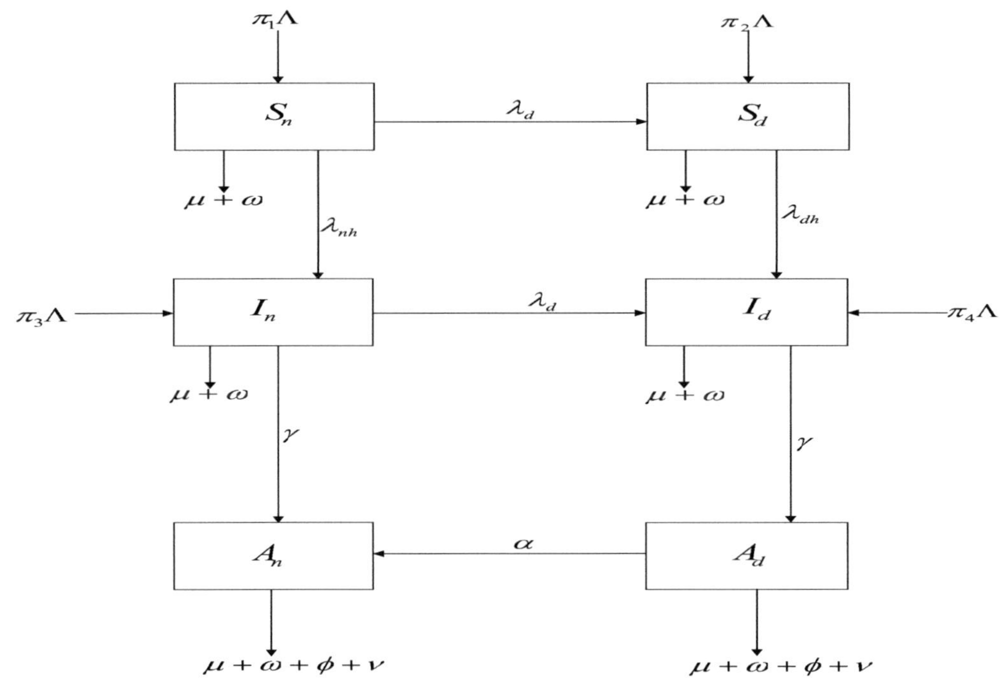

Fig. 1. Structure of the model.

Lemma 1. *The equations preserve positivity of solutions.*

Proof. The vector field given by the right hand side of (5) points inward on the boundary of $\mathbb{R}^6_+ \setminus \{0\}$. For example, if $S_n = 0$ then $S_n' = \pi_1\Lambda \geq 0$. All the other components are similar. □

Lemma 2. *Each non-negative solution is bounded in* L^1*-norm by* $\max\{N(0), \Lambda/\mu\}$.

Proof. The norm L^1 norm of each non-negative solution is N and it satisfies the inequality $N' \leq \Lambda - \mu N$. Solutions to the equation $M' = \Lambda - \mu M$ are monotone increasing and bounded by Λ/μ if $M(0) < \Lambda/\mu$. They are monotone decreasing and bounded above if $M(0) \geq \Lambda/\mu$. Since $N' \leq M'$ the claim follows. □

Corollary 1. *The region*

$$\Phi = \left\{ (S_n, I_n, A_n, S_d, I_d, A_d) \in \mathbb{R}^6_+ : N \leq \frac{\Lambda}{\mu} \right\}. \tag{6}$$

is invariant and attracting for system (5).

Theorem 1. *For every non-zero, non-negative initial value, solutions of model system (5) exist for all times*

Proof. Local existence of solutions follow from standard arguments since the right hand side of (5) is locally Lipschitz. Global existence follows from the a-priori bounds. □

3. Disease-free equilibrium and stability analysis

The disease free equilibrium of model system (5), $\mathcal{E}^0$ is given by

$$\mathcal{E}^0 = \left(S_n^0, I_n^0, A_n^0, S_d^0, I_d^0, A_d^0\right) = \left(\frac{\pi_1 \Lambda}{\mu + \omega + \beta_{d_1} c_{d_1}}, 0, 0, \frac{\Lambda(\pi_2(\mu + \omega) + \beta_{d_1} c_{d_1})}{(\mu + \omega)(\mu + \omega + \beta_{d_1} c_{d_1})}, 0, 0\right). \quad (7)$$

Following van den Driessche and Watmough (27), the effective reproduction number of model system (5) is given as

$$\begin{aligned} \mathcal{R}_{SD} &= \tfrac{c_{d_2}\beta_{d_2} + c_d p_{d_d} \beta_d}{2a_3} + c_n \left(\tfrac{\pi_1 p_{n_d} a_1 c_{d_1} \beta_{d_1} \beta_d}{2a_3 a_4 a_6} + \tfrac{p_{nn}\beta_n}{2a_4}\right) \\ &+ \sqrt{\left(\tfrac{c_{d_2}\beta_{d_2} + c_d p_{d_d} \beta_d}{2a_3} + c_n \left(\tfrac{\pi_1 p_{n_d} a_1 c_{d_1} \beta_{d_1} \beta_d}{2a_3 a_4 a_6} + \tfrac{p_{nn}\beta_n}{2a_4}\right)\right)^2 - \tfrac{c_n \beta_n (c_{d_2} p_{nn} \beta_{d_2} + c_d \beta_d (p_{nn} p_{d_d} - p_{n_d} p_{dn}))}{a_3 a_4}} \end{aligned} \quad (8)$$

with $a_1 = \mu + \omega$, $a_2 = \mu + \omega + \phi + \nu$, $a_3 = \mu + \omega + \gamma$, $a_4 = \mu + \omega + \gamma + c_{d_1}\beta_{d_1}$, $a_5 = \mu + \omega + \phi + \nu$, $a_6 = \pi_2(\mu + \omega) + c_{d_1}\beta_{d_1}$ throughout the manuscript. The reproduction number $\mathcal{R}_{SD}$ is defined as the number of secondary HIV infections produced by one HIV infected individual during his/ her entire infectious period in a mixed population of non-drug users and intravenous drug male prisoners. Theorem 2 follows from van den Driessche and Watmough (27).

Theorem 2. *The disease free equilibrium $\mathcal{E}^0$ of model system (5) is locally asymptotically stable if $\mathcal{R}_{S_D} < 1$ and unstable otherwise.*

Analysis of the effective reproduction number, $\mathcal{R}_{SD}$
The reproduction number is differentiated into categories:
Case 1: No intravenous drug users in the community
In this case $\beta_d = \beta_{d_c} c_{d_c} = \beta_d c_d = p_{n_d} = p_{d_n} = 0$, $p_{n_n} = 1$ so that $\mathcal{R}_{S_D}$ becomes $\mathcal{R}_{0_S}$ which is given by

$$\mathcal{R}_{0_S} = \frac{\beta_n c_n}{a_3}, \quad (9)$$

which is the number of secondary HIV infections produced by one HIV infected individual through homosexual tendencies in a male prison. It is important to note $\mathcal{R}_{0_S}$ is a decreasing function of ω, suggesting that increasing the number of prisoners leaving the prison reduces the concentration of HIV cases in prison. Theoretically this is feasible, in reality this begs more questions than answers as sentences communicated cannot be reversed because of HIV. Perhaps, it may be necessary to consider the use of open prison systems where prisoners with less serious crimes can serve their sentences while staying at their homes. This has a further advantage of reducing the high levels of raping of man by man in prisons and the homosexual tendencies which male prisoners resort to in enclosed prisons which is one of the major forces driving HIV/AIDS in male prisons.
Increase in intravenous drug users
In this case $(p_{p_p}, \beta_{d_1} c_{d_1}) \to (1, \infty)$ so that $\mathcal{R}_{S_D}$ becomes $\mathcal{R}_{0_D}$ which is given by

$$\mathcal{R}_{0_D} = \frac{\beta_d c_d + \beta_{d_1} c_{d_1}}{a_3}. \quad (10)$$

$\mathcal{R}_{0_D}$ just like is $\mathcal{R}_{0_S}$ is a decreasing function of ω, meaning that use of open prison systems will be beneficial in the control of HIV among male prisoners. It is important to note that levels of sexual contact are higher among intravenous drug users than non-drug users, with it increased risk of contracting HIV, so $c_n\beta_n < c_d\beta_d$ and this translates $\mathcal{R}_{0_S} < \mathcal{R}_{0_D}$. This suggest that intravenous drug use enhances HIV transmission in male prisons. Drug using prisoners are at an increased risk of HIV infection than their non-drug using counterparts. May be introducing drug substitution treatment together with introducing needle free exchange programmes will reduce the epidemic in prisons. A reduction in needle in sharing among prisoners result in HIV/AIDS prevalence as the sharing of unsterile needles in a major source of HIV transmission among male prisoners.

4. Numerical simulations

In this section, we carry out detailed numerical simulations using MatLab programming language to assess the effects of HIV transmission among male prisoners in the absence any interventional strategy which is more common in developing countries in Africa for different initial conditions. The parameter values that we use for numerical simulations are in Table 1. In Table 1, NPA denotes National Prison Administration (Zimbabwe). For influence of peer pressure forces influencing one to become an IDU, we used values adapted from Bhunu et al. (4) which are peer pressure forces necessary for one to start smoking, for the sake of illustration. For influence of peer pressure forces influencing one to become an IDU, we used values adapted from Bhunu et al. (2010) (4) which are peer pressure forces necessary for one to start smoking.

Parameter	Symbol	Value	Source
Recruitment rate	Λ	$0.00163\text{yr}^{-1} * 3000000$	NPA
Natural mortality rate	μ	0.02yr^{-1}	(5)
Natural rate of progression to AIDS	γ	0.1yr^{-1}	(5)
Rate of leaving prison due to AIDS related sickness	ϕ	0.25	Assumed
AIDS related death rate	ν	0.4yr^{-1}	(5)
Product of effective contact rate for HIV infection and probability of HIV transmission per drug injection	$c_{d_2}\beta_{d_2}$	0.562yr^{-1}	(16)
Probability of HIV transmission per sexual contact	β_n, β_d	$0.125\ (0.01\text{-}0.95)\text{yr}^{-1}$	(5)
Sexual acquistion rate	c_n, c_d	3yr^{-1}	(5)
Product of effective contact rate for becoming a drug user and probability of becoming a drug misuser per contact with a misuser	$c_{d_1}\beta_{d_1}$	0.4yr^{-1}	(4)
Rate of quitting drug misuse of sickness	α	0.3yr^{-1}	(4)
Rate of release from prison	ω	0.25yr^{-1}	Assumed
Proportion recruited into S_n, S_d, I_n, I_d classes	$\pi_1, \pi_2, \pi_3, \pi_4$	0.375,0.375,0.125,0.125	Assumed

Table 1. Model parameters and their interpretations.

Figure 2 is a graphical representation showing the effect of varying initial conditions when $\mathcal{R}_{S_D} > 1$. In Figures 2(a) and 2(b) show the effects of varying the HIV-infected not yet showing sysmptoms on HIV-infected only and AIDS, respectively. Both graphs show a higher number of HIV-only and AIDS among intravenous drug using male prisoners than non-drug users. This tends to show intravenous drug using male prisoners are at increased risk of HIV infection due to sharing of unsterile needles and increased rates of homosexual sex habits.

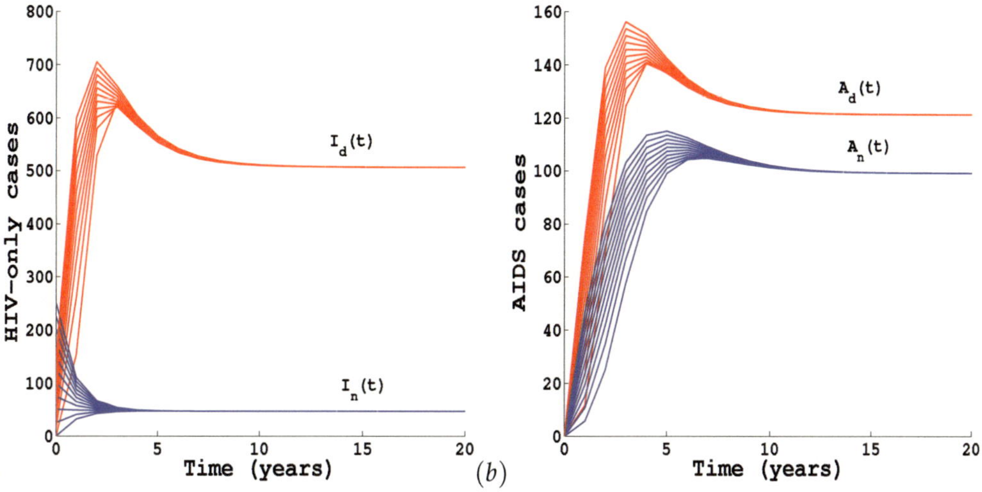

(*a*) (*b*)

Fig. 2. Effects of varying the HIV infected-only initial conditions when $\mathcal{R}_{S_D} > 1$. Parameter values used are in Table 1.

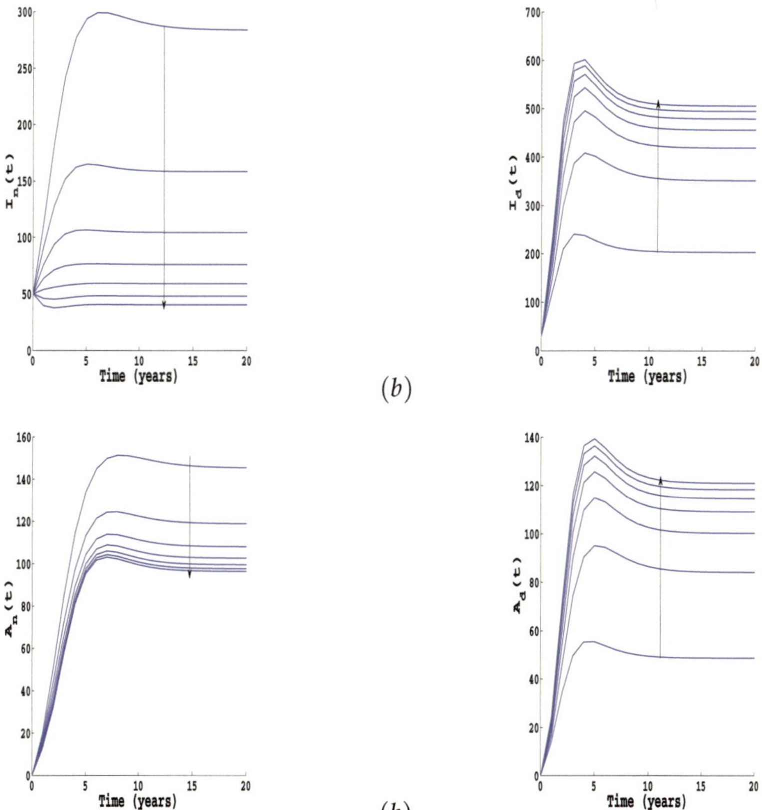

(*a*) (*b*)

(*a*) (*b*)

Fig. 3. Simulations showing the effects of varying the rate at which non-drug using prisoners become intravenous drug users on the population on drug using HIV-infected prisoners. Parameter values used are in Table 1.

Figure 3 shows the effects of intravenous drug use on HIV/AIDS transmission dynamics among male prisoners is illustrated by varying the rate a male prisoner becoming an intravenous drug user while in prison. It shows an increase in the number of HIV/AIDS cases among drug users cases with increase in drug use while the opposite will be happening among non-drug users. This suggest that effective control of HIV among male prisoners to some extent on the control of intravenous drug use.

5. Discussion

A mathematical model have been presented in attempt to understand the transmission dynamics of HIV/AIDS among male prisoners. Male prisoners are infected with HIV while in prison through intravenous drug use using unsterile needles (syringes) and homosexual tendencies. Intravenous drug use in male prisons act in two way: (i) sharing of unsterile needles/ syringes enhance the transmission of HIV; (ii) flashing blood that drawing is blood from someone who would have injected himself with a drug and inject it into one self which on its own exposes the injector to the HIV infection. Also intravenous drug using prisoners are more likely to engage in homosexual relations with other male prisoners and with it increased risky of HIV transmission. Analysis of the reproduction number have shown that (i) a reduction in drug use results in a decrease of HIV/ AIDS prevalence among male prisoners, (ii) release of prisoners may also act in reducing the concentration HIV/AIDS cases in prisons. The later fact is not feasible, but perhaps implementing opening prison systems where prisoners of less serious crimes are allowed to save their crimes while staying with their families enables male prisoners to cope up with stressful prison conditions. Open prison systems will reduce the influence of peer pressure among prisoners as they will have moral and pyschological support from the family which does not exist in enclosed prison systems. Numerical simulations carried also support the analytic results that increase in drug use and tattooing increases HIV/ AIDS prevalence among male prisoners. The result of this study have a public health implication considering high rates of syringe lending and borrowing in prisons. This might explain why there are more HIV cases in prisons than the general population in the case of the USA (8) and this might be the case world wide. HIV infected men in prison pose a risk to their communities upon release from prison, especially in Africa where partners in marriage rarely discuss safe sex so in the absence open prison systems, it may be best to have mandatory HIV/ AIDS screening and specific educational programmes for prisoners. This will reduce the prevalence of high-risk behaviours and lower HIV transmission in male prisons, thus reducing post-release public health threat. Given the high levels of HIV in prisons about three and half times higher among prisoners than the general population, it may be best to consider the introduction of needle/ syringe free exchange programme and drug substitution treatment as a way of keeping in check HIV transmission in men prisons. Additionally provision of condoms might also help given the high levels of homosexuality in male prisons.

6. References

[1] Amnesty International. Abuse of Women in Custody: Sexual Misconduct and Shackling of Pregnant Women, 2001.
[2] Anderson, May RM. Infectious Diseases of Humans, Dynamics and Control, Oxford University Press, 1991.
[3] Bailey N, The Mathematical Theory of Infectious Diseases, Charles Griffin, 1975.

[4] Bhunu CP, Mushayabasa S, Tchuenche JM. A theoretical assessment of the effects of smoking on the transmission dynamics of tuberculosis. *Bulletin of Mathematical Biology* DOI 10.1007/s11538-010-9568-6, 2010(a). Available at (http://www.springerlink.com/content/4n410216p3555249/fulltext.pdf)

[5] Bhunu CP, Garira W, Mukandavire Z. Modelling HIV/AIDS and tuberculosis coinfection. *Bulletin of Mathematical Biology* 71: 1745-1780, 2009.

[6] Brauer F, C. Castillo-Chavez. Mathematical Models in Population Biology and Epidemiology, Springer, 2000.

[7] Buavirat A, Page-Shafer K, van Griensven GJP, Mandel JS, Evans J, Chuaratanaphong J, Chiamwongpat S, Sacks R, Moss A. Risk of prevalent HIV infection associated with incarceration among injecting drug users in Bangkok, Thailand: case-control study. *BMJ 326*(7384): 308, 2003.

[8] Centers for Disease Control and Prevention (CDC). HIV transmission among male inmates in a state prison system-Georgia, 1992-2005. *MMWR Morb Mortal Wkly Rep* 55(15): 421–426, 2006.

[9] Centers for Disease Control and Prevention (CDC). National Center for HIV/AIDS, Viral Hepatitis, STD, and TB Prevention. Prevention and control of tuberculosis in correctional and detention facilities: recommendations from CDC, endorsed by the Advisory Council for the Elimination of Tuberculosis, the National Commission on Correctional Health Care, and the American Correctional Association. *MMWR Recomm Rep* 55(RR-9): 1–44, 2006.

[10] Centers for Disease Control and Prevention. Tuberculosis outbreaks in prison housing units for HIV-infected inmatesŮCalifornia, 1995–1996. *MMWR Morb Mortal Wkly Rep* 48(4):79–82, 1999.

[11] Crofts N, Stewart T, Hearne P, Ping XY, Breschkin AM, Locarnini SA. Spread of bloodborne viruses among Australian prison entrants. *BMJ* 310(6975): 285–288, 1995.

[12] Doll D. Tattooing in prison and HIV infection. *The Lancet* 2(9): 66-67, 1988.

[13] Dolan J, Kite B, Aceijas C, Stimson GV. HIV in prison in low income and middle-income countries. *Lancet Infectious Diseases* 7: 32-43, 2007.

[14] Dolan KA, Wodak A. HIV transmission in a prison system in an Australian state. *Med J Aust* 171(1):14–17, 1999.

[15] Flanigan TP, Rich JD, Spaulding A. HIV care among incarcerated persons: a missed opportunity. *AIDS* 13(17): 2475, 1999.

[16] Green D, Al-Fwzan W. An improved optimistic three-stage model for the spread of HIV amongst injecting intravenous drug users. *J Discrete Contin Dyn Sys* (Supplement 2009): 286-299, 2009.

[17] Human Rights Watch. HIV/AIDS in prisons, 2006.

[18] Human Rights Watch. World Report; Special Programs and CampaignsŮPrisons, 2002.

[19] Human Rights Watch. No Escape: Male Rape in USA Prisons, 1991.

[20] International Centre for Prison Studies. The World Female Imprisonment List. KingŠs College, London, UK, 2006.

[21] International Centre for Prison Studies. The World Prison Population List. KingŠs College, London, UK, 2007.

[22] Martin RE, Gold F, Murphy W, Remple V, Berkowitz J, Money D. Drug use and risk of bloodborne infections: a survey of female prisoners in British Columbia. *Can J Public Health* 96(2):97–101, 2005.

[23] Sarang A, Rhodes T, Platt L, Kirzhanova, V, Shelkovnikova O, Volnov V, Blagovo D, Rylkov A. Drug injecting and syringe use in the HIV risk environment of Russian penitentiary institutions: qualitative study. *Addiction* 101(12): 1787-1796, 2006.
[24] United Nations Office On Drugs and Crime (UNODC). Women and HIV in prison settings. http://www.unodc.org/documents/hiv-aids/Women and HIV in prison settings.pdf, 2008.
[25] United Nations Office On Drugs and Crime (UNODC). HIV/AIDS prevention and care for female injecting drug users. http://www.unodc.org/pdf/HIV-AIDS_femaleIDUs_Aug06.pdf, 2006.
[26] UNAIDS. AIDS Epidemic Update. Geneva, UNAIDS, 2006.
[27] van den Driessche P, Watmough J. Reproduction numbers and sub-threshold endemic equilibria for the compartmental models of disease transmission. *Math Biosci* 180: 29-48, 2002.

Part 3

Prevention and Treatment of AIDS-Related Diseases

5

Individuals with HIV/AIDS: Clinical Manifestations in the Oral Cavity in the Post-HAART Era

Ranjitha Krishna, Saiprasad Zemse and Scott Derossi
Georgia Health Sciences University, College of Dental Medicine
United States of America

1. Introduction

Oral lesions are very common in individuals with HIV (human immunodeficiency virus) infection and AIDS (acquired immune deficiency syndrome). They are reported to occur in 50% of people infected with HIV and in about 80% of people diagnosed with AIDS (Palmer, et al., 1996). Introduction of HAART (highly active anti-retroviral therapy) in 1996 has reduced the mortality and morbidity in people affected with HIV and AIDS as well as improved their quality of life. It has also resulted in a decrease, to a certain extent, in the incidence and prevalence of oral lesions.

Since HIV infection was first diagnosed in 1981, a variety of oral lesions has been associated with infected individuals, and they can be good indicators of the disease in otherwise healthy people. Oral lesions can also help determine the progression of the disease. In developed countries, CD4 lymphocyte counts and HIV viral load are the two main laboratory markers that are used to determine disease progression. However, in certain developing countries, people do not always have access to these tests, and severity of the oral lesions can serve as good indicators of disease progression.

Table 1 highlights the importance of diagnosing and treating oral lesions in individuals with HIV (Coogan, et al., 2005)

1.	Can help diagnose the presence of HIV infection in otherwise healthy individuals
2.	Develop early in an infection
3.	Help determine the progression of HIV infection to AIDS
4.	Entry and end-points in vaccine trials
5.	Used in staging and classification of HIV diseases as determinants of opportunistic infection and anti-HIV therapy

Table 1. Importance of oral manifestations of HIV disease

1.1 Classification of oral lesions associated with HIV

The EC-Clearinghouse on oral problems related to HIV infection and WHO Collaborating Centre on Oral manifestations of the immunodeficiency virus proposed the classification of oral manifestations of HIV infection in September of 1992 based on their strength of association with the presence of HIV infection: ("Classification and Diagnostic Criteria for Oral Lesions in HIV Infection. EC-Clearinghouse on Oral Problems Related to HIV Infection and WHO Collaborating Centre on Oral Manifestations of the Immunodeficiency Virus," 1993). More recently in 2002, an international workshop was convened to discuss the classification of oral lesions associated with HIV/AIDS almost 2 decades after the virus was first identified (Patton, et al., 2002) and it was agreed that the original EC-Clearinghouse classification could still be used in current times. Table 2 summarizes the classification of oral lesions associated with HIV.

Group 1: Lesions strongly associated with HIV infection	Group 2: Lesions less commonly associated with HIV infection	Group 3: Lesions seen in HIV infection
Candidiasis Hairy leukoplakia Kaposi's sarcoma Non-Hodgkin's lymphoma Periodontal disease (linear gingival erythema, necrotizing ulcerative gingivitis, necrotizing ulcerative periodontitis)	**Bacterial infections:** *Mycobacterium avium-intracellularae* *Mycobacterium tuberculosis* Melanogic hyperpigmentation Necrotizing (ulcerative) stomatitis Salivary gland disease Dry mouth due to decreased salivary flow Unilateral/bilateral swelling of salivary glands Thrombocytopenia purpura Non-specific ulcerations **Viral infections:** Herpes simplex virus Human papillomavirus Condyloma acuminatum Focal epithelial hyperplasia Verruca vulgaris Varicella-zoster virus	**Bacterial infections:** *Actinomyces israelii* *Escherichia coli* *Klebsiella pneumonia* Cat-scratch disease Drug reactions (ulcerative, erythema multiforme, lichenoid, toxic epidermolysis) Epitheliod (bacillary) angiomatosis **Fungal infection other than candidiasis** *Cryptococcus neoformans* *Geotrichum candidum* *Histoplasma capsulatum* *Mucoraceae (mucomycosis zygomycosis)* *Aspergilus flavus* **Neurological disturbances:** Facial palsy Trigeminal neuralgia

Table 2. Classification of oral lesions associated with HIV

In this chapter, we will discuss only those lesions that are commonly seen in persons infected with HIV.

2. Candidiasis

2.1 Background

Candidiasis is a common opportunistic infection caused by an overgrowth of the *Candida* microorganisms already present in the oral cavity. Incidence of oral candidiasis has been high in developing countries (Tukutuku, et al., 1990). Since the discovery of HIV in 1981, candidiasis has been shown to be associated with HIV-infected individuals (Gottlieb, et al., 1981). Previous reports show that oral candidiasis occurs in 54-93% of individuals with AIDS (Schmidt-Westhausen, et al., 1991). In recent reports, due to the introduction of anti-retroviral therapy only 20% of individuals infected with HIV showed oral candidiasis (Davies, et al., 2006).

2.2 Pathogenesis

Oral candidiasis is primarily caused by a dimorphic ubiquitous *Candida albicans*. The cell wall of *Candida* is primarily made up of three polysaccharides, mannan, glucan and chitin. *Candida* attaches to oral tissues and dentures with the help of adhesins such as Als1p, Als5p, Int1p and Hwp1p (Chaffin, et al., 1998, Hostetter, 1994). These glycoproteins bind to the extracellular matrix of mammalian cells such as fibrinogen, laminin and collagen (Chaffin, et al., 1998). Candidal adhesion to endothelial surfaces is achieved by the cell surface polysaccharide mannan, which binds to complement receptor 3 (CR3), an integrin found on human cells (Calderone and Braun, 1991). There is increased association of integrin analogs (iC3B and CR3d receptor) and fibronectin receptor with most of the virulent forms of *Candida* (Ollert, et al., 1990). Thus, CR3-like proteins promote adherence of *Candida albicans* to host cells.

2.3 Clinical features

There are three clinical forms of candidiasis: pseudo-membranous (thrush), erythematous (atrophic) and perioral angular chelitis. Proliferation of pseudo-membranous fungi forms a gray-white structure composed of inflammatory substrate and matted organisms resting on an erythematous base. These lesions are most commonly evident on the tongue, buccal mucosa, hard and soft palate and pharyngeal tissues. The erythematous form shows mucosal hyperemia and inflammation with a reddened erythematous patches (Calderone and Fonzi, 2001). The mucous membrane appears dry, red and glazed. Affected individuals show burning sensitivity and pain sensation of dry mouth, odynophagia, dysgeusia and smell of yeast infection. Angular chelitis shows commissural involvement as erythematous/hyperkeratotic with fissuring and sensitivity. Individuals receiving HAART show low occurrence of these clinical features. Before the emergence of HAART, the incidence of oral candidiasis was relatively high in persons with AIDS.

2.4 Treatment

An early study for treatment of *Candida* infections was carried out by Williams in 1977, where nystatin was compared to no treatment in 56 patients (Williams, et al., 1977). Since then ketoconazole, fluconazole, clotrimazole, itraconazole, neomycin sulphate, colistin, trimethoprin and sulphamethoxazole have been tried in combination and at different concentrations for treatment of oral candidiasis (Hann, et al., 1982, Owens, et al., 1984, Palmblad, et al., 1992, Philpott-Howard, et al., 1993, Rozenberg-Arska, et al., 1991, Vogler, et al., 1987). Most recently ketoconazole and clotrimazole were found most effective in treatment of oral candidiasis (Worthington, et al., 2002). Initial local treatments are first line of therapy (Bensadoun, et al., 2008). Mucosal contact for 2 minutes is recommended either by rinsing, gargling or swallowing.

Systemic treatments are considered in high-risk patients only when local therapy fails (Charlier, et al., 2006). When topical and systemic therapy fails, intravenously administered amphotericin B and echinocandins are considered in high-risk patients. Intermittent use of antifungal agents has been advocated to prevent development of resistant fungal infections (Samaranayake, et al., 2002). Recently, gel formulation of fluconazole has proven to be a better alternative treatment form than tablet formulation (Nairy, et al.).

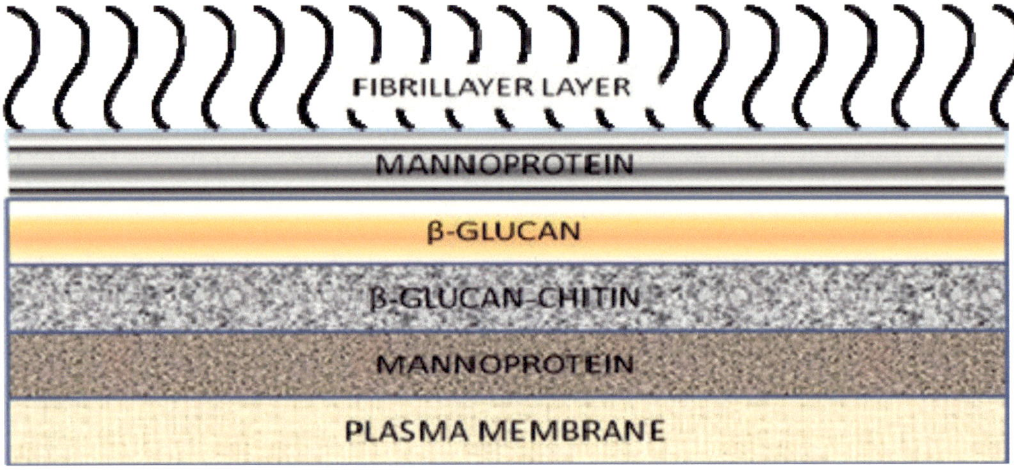

Fig. 1. Cell wall of *Candida albicans*

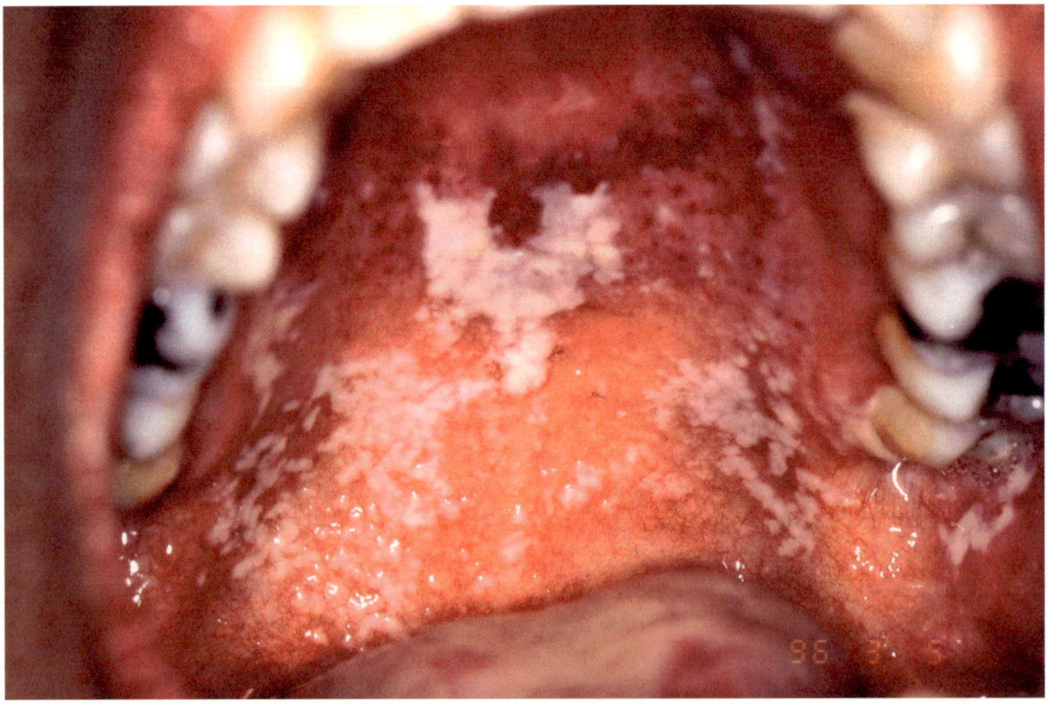

Fig. 2. Hypertrophic Candidiasis

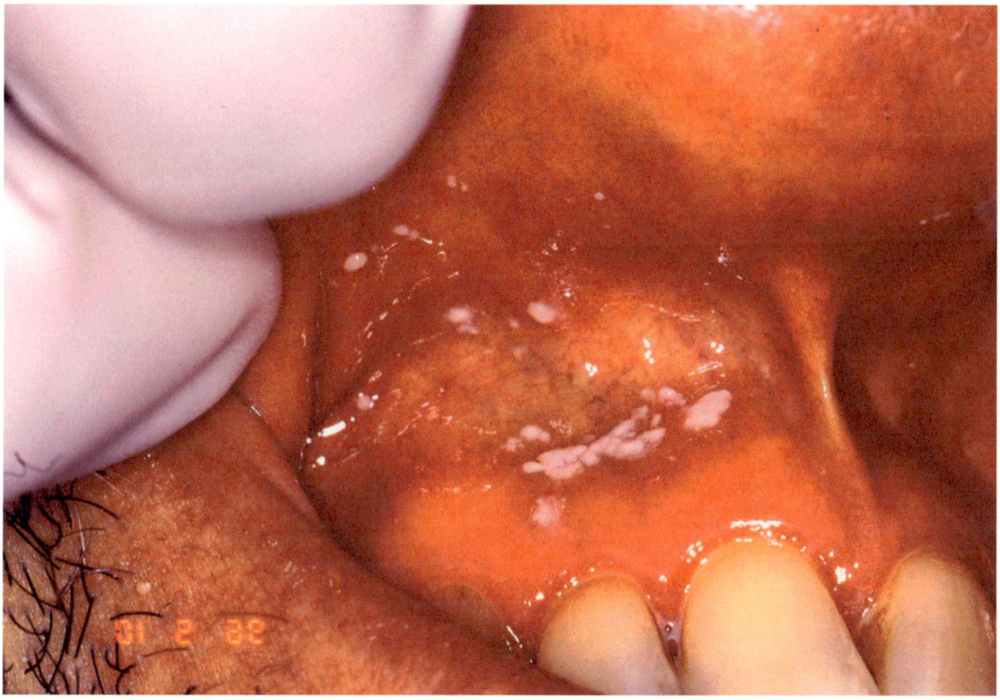

Fig. 3. Pseudo-membranous Candidiasis

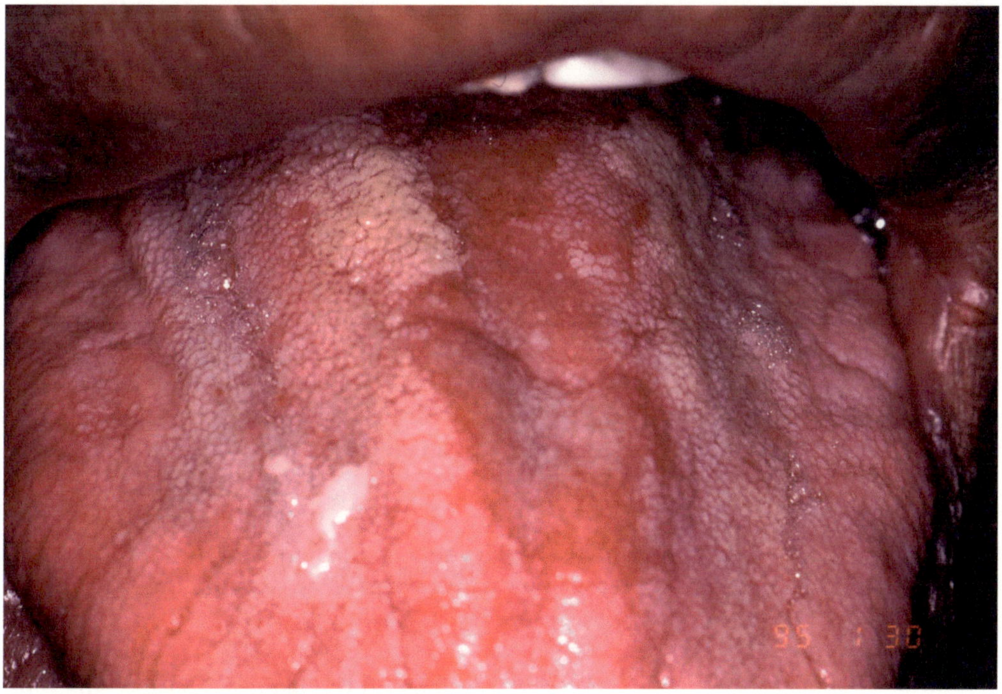

Fig. 4. Atrophic/Erythematous Candidiasis

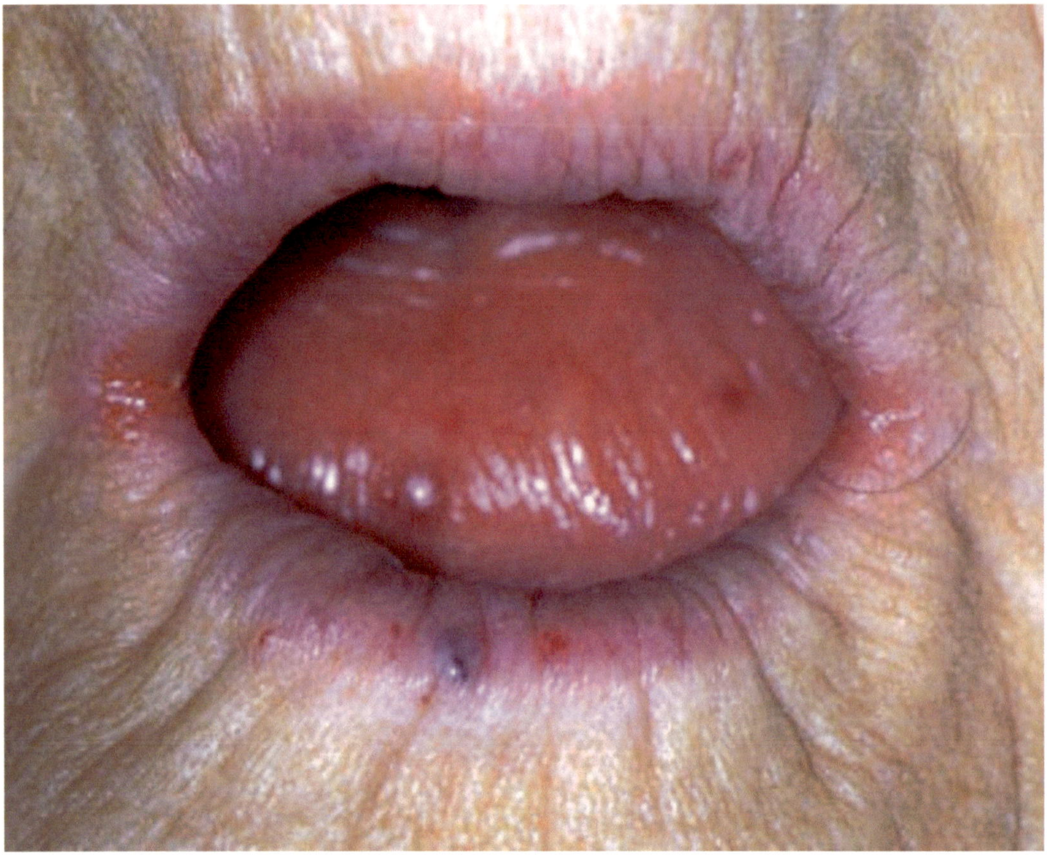

Fig. 5. Angular Chelitis

3. Hairy leukoplakia

3.1 Background

OHL (Oral hairy leukoplakia) is caused by Epstein-Barr virus and was first described in 1984. 50% of individuals with HIV present with this condition and it is a very good indicator of immunosuppression. The lesion usually presents itself when the CD4 cell counts fall below $0.3*10^9/L$ (Bravo, et al., 2006). According to the CDC (Centers for Disease Control and Prevention), this condition has a clear prognostic value in predicting the future development of AIDS ("1993 Revised Classification System for HIV Infection and Expanded Surveillance Case Definition for AIDS among Adolescents and Adults," 1992).

3.2 Pathogenesis

The pathogenesis of OHL is due to the replication of Epstein-Barr virus and increased virulence in conjunction with a decrease in local and systemic host immunity.

3.3 Clinical features

OHL present themselves as white, corrugated lesions on the lateral surface of the tongue and are not painful. There has been a decrease in the incidence of OHL due to the potent anti-retroviral drugs. However, if OHL is seen in an HIV-infected person, it may indicate failure of current therapy. Differential diagnosis of this condition includes oral candidiasis, lichen planus, other forms of leukoplakia, HPV (human papilloma virus) associated intraepithelial neoplasia, and oral squamous cell carcinoma.

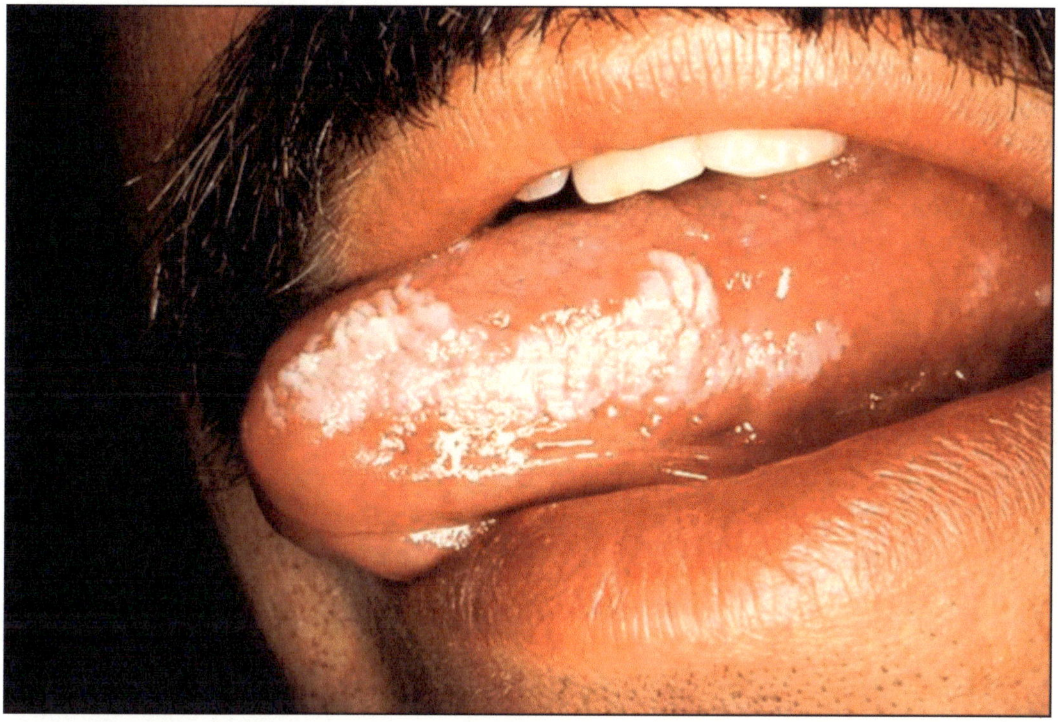

Fig. 6. Oral Hairy Leukoplakia

3.4 Treatment

OHL is a relatively benign condition with low morbidity and does not require any specific treatment. Most of the time, these lesions resolve spontaneously. However, several treatment options are available for those who feel uncomfortable or have cosmetic concerns due to the lesion. Since the lesion is caused by multiplication of the Epstein-Barr virus topical and systemic anti-viral agents work effectively in resolving the lesion. High doses of Acyclovir (800 mg 5 times a day) (Resnick, et al., 1988), Valacyclovir (1000 mg 3 times a day), and Famciclovir (500 mg 3 times a day) have all been shown to resolve the lesions in 1-2 weeks (Schofer, et al., 1987). However, once the effect of the anti-viral agent wears off, the lesions can recur several weeks later.

Topical application of Podophyllin resin in 25% solution has produced resolution of the lesion in 1-2 weeks (Gowdey, et al., 1995). Topical therapy with retinoic acid has also been shown to cause resolve the lesions due to inhibition of Epstein-Barr virus replication. Ablative and cryotherapy have also had success in treatment of the lesions. Although the above treatment options are effective in resolving the lesion, OHL can recur several weeks after treatment since none of these agents eliminate the latent state of infection.

4. Kaposi's sarcoma

4.1 Background

KS (Kaposi's sarcoma) is an angioproliferative tumor described by the Hungarian pathologist Moritz Kaposi in 1872. It is caused by KSHV (Kaposi's sarcoma-associated herpes virus) or γ2-herpes virus. KSHV belongs to the genus Rhadinovirus and has a DNA sequence similar to other rhadinoviruses (Albrecht, et al., 1992). With the introduction of HAART in 1996, the incidence of AIDS-related cancers such as KS and NHL (non - Hodgkin's lymphoma) has decreased (Shiels, et al., 2008). During the 1980s and early 1990s, US population rates of KS increased 30 fold (Eltom, et al., 2002). There were no KS cases during 1975-1979, before the advent of AIDS. In an HIV cancer match study, 81% of KS cases matched to HIV registries during 1980-2007 (Shiels, et al., 2011). AIDS occurred in a higher proportion of patients with Kaposi's sarcoma in age groups of 0-29 and 30-59 years (Shiels, et al., 2011).

4.2 Pathogenesis

KS lesions show varying cell diversity. Lesions are flat, comprising of inflammatory cells (T, B cells and monocytes). Neovascularization develops prior to development of these lesions and contain spindle-shaped cells. This dermal stage progresses to the plaque stage, in which the lesions are more indurated, edematous, and red or violet in color. The lesion eventually reaches the nodular stage and is characterized by visible masses with dominant spindle cells and inflammatory cells. These spindle cells express lymphatic-specific markers (e.g., Podoplanin and lymphatic vessel hyaluronan receptor LYVE-1) as well as participate in the signaling process during lymphangiogenesis (Skobe, et al., 1999, Weninger, et al., 1999).

4.3 Clinical features

There are four types of KS: classic type, endemic African KS, KS in organ transplant recipients, and HIV-infection/AIDS associated KS (Trattner, et al., 1993). KS is the most common neoplasm (20-50%) found in HIV-infected individuals (mostly homosexual and bisexual men) (Scully, et al., 1991).Oral lesions are evident in 40% of KS (Greenspan and Greenspan, 1990).Red or purplish macules, papules or nodules appear most frequently on the hard palate (Greenspan and Greenspan, 1990). Unless infected or ulcerated, these lesions do not blanch on pressure (Greenspan and Greenspan, 1990). Laryngeal involvement is also evident in individuals with KS (Pantanowitz and Dezube, 2006). Primary symptoms are hoarseness, throat discomfort, urge to cough, aphonia, dysphagia, stridor, and complete airway obstruction.

4.4 Treatment

The extent and bulk of the disease determines the therapeutic alternative that needs to be considered. Individuals with fewer than five cutaneous lesions are kept on watch until rapid proliferation, widespread dissemination or KS-related symptoms become more apparent. Treatment with HAART or other anti-retroviral therapies are beneficial and have shown histologic regression of existing lesions (Eng and Cockerell, 2004). HAART therapy causes inhibition of HIV replication, diminishes the HIV-1 transactivating protein Tat, ameliorates the immune response against KSHV, and shows direct anti-angiogenic activity (Cattelan, et al., 1999, Pati, et al., 2002, Sgadari, et al., 2002). Radiotherapy is indicated for lesions on the face, hands and upper extremities, obstructive lymphadenopathy, periorbital edema, lesions on soles of the feet, anorectal or genital lesions, oral lesions and ulcerating cutaneous lesions. Radiotherapy shows merits in symptomatic disease where systemic treatment is not necessary and expensive chemotherapy can be avoided (Swift, 1996). If an active opportunistic infection is observed, chemotherapeutic agents should be considered. Systemic chemotherapeutic treatment is indicated in extensive KS of oral cavity, widespread skin involvement, pedal or scrotal edema, symptomatic visceral involvement and flare induced by immune reconstitution inflammatory syndrome (Osoba, et al., 2001). Individuals may suffer from neutropenia and thrombocytopenia and hence controlled therapy should be the choice of treatment. Only nodular and symptomatic lesions of oropharynx should be treated with radiation. Recombinant and non-recombinant alpha interferons can be used for treatment of epidemic KS (De Wit, et al., 1988).

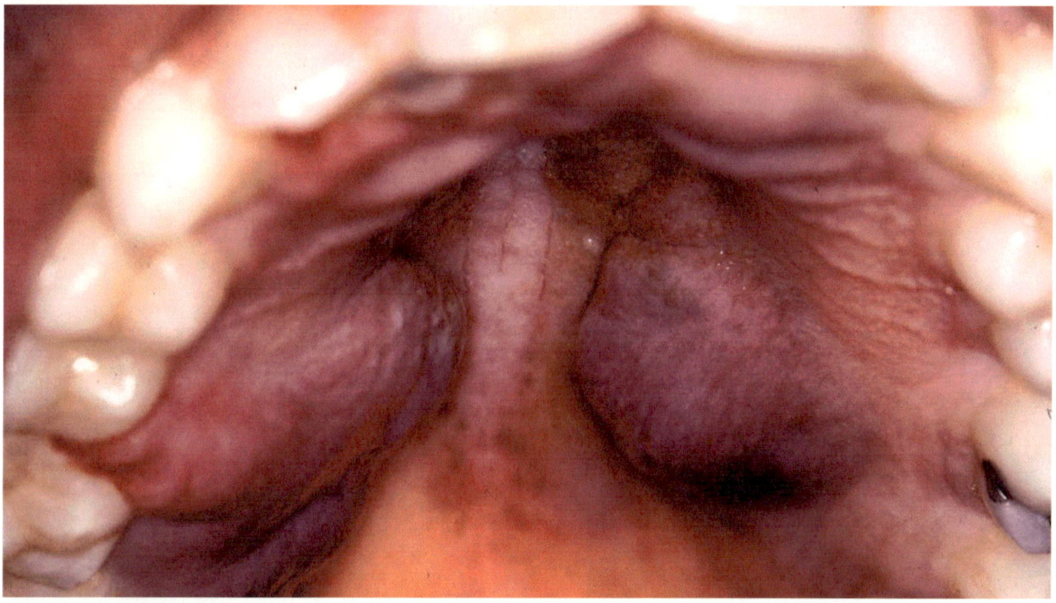

Fig. 7. Kaposi's Sarcoma

5. Human Papilloma Virus (HPV) infections

5.1 Background

HPV is the leading cause of orpharyngeal carcinomas (D'Souza, et al., Rosenquist, 2005). HPV16 is a common cause for the majority of oropharyngeal carcinomas (Kreimer, et al., 2005) . HPV-positive individuals are most frequently Caucasian and belong to high socioeconomic status (Gillison, et al., 2008). HIV-infected individuals have two to four-fold increase in risk for developing HPV-related oral cancers (Gilbert, et al.). HPV has also been considered as one of the etiologic factors for OHL (oral hairy leukoplakia) (Fejerskov, et al., 1977), as shown by identification of HPV antigens and HPV DNA (Loning, et al., 1985). HPV-induced OL shows prevalence ranged from 17% to 68.6% (Shroyer, et al., 1993, Sugiyama, et al., 2003).

5.2 Pathogenesis

HPV is mainly infectious through expression of oncogenes such as E6/E7 (Al-Bakkal, et al., 1999), which cause phosphorylation of CHK2, leading to caspase activation (Al-Bakkal, et al., 1999, Moody and Laimins, 2009, Tominaga, et al., 1999). The intrinsic apoptotic pathway of caspase activation plays an important role in HPV replication (Moody, et al., 2007). HPV proteins flourish and regulate amplification primarily by caspase activation, leading to immortalization of the suprabasal layer of epithelium, specifically the keratinocytes (Sakai, et al., 1996).

5.3 Clinical features

HPV induced oral and pharyngeal cancers are most evident in younger females (<40 years). OSCC (oral squamous cell carcinoma) normally occur on the buccal mucosa (2-10%), lip (4-40%), alveolar ridge (2-18%) retromolar trigonous (2-6%), hard palate (3-6%), floor of mouth (25%), ventral two third of tongue (50%), alveolar ridge (2-18%), floor of mouth (25%) and oropharynx (25%). Squamous cell carcinoma of the oropharynx most commonly originates in the tonsils and tongue base (the two most common sites), pharyngeal walls, and soft palate.

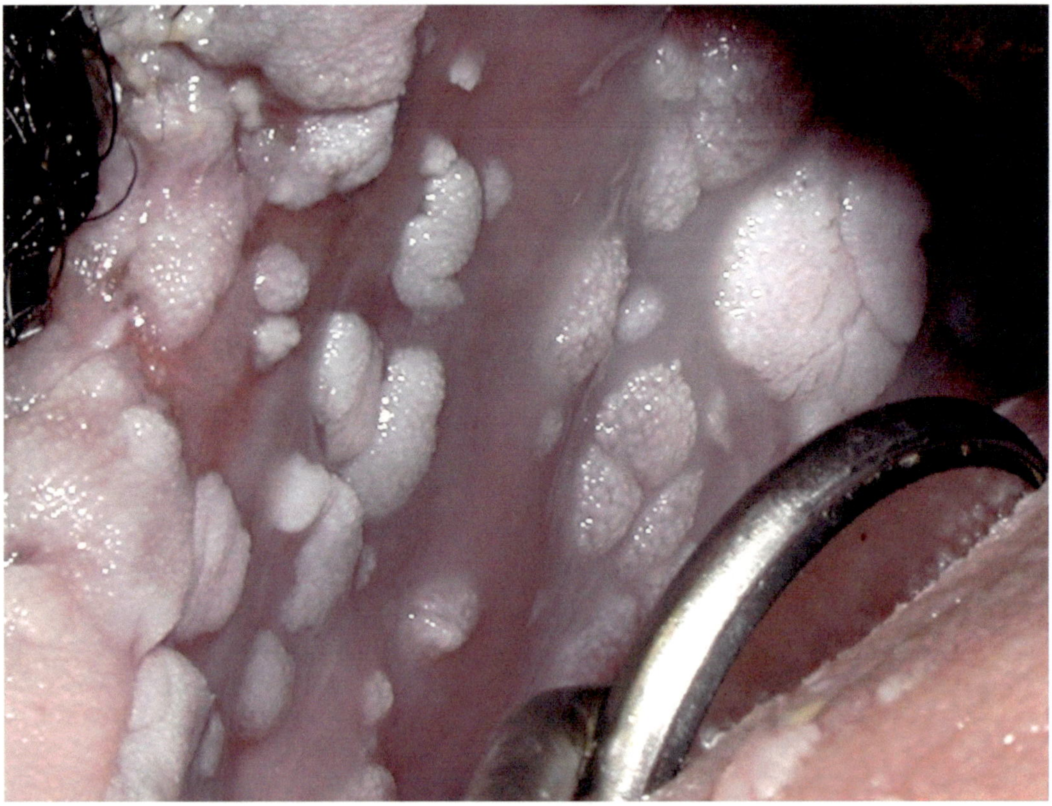

Fig. 8. Human Papilloma Virus Lesions

5.4 Treatment

Treatment of HPV infection can be achieved either by use of targeted therapy against the virus or immune-stimulating therapy. Most dysplastic tissue can be treated by ablative and excisional therapy. Use of radiochemotherapy in the form of radiation ± cisplatin or cetuximal has shown beneficial results in treatment of oropharyngeal carcinoma. The overall survival rate was 60 % in HPV-positive individuals and 73 % in HPV-negative individuals (Lill, et al.).

6. Periodontal lesions associated with HIV

6.1 Linear Gingival Erythema (LGE)

6.1.1 Background

This lesion is also known as 'red-band gingivitis' or 'HIV-associated gingivitis'. LGE is commonly seen in immune-compromised individuals and is considered to be a potential precursor for necrotizing ulcerative gingivitis (NUG)/ necrotizing ulcerative periodontitis (NUP). According to the recent classification of periodontal diseases (Armitage, 1999), LGE is classified under 'Gingival diseases of fungal origin.'

6.1.2 Pathogenesis

There is an increased number of bacteria and *Candida* species in the gingival sulcus associated with LGE. The bacteria seen include those commonly observed in periodontal disease such as *Bacteriodes gingivalis, Bacteriodes intermedius, Actinomyces viscosus, Fusobacterium nucleatum,* and *Aggregatibacter actinomycetemcomitans.*

6.1.3 Clinical features

The lesions present themselves as 2-3 mm wide red band around the marginal gingival of the teeth. These lesions are not typically painful, but bleed readily.

6.1.4 Treatmen

Typically, no treatment is needed for this condition. Although LGE is listed under 'Lesions of fungal origin', it is not typically treated with anti-fungal medications. Mechanical removal of plaque and calculus helps reduce inflammation and excessive bleeding. Chlorhexidine gluconate (0.12%) mouth rinses can be used twice daily. If the lesion persists, systemic antibiotics (metronidazole) may be prescribed to reduce the bacterial load.

6.2 Necrotizing Ulcerative Gingivitis and Periodontitis (NUG and NUP)

6.2.1 Background

NUG is a painful condition of the gingiva characterized by ulcerations, bleeding, and foul breath. It is also called Vincent's infection, Vincent's angina, or trench mouth. When the infection spreads to the alveolar bone, it is called NUP. Prevalence of NUP in HIV-infected individuals has been reported by various researchers. Its prevalence with HIV was reported in 1994 as 6% (Glick, et al., 1994). Over a period of a decade, the incidence of HIV in NUP patients increased to 69.6% (Shangase, et al., 2004). Recent reports suggest 43% of patients with NUP were HIV-seropositive (Phiri, et al.). Studies have shown that HIV-infected individuals with NUP are 20.8% more likely to have a CD4+ count lower than 200 (Glick, et al., 1994).

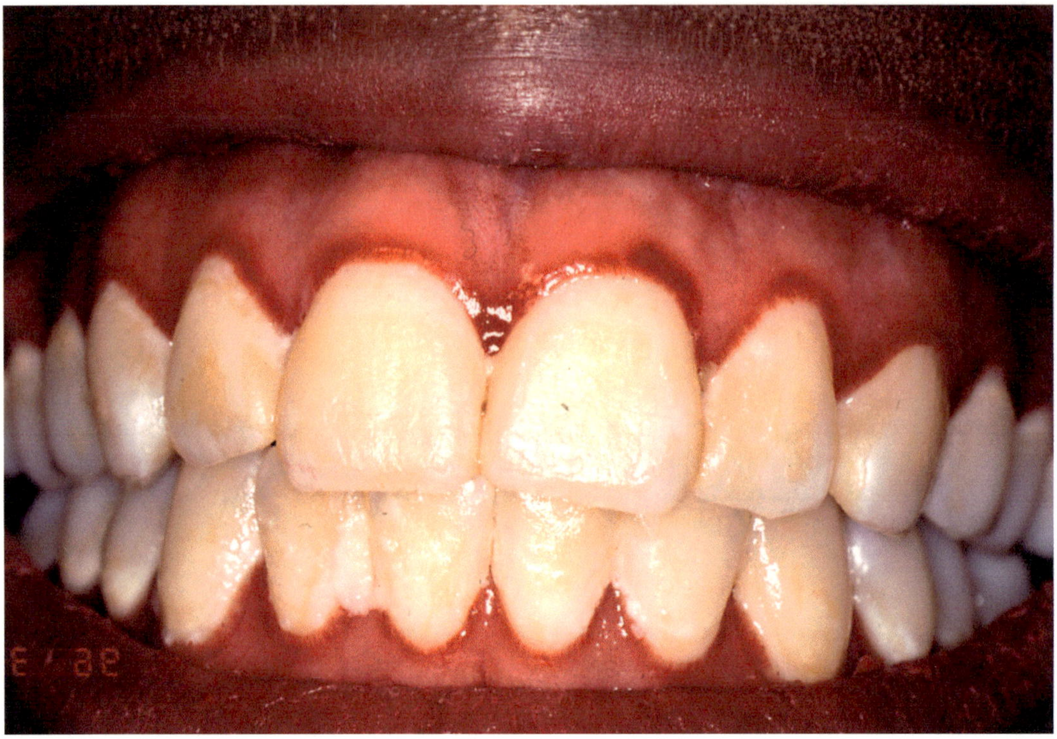

Fig. 9. Linear Gingival Erythema

6.2.2 Pathogenesis

NUP is commonly a progression of NUG that demonstrates bone loss and clinical attachment levels (MacCarthy and Claffey, 1991). Both are primarily caused by bacterial infection with microflora consisting of Treponema and Selenomonas species, *Prevotella intermedia, Fusobacterium nucleatum* and *Porphyromonas gingivalis* (Falkler, et al., 1987, Loesche, et al., 1982). Malnutrition, smoking, stress, trauma and preexisting gingivitis are other etiologic factors (Peruzzo, et al., 2007, Taiwo, 1993). Most persons with NUG have alterations in the immune system making them more prone to microbial infections (Cogen, et al., 1983). This immunosuppression is also evident in infection by HIV (Goedert, et al., 1984). *Treponema denticola* (*T. denticola*) is the principal oral helical-shaped anaerobic spirochete that plays an essential role in immunosuppression. The disease process is mediated through adherence to mucosal surfaces, specific cleavage of cell surface receptors, inhibition of host defense mechanisms, penetration in epithelial cells, and induction of gingival inflammation and bone resorption. Proteases such as chymotrypsin, phospholipase C, oligopeptidase and cystalysin play an important role in pathogenicity (Chi, et al., 2003, Ellen and Galimanas, 2005, Fenno and McBride, 1998) and is induced by a range of pro-inflammatory cytokines such as IL-1α, IL-1β, tumor necrosis factor-α, IL-6 and IL-8 (Gemmell and Seymour, 1998, Nixon, et al., 2000). These cytokines affect connective tissue destruction and alveolar bone desorption (Gemmell and Seymour, 1998). Phosphorylation of intracellular receptors such as Fos-c, MKK1, MAP kinase and nuclear factor κB molecules by *T. denticola* affect these changes (Tanabe, et al., 2008).

6.2.3 Clinical features

The clinical characteristics of NUG includes ulcerated and necrotic papillary and marginal gingival covered by a yellowish-white or grayish slough or "pseudomembrane", blunting and cratering of papillae, spontaneous bleeding or bleeding on probing, pain and fetid breath (Barnes, et al., 1973, Falkler, et al., 1987, Horning and Cohen, 1995). It may be accompanied by fever, lymphadenopathy, and malaise. Progression of gingivitis to NUP is commonly associated with clinical attachment loss and alveolar bone destruction.

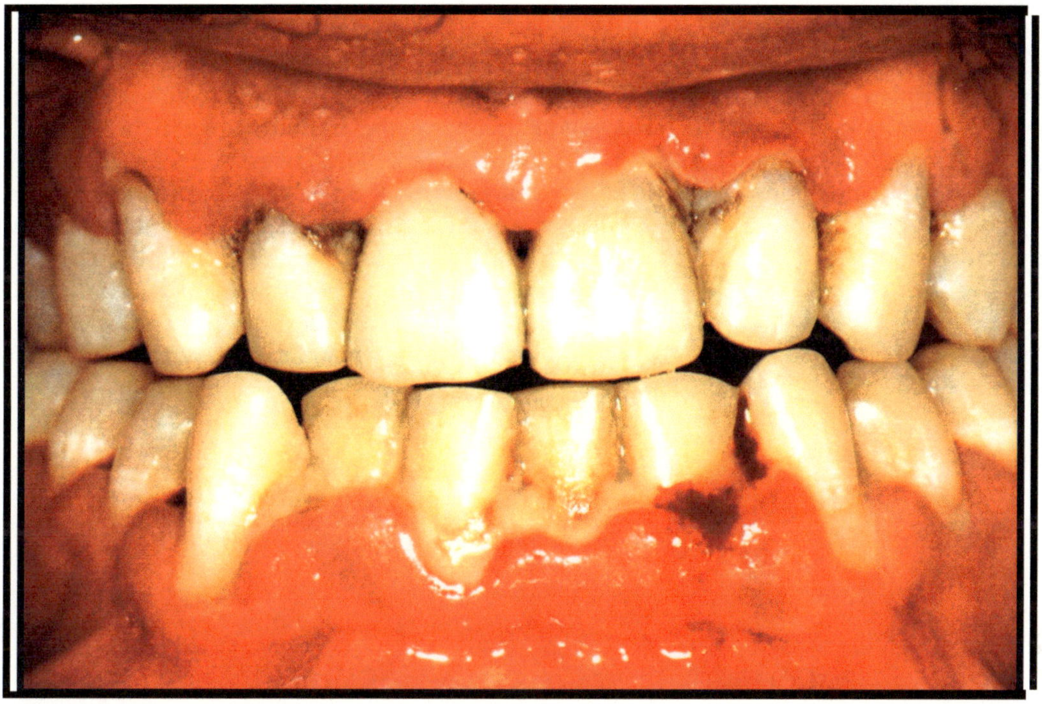

Fig. 10. Necrotizing Ulcerative Periodontitis

6.2.4 Treatment

The first treatment for NUG was devised by Dr. S. Schluger in 1949 (Schluger, 1949).Bacterial pathogens were controlled or eliminated by mechanical debridement or use of antibiotics in earlier days (Johnson and Engel, 1986). Aureomycin and penicillin were the first antibiotics considered for treatment of NUG in 1950 (Goldman and Bloom, 1950, Montis, 1950). Mechanical treatment consists of scaling and root planing. In addition to mechanical debridement, antibiotic and antimicrobial therapies are essential for management of NUP. Oxidizing mouthwash such as 3% hydrogen peroxide has also shown to have beneficial effects in management of NUG and NUP.

7. Non-Hodgkin lymphoma

7.1 Background

There are three subtypes of on-Hodgkin's lymphoma (NHL): diffuse large B cell lymphoma (DLBCL), Burkitt's lymphoma (BL) and central nervous system lymphoma (CNSL)(Engels, et al., 2006). An increase in occurrence of DLBCL (10.2%), BL (27.8%) and CNSL (48.3%) was seen in individuals with AIDS during 1990-1995 (Shiels, et al., 2011). The 5-year survival rate improved from 1960 to the mid 1970s, but not much after that in the USA (Shiels, et al., 2011). NHL relates to congenital and acquired immunodeficiency diseases (Filipovich, et al., 1992). The relative risk of NHL in individuals with AIDS is about 150-250 in Western countries and over 1000 in children (Goedert, 2000).

7.2 Pathogenesis

The head and neck regions are the most common sites for NHL, showing in 30-40% of cases (Economopoulos, et al., 1996). The neoplastic cells express CD20, CD79, BCL-2 and BCL-6, most of which are B-cell antigens (Hoefnagel, et al., 2003). The hallmark of B-cell malignancies is chromosomal translocation involving the immunoglobulin heavy chain (IGH) gene at band 14q32.33 with specific oncogene loci, referred to as the 14q32 translocation. Among these specific 14q32 translocations, *de novo* acute leukemia/lymphoma with c-MYC and/or BCL6 abnormalities in addition to t(14;18) was characterized by an extremely aggressive clinical course with nodal and/or extranodal involvement, and massive bone marrow infiltration(Kramer, et al., 1991). Incidence of IGH translocation on B-cell NHL has been reported in previous studies (Kramer, et al., 1998). Thus multiple involvement of the IGH gene in chromosomal rearrangements is associated with the pathogenesis and the progression of NHL.

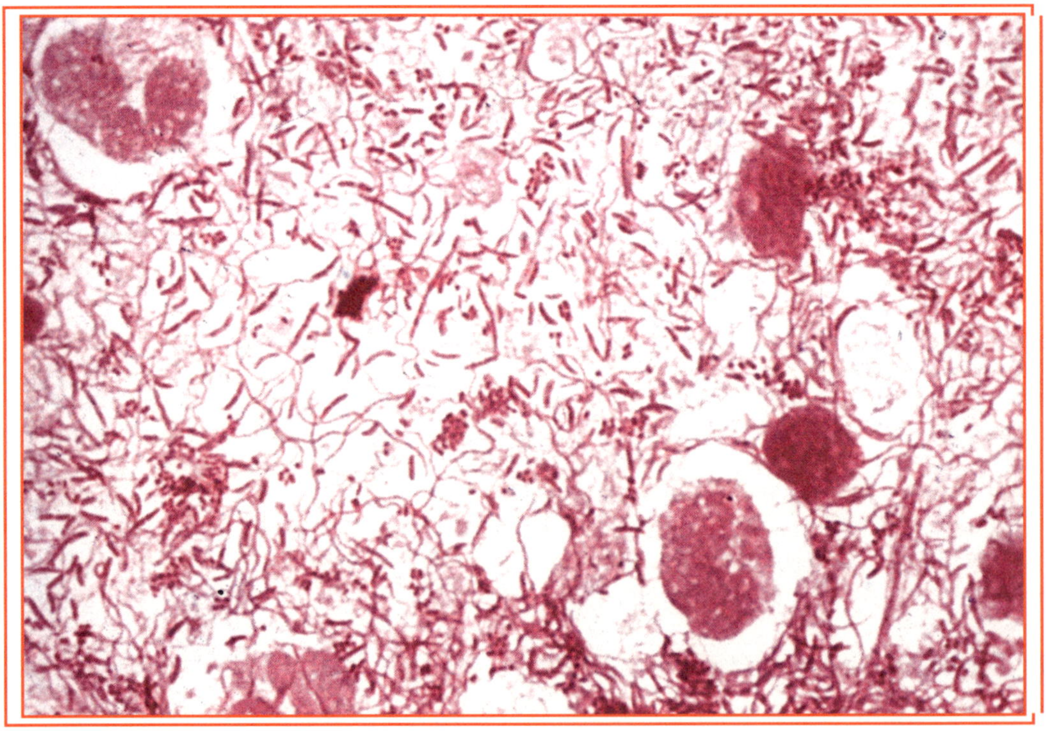

Fig. 11. Histology of NUP lesion- Infiltration of Spirochetes into the Connective Tissue

Stage I	Involvement of a single lymph node region (I) or a single extralymphatic organ or site (IE)
Stage II	Involvement of two or more lymph node regions on the same side of the diaphragm (II) alone or with localized involvement of an extralymphatic organ or site (IIE)
Stage III	Involvement of lymph node regions on both sides of the diaphragm (III) alone or with localized involvement of an extralymphatic organ or site (IIIE) or spleen (IIIS) or both (IIISE)
Stage IV	Diffuse or disseminated involvement of one or more extralymphatic organs with or without associated lymph node involvement

Table 3. Ann Arbor Classification of Non-Hodgkin's Lymphomas (Rupniewska, 1979)

7.3 Clinical features

Oral NHL lesions are often in disseminated disease states. The most common oral sites of involvement are the palate, tonsil, buccal mucosa, floor of the mouth, and the retromolar region. These lesions are non-tender, diffuse swellings usually involving the gingiva, buccal vestibule and posterior hard palate. Gnathic lesions arise from soft tissue invading the bony skeleton. One third of patients show fever, weight loss, adenopathy, night sweats, or hepatosplenomegaly. Oral lesions are fluctuant swellings showing ulceration, pain, tooth mobility and paresthesia when peripheral nerves are involved (Vega, et al., 2005). Salivary gland lymphomas account for approximately 3% of all salivary gland tumors (Barnes, et al., 1998). About 80% of the cases are reported in parotid gland, 16% in submandibular, 2% in sublingual and 2% in minor salivary glands. Affected bony areas show a "punched out" pattern that is due to multiple areas of destruction with ill defined radiolucent lesion. Involvement of the maxillary sinus will cause opacification with eroded cortical walls and associated sinus mass (Fukuda, et al., 1987). The Ann Arbor staging system, originally designed for Hodgkin's disease, is used for NHL as evident above.

7.4 Treatment

A prognostic index has been developed by the International NHL prognostic factors project based on data from 2,031 patients with aggressive lymphomas treated with regimens containing doxorubicin ("A Predictive Model for Aggressive Non-Hodgkin's Lymphoma," 1993). Analysis of 1274 patients younger than 60 years showed three clinical features independently associated with survival: serum LDL (lactate dehydrogenase) levels, tumor stage, and their performance status ("A Predictive Model for Aggressive Non-Hodgkin's Lymphoma," 1993). Past studies showed the importance of gallium-67 uptake in lymphomas as a useful prognostic indicator (Janicek, et al., 1997). The importance of prognostic index is that good-risk patients can be identified for standard therapy and poor-risk patients can be identified for new research protocols to improve the rate of therapy. With conventional therapy only 25% of patients who were gallium-positive midway through therapy had durable responses , while 70% of those who were gallium-negative remained free of disease (Janicek, et al., 1997). In patients with stage I or II disease, regional therapy leads to long-term control, with relapse rate of 44%-47% at 10 years and survival rates of 75% for patients younger than 60 years (Vaughan Hudson, et al., 1994). Stage III and IV patients can be treated by alkylating agents, combination chemotherapy regimens with 2-4 drugs, and high dose therapy with bone marrow transplant reinfusion(Freedman, et al., 1996, Govindan, et al., 2009).

8. Conclusions

Thorough examination of the oral cavity should be part of the physical examination for everybody, but especially in HIV-positive individuals and those who are at a high risk for acquiring HIV infection. Oral lesions can not only compromise the quality of life and increase morbidity in patients with HIV/AIDS, but can also serve as indicators for the presence of the disease and disease progression. It is also very important for health care providers and medical practitioners from different specialties to collaborate in providing the overall care for these immune-compromised patients.

9. References

"1993 Revised Classification System for Hiv Infection and Expanded Surveillance Case Definition for Aids among Adolescents and Adults." *MMWR Recomm Rep* 41, no. RR-17 (1992): 1-19.

Al-Bakkal, Ghasaq, Giuseppe Ficarra, Karol McNeill, Lewis R. Eversole, Gaetana Sterrantino, and Catalena Birek. "Human Papilloma Virus Type 16 E6 Gene Expression in Oral Exophytic Epithelial Lesions as Detected by in Situ Rtpcr." *Oral surgery, oral medicine, oral pathology, oral radiology, and endodontics* 87, no. 2 (1999): 197-208.

Albrecht, J. C., J. Nicholas, D. Biller, K. R. Cameron, B. Biesinger, C. Newman, S. Wittmann, M. A. Craxton, H. Coleman, and B. Fleckenstein. "Primary Structure of the Herpesvirus Saimiri Genome." *J. Virol.* 66, no. 8 (1992): 5047-58.

Armitage, G. C. "Development of a Classification System for Periodontal Diseases and Conditions." *Ann Periodontol* 4, no. 1 (1999): 1-6.

Banin, S., L. Moyal, S. Y. Shieh, Y. Taya, C. W. Anderson, L. Chessa, N. I. Smorodinsky, C. Prives, Y. Reiss, Y. Shiloh, and Y. Ziv. "Enhanced Phosphorylation of P53 by Atm in Response to DNA Damage." *Science* 281, no. 5383 (1998): 1674-77.

Barnes, G. P., W. F. Bowles, 3rd, and H. G. Carter. "Acute Necrotizing Ulcerative Gingivitis: A Survey of 218 Cases." *J Periodontol* 44, no. 1 (1973): 35-42.

Barnes, Leon, Eugene N. Myers, and Emanuel P. Prokopakis. "Primary Malignant Lymphoma of the Parotid Gland." *Arch Otolaryngol Head Neck Surg* 124, no. 5 (1998): 573-77.

Bensadoun, Rene-Jean, Jamel Daoud, Brahim El Gueddari, Laurent Bastit, Rene Gourmet, Andrzej Rosikon, Christophe Allavena, Philippe Céruse, Gilles Calais, and Pierre Attali. "Comparison of the Efficacy and Safety of Miconazole 50-Mg Mucoadhesive Buccal Tablets with Miconazole 500-Mg Gel in the Treatment of Oropharyngeal Candidiasis." *Cancer* 112, no. 1 (2008): 204-11.

Bravo, I. M., M. Correnti, L. Escalona, M. Perrone, A. Brito, V. Tovar, and H. Rivera. "Prevalence of Oral Lesions in Hiv Patients Related to Cd4 Cell Count and Viral Load in a Venezuelan Population." *Med Oral Patol Oral Cir Bucal* 11, no. 1 (2006): E33-9.

Calderone, R. A., and P. C. Braun. "Adherence and Receptor Relationships of Candida Albicans." *Microbiol. Mol. Biol. Rev.* 55, no. 1 (1991): 1-20.

Calderone, Richard A., and William A. Fonzi. "Virulence Factors of Candida Albicans." *Trends in Microbiology* 9, no. 7 (2001): 327-35.

Cattelan, A. M., M. L. Calabro, S. M. L. Aversa, M. Zanchetta, F. Meneghetti, A. De Rossi, and L. Chieco-Bianchi. "Regression of Aids-Related Kaposi's Sarcoma Following Antiretroviral Therapy with Protease Inhibitors: Biological Correlates of Clinical Outcome." *European Journal of Cancer* 35, no. 13 (1999): 1809-15.

Chaffin, W. Lajean, Jose Luis Lopez-Ribot, Manuel Casanova, Daniel Gozalbo, and Jose P. Martinez. "Cell Wall and Secreted Proteins of Candida Albicans: Identification, Function, and Expression." *Microbiol. Mol. Biol. Rev.* 62, no. 1 (1998): 130-80.

Charlier, C., E. Hart, A. Lefort, P. Ribaud, F. Dromer, D. W. Denning, and O. Lortholary. "Fluconazole for the Management of Invasive Candidiasis: Where Do We Stand after 15 Years?" *Journal of Antimicrobial Chemotherapy* 57, no. 3 (2006): 384-410.

Chi, Bo, Mingshan Qi, and Howard K. Kuramitsu. "Role of Dentilisin in Treponema Denticola Epithelial Cell Layer Penetration." *Research in Microbiology* 154, no. 9 (2003): 637-43.

"Classification and Diagnostic Criteria for Oral Lesions in Hiv Infection. Ec-Clearinghouse on Oral Problems Related to Hiv Infection and Who Collaborating Centre on Oral Manifestations of the Immunodeficiency Virus." *J Oral Pathol Med* 22, no. 7 (1993): 289-91.

Cogen, R. B., A. W. Stevens, Jr., S. Cohen-Cole, K. Kirk, and A. Freeman. "Leukocyte Function in the Etiology of Acute Necrotizing Ulcerative Gingivitis." *J Periodontol* 54, no. 7 (1983): 402-7.

Coogan, M. M., J. Greenspan, and S. J. Challacombe. "Oral Lesions in Infection with Human Immunodeficiency Virus." *Bull World Health Organ* 83, no. 9 (2005): 700-6.

D'Souza, Gypsyamber, Hao H. Zhang, Warren D. D'Souza, Robert R. Meyer, and Maura L. Gillison. "Moderate Predictive Value of Demographic and Behavioral Characteristics for a Diagnosis of Hpv16-Positive and Hpv16-Negative Head and Neck Cancer." *Oral Oncology* 46, no. 2: 100-04.

Davies, Andrew N., Susan R. Brailsford, and David Beighton. "Oral Candidosis in Patients with Advanced Cancer." *Oral Oncology* 42, no. 7 (2006): 698-702.

De Wit, Ronald, CharlesA B. Boucher, KeesH N. Veenhof, JanK M. E. Schattenkerk, PietJ M. Bakker, and SvenA Danner. "Clinical and Virological Effects of High-Dose Recombinant Interferon-? In Disseminated Aids-Related Kaposi's Sarcoma." *The Lancet* 332, no. 8622 (1988): 1214-17.

Economopoulos, Theofanis, Niki Asprou, Nicholas Stathakis, Efstathios Papageorgiou, John Dervenoulas, Katiana Xanthaki, and Sotos Raptis. "Primary Extranodal Non-Hodgkin's Lymphoma in Adults: Clinicopathological and Survival Characteristics." *Leukemia & Lymphoma* 21, no. 1-2 (1996): 131-36.

Ellen, Richard P., and Vaia B. Galimanas. "Spirochetes at the Forefront of Periodontal Infections." *Periodontology 2000* 38, no. 1 (2005): 13-32.

Eltom, Mohamed A., Ahmedin Jemal, Sam M. Mbulaiteye, Susan S. Devesa, and Robert J. Biggar. "Trends in Kaposi's Sarcoma and Non-Hodgkin's Lymphoma Incidence in the United States from 1973 through 1998." *Journal of the National Cancer Institute* 94, no. 16 (2002): 1204-10.

Eng, W., and C. J. Cockerell. "Histological Features of Kaposi Sarcoma in a Patient Receiving Highly Active Antiviral Therapy." *Am J Dermatopathol* 26, no. 2 (2004): 127-32.

Engels, E. A., R. M. Pfeiffer, J. J. Goedert, P. Virgo, T. S. McNeel, S. M. Scoppa, and R. J. Biggar. "Trends in Cancer Risk among People with Aids in the United States 1980-2002." *AIDS* 20, no. 12 (2006): 1645-54.

Falkler, W. A., Jr., S. A. Martin, J. W. Vincent, B. D. Tall, R. K. Nauman, and J. B. Suzuki. "A Clinical, Demographic and Microbiologic Study of Anug Patients in an Urban Dental School." *J Clin Periodontol* 14, no. 6 (1987): 307-14.

Fejerskov, O., B. Roed-Petersen, and J. J. Pindborg. "Clinical, Histological and Ultrastructural Features of a Possibly Virus-Induced Oral Leukoplakia." *Acta Pathol Microbiol Scand A* 85, no. 6 (1977): 897-906.

Fenno, J. Christopher, and Barry C. McBride. "Virulence Factors of Oral Treponemes." *Anaerobe* 4, no. 1 (1998): 1-17.

Filipovich, A. H., A. Mathur, D. Kamat, and R. S. Shapiro. "Primary Immunodeficiencies: Genetic Risk Factors for Lymphoma." *Cancer Research* 52, no. 19 Supplement (1992): 5465s-67s.

Freedman, A. S., J. G. Gribben, D. Neuberg, P. Mauch, R. J. Soiffer, K. C. Anderson, L. Pandite, M. J. Robertson, M. Kroon, J. Ritz, and L. M. Nadler. "High-Dose Therapy and Autologous Bone Marrow Transplantation in Patients with Follicular Lymphoma During First Remission." *Blood* 88, no. 7 (1996): 2780-86.

Fukuda, Y., T. Ishida, M. Fujimoto, T. Ueda, and K. Aozasa. "Malignant Lymphoma of the Oral Cavity: Clinicopathologic Analysis of 20 Cases." *J Oral Pathol* 16, no. 1 (1987): 8-12.

Gemmell, E., and G. J. Seymour. "Cytokine Profiles of Cells Extracted from Humans with Periodontal Diseases." *Journal of Dental Research* 77, no. 1 (1998): 16-26.

Gilbert, P. A., N. T. Brewer, and P. L. Reiter. "Association of Human Papillomavirus-Related Knowledge, Attitudes, and Beliefs with Hiv Status: A National Study of Gay Men." *J Low Genit Tract Dis* 15, no. 2: 83-8.

Gillison, Maura L., Gypsyamber D'Souza, William Westra, Elizabeth Sugar, Weihong Xiao, Shahnaz Begum, and Raphael Viscidi. "Distinct Risk Factor Profiles for Human Papillomavirus Type 16â€"Positive and Human Papillomavirus Type 16â€"Negative Head and Neck Cancers." *Journal of the National Cancer Institute* 100, no. 6 (2008): 407-20.

Glick, M., B. C. Muzyka, L. M. Salkin, and D. Lurie. "Necrotizing Ulcerative Periodontitis: A Marker for Immune Deterioration and a Predictor for the Diagnosis of Aids." *J Periodontol* 65, no. 5 (1994): 393-7.

Goedert, J. J. "The Epidemiology of Acquired Immunodeficiency Syndrome Malignancies." *Semin Oncol* 27, no. 4 (2000): 390-401.

Goedert, J. J., M. G. Sarngadharan, R. J. Biggar, S. H. Weiss, D. M. Winn, R. J. Grossman, M. H. Greene, A. J. Bodner, D. L. Mann, D. M. Strong, and et al. "Determinants of

Retrovirus (Htlv-Iii) Antibody and Immunodeficiency Conditions in Homosexual Men." *Lancet* 2, no. 8405 (1984): 711-6.

Goldman, H. M., and J. Bloom. "Topical Application of Aureomycin for the Treatment of the Acute Phase of Ulcerative Necrotizing Gingivitis (Vincent's Infection)." *Oral Surg Oral Med Oral Pathol* 3, no. 9 (1950): 1148-50.

Gottlieb, Michael S., Robert Schroff, Howard M. Schanker, Joel D. Weisman, Peng Thim Fan, Robert A. Wolf, and Andrew Saxon. "Pneumocystis Carinii Pneumonia and Mucosal Candidiasis in Previously Healthy Homosexual Men." *New England Journal of Medicine* 305, no. 24 (1981): 1425-31.

Govindan, Ramaswamy, Inc Ovid Technologies, Books@Ovid, and Collection Electronic Books. *Devita, Hellman, and Rosenberg's Cancer Principles & Practice of Oncology Review* Lippincott William & Wilkins, 2009 [cited.

Gowdey, G., R. K. Lee, and W. M. Carpenter. "Treatment of Hiv-Related Hairy Leukoplakia with Podophyllum Resin 25% Solution." *Oral Surg Oral Med Oral Pathol Oral Radiol Endod* 79, no. 1 (1995): 64-7.

Greenspan, D., and J. S. Greenspan. "Oral Lesions of Hiv Infections: Features and Therapy." *AIDS Clin Rev* (1990): 81-93.

Hann, I. M., R. Corringham, M. Keaney, P. Noone, J. Fox, M. Szawatkowski, H. G. Prentice, H. A. Blacklock, M. Shannon, E. Gascoigne, E. Boesen, and A. V. Hoffbrand. "Ketoconazole Versus Nystatin Plus Amphotericin B for Fungal Prophylaxis in Severely Immunocompromised Patients." *The Lancet* 319, no. 8276 (1982): 826-29.

Hoefnagel, J. J., M. H. Vermeer, P. M. Jansen, G. J. Fleuren, C. J. L. M. Meijer, and R. Willemze. "Bcl-2, Bcl-6 and Cd10 Expression in Cutaneous B-Cell Lymphoma: Further Support for a Follicle Centre Cell Origin and Differential Diagnostic Significance." *British Journal of Dermatology* 149, no. 6 (2003): 1183-91.

Horning, G. M., and M. E. Cohen. "Necrotizing Ulcerative Gingivitis, Periodontitis, and Stomatitis: Clinical Staging and Predisposing Factors." *J Periodontol* 66, no. 11 (1995): 990-8.

Hostetter, M. K. "Adhesins and Ligands Involved in the Interaction of Candida Spp. With Epithelial and Endothelial Surfaces." *Clin. Microbiol. Rev.* 7, no. 1 (1994): 29-42.

"Human Papillomaviruses." *IARC Monogr Eval Carcinog Risks Hum* 90 (2007): 1-636.

Janicek, M., W. Kaplan, D. Neuberg, G. P. Canellos, L. N. Shulman, and M. A. Shipp. "Early Restaging Gallium Scans Predict Outcome in Poor-Prognosis Patients with Aggressive Non-Hodgkin's Lymphoma Treated with High-Dose Chop Chemotherapy." *Journal of Clinical Oncology* 15, no. 4 (1997): 1631-37.

Johnson, B. D., and D. Engel. "Acute Necrotizing Ulcerative Gingivitis. A Review of Diagnosis, Etiology and Treatment." *J Periodontol* 57, no. 3 (1986): 141-50.

Kramer, M. H. H., J. Hermans, E. Wijburg, K. Philippo, E. Geelen, J. H. J. M. van Krieken, D. de Jong, E. Maartense, E. Schuuring, and P. M. Kluin. "Clinical Relevance of Bcl2, Bcl6, and Myc Rearrangements in Diffuse Large B-Cell Lymphoma." *Blood* 92, no. 9 (1998): 3152-62.

Kramer, M. H., S. Raghoebier, G. C. Beverstock, D. de Jong, P. M. Kluin, and J. C. Kluin-Nelemans. "De Novo Acute B-Cell Leukemia with Translocation T(14;18): An Entity with a Poor Prognosis." *Leukemia* 5, no. 6 (1991): 473-8.

Kreimer, Aimee R., Gary M. Clifford, Peter Boyle, and Silvia Franceschi. "Human Papillomavirus Types in Head and Neck Squamous Cell Carcinomas Worldwide: A Systematic Review." *Cancer Epidemiology Biomarkers & Prevention* 14, no. 2 (2005): 467-75.

Lill, Claudia, Gabriela Kornek, Barbara Bachtiary, Edgar Selzer, Christian Schopper, Martina Mittlboeck, Martin Burian, Friedrich Wrba, and Dietmar Thurnher. "Survival of Patients with Hpv-Positive Oropharyngeal Cancer after Radiochemotherapy Is Significantly Enhanced." *Wiener Klinische Wochenschrift.*

Loesche, W. J., S. A. Syed, B. E. Laughon, and J. Stoll. "The Bacteriology of Acute Necrotizing Ulcerative Gingivitis." *J Periodontol* 53, no. 4 (1982): 223-30.

Loning, Thomas, Hans Ikenberg, Jurgen Becker, Lutz Gissmann, Ilsetraut Hoepfer, and Harald zur Hausen. "Analysis of Oral Papillomas, Leukoplakias, and Invasive Carcinomas for Human Papillomavirus Type Related DNA." *J Investig Dermatol* 84, no. 5 (1985): 417-20.

MacCarthy, D., and N. Claffey. "Acute Necrotizing Ulcerative Gingivitis Is Associated with Attachment Loss." *J Clin Periodontol* 18, no. 10 (1991): 776-9.

Montis. "[Treatment of Vincent's Angina with Penicillin]." *Medicina (Madr)* 18, no. 5 (1950): 376-8.

Moody, Cary A., Amelie Fradet-Turcotte, Jacques Archambault, and Laimonis A. Laimins. "Human Papillomaviruses Activate Caspases Upon Epithelial Differentiation to Induce Viral Genome Amplification." *Proceedings of the National Academy of Sciences* 104, no. 49 (2007): 19541-46.

Moody, Cary A., and Laimonis A. Laimins. "Human Papillomaviruses Activate the Atm DNA Damage Pathway for Viral Genome Amplification Upon Differentiation." *PLoS Pathog* 5, no. 10 (2009): e1000605.

Moore, Patrick S., and Yuan Chang. "Molecular Virology of Kaposi's Sarcoma "Associated Herpesvirus." *Philosophical Transactions of the Royal Society of London. Series B: Biological Sciences* 356, no. 1408 (2001): 499-516.

Nairy, Harish, Charyulu Narayana, Veena Shetty, and Prabhu Prabhakara. "A Pseudo-Randomised Clinical Trial of in Situ Gels of Fluconazole for the Treatment of Oropharngeal Candidiasis." *Trials* 12, no. 1: 99.

Nixon, C. S., M. J. Steffen, and J. L. Ebersole. "Cytokine Responses to Treponema Pectinovorum and Treponema Denticola in Human Gingival Fibroblasts." *Infect Immun* 68, no. 9 (2000): 5284-92.

Ollert, M. W., E. Wadsworth, and R. A. Calderone. "Reduced Expression of the Functionally Active Complement Receptor for Ic3b but Not for C3d on an Avirulent Mutant of Candida Albicans." *Infect. Immun.* 58, no. 4 (1990): 909-13.

Osoba, David, Donald W. Northfelt, David W. Budd, and David Himmelberger. "Effect of Treatment on Health-Related Quality of Life in Acquired Immunodeficiency Syndrome (Aids)-Related Kaposi's Sarcoma: A Randomized Trial of Pegylated-

Liposomal Doxorubicin Versus Doxorubicin, Bleomycin, and Vincristine." *Cancer Investigation* 19, no. 6 (2001): 573-80.

Owens, Norma J., Charles H. Nightingale, Robert T. Schweizer, Peter K. Schauer, Paul T. Dekker, and Richard Quintiliani. "Prophylaxis of Oral Candidiasis with Clotrimazole Troches." *Arch Intern Med* 144, no. 2 (1984): 290-93.

Palmblad, J., B. LÖNnqvist, B. Carlsson, G. Grimfors, M. JÄRnmark, R. Lerner, P. Ljungman, C. NystrÖM-Rosander, B. Petrini, and G. ÖBerg. "Oral Ketoconazole Prophylaxis for Candida Infections During Induction Therapy for Acute Leukaemia in Adults: More Bacteraemias." *Journal of Internal Medicine* 231, no. 4 (1992): 363-70.

Palmer, G. D., P. G. Robinson, S. J. Challacombe, W. Birnbaum, D. Croser, P. L. Erridge, T. Hodgson, D. Lewis, A. McLaren, and J. M. Zakrzewska. "Aetiological Factors for Oral Manifestations of Hiv." *Oral Dis* 2, no. 3 (1996): 193-7.

Pantanowitz, L., and B. J. Dezube. "Kaposi Sarcoma of the Larynx." *AIDS Read* 16, no. 4 (2006): 194-5.

Pati, Shibani, Colleen B. Pelser, Joseph Dufraine, Joseph L. Bryant, Marvin S. Reitz, and Frank F. Weichold. "Antitumorigenic Effects of Hiv Protease Inhibitor Ritonavir: Inhibition of Kaposi Sarcoma." *Blood* 99, no. 10 (2002): 3771-79.

Patton, L. L., J. A. Phelan, F. J. Ramos-Gomez, W. Nittayananta, C. H. Shiboski, and T. L. Mbuguye. "Prevalence and Classification of Hiv-Associated Oral Lesions." *Oral Dis* 8 Suppl 2 (2002): 98-109.

Peruzzo, Daiane C., Bruno B. Benatti, Glaucia M. B. Ambrosano, GetÃºlio R. Nogueira-Filho, Enilson A. Sallum, MÃ¡rcio Z. Casati, and Francisco H. Nociti. "A Systematic Review of Stress and Psychological Factors as Possible Risk Factors for Periodontal Disease." *Journal of Periodontology* 78, no. 8 (2007): 1491-504.

Philpott-Howard, J. N., J. J. Wade, G. J. Mufti, K. W. Brammer, G. Ehniniger, and Group Multicentre Study. "Randomized Comparison of Oral Fluconazole Versus Oral Polyenes for the Prevention of Fungal Infection in Patients at Risk of Neutropenia." *Journal of Antimicrobial Chemotherapy* 31, no. 6 (1993): 973-84.

Phiri, R., L. Feller, and E. Blignaut. "The Severity, Extent and Recurrence of Necrotizing Periodontal Disease in Relation to Hiv Status and Cd4+ T Cell Count." *J Int Acad Periodontol* 12, no. 4: 98-103.

"A Predictive Model for Aggressive Non-Hodgkin's Lymphoma." *New England Journal of Medicine* 329, no. 14 (1993): 987-94.

Resnick, L., J. S. Herbst, D. V. Ablashi, S. Atherton, B. Frank, L. Rosen, and S. N. Horwitz. "Regression of Oral Hairy Leukoplakia after Orally Administered Acyclovir Therapy." *JAMA* 259, no. 3 (1988): 384-8.

Rosenquist, K. "Risk Factors in Oral and Oropharyngeal Squamous Cell Carcinoma: A Population-Based Case-Control Study in Southern Sweden." *Swed Dent J Suppl*, no. 179 (2005): 1-66.

Rozenberg-Arska, M., A. W. Dekker, J. Branger, and J. Verhoef. "A Randomized Study to Compare Oral Fluconazole to Amphotericin B in the Prevention of Fungal Infections in Patients with Acute Leukaemia." *Journal of Antimicrobial Chemotherapy* 27, no. 3 (1991): 369-76.

Rupniewska, Z. M. "[Role of the Ann Arbor Classification in the Staging of Non-Hodgkin's Lymphomas]." *Pol Arch Med Wewn* 61, no. 4 (1979): 317-21.

Sakai, H., T. Yasugi, J. D. Benson, J. J. Dowhanick, and P. M. Howley. "Targeted Mutagenesis of the Human Papillomavirus Type 16 E2 Transactivation Domain Reveals Separable Transcriptional Activation and DNA Replication Functions." *J. Virol.* 70, no. 3 (1996): 1602-11.

Samaranayake, L. P., P. L. Fidel, J. R. Naglik, S. P. Sweet, R. Teanpaisan, M. M. Coogan, E. Blignaut, and P. Wanzala. "Fungal Infections Associated with Hiv Infection." *Oral Dis* 8 Suppl 2 (2002): 151-60.

Schluger, S. "Necrotizing Ulcerative Gingivitis in the Army; Incidence, Communicability and Treatment." *J Am Dent Assoc* 38, no. 2 (1949): 174-83.

Schmidt-Westhausen, A., R. A. Schiller, H. D. Pohle, and P. A. Reichart. "Oral Candida and Enterobacteriaceae in Hiv-1 Infection: Correlation with Clinical Candidiasis and Antimycotic Therapy." *J Oral Pathol Med* 20, no. 10 (1991): 467-72.

Schofer, H., F. R. Ochsendorf, E. B. Helm, and R. Milbradt. "Treatment of Oral 'Hairy' Leukoplakia in Aids Patients with Vitamin a Acid (Topically) or Acyclovir (Systemically)." *Dermatologica* 174, no. 3 (1987): 150-1.

Scully, C., G. Laskaris, J. Pindborg, S. R. Porter, and P. Reichart. "Oral Manifestations of Hiv Infection and Their Management. I. More Common Lesions." *Oral Surg Oral Med Oral Pathol* 71, no. 2 (1991): 158-66.

Sgadari, Cecilia, Giovanni Barillari, Elena Toschi, Davide Carlei, Ilaria Bacigalupo, Sara Baccarini, Clelia Palladino, Patrizia Leone, Roberto Bugarini, Laura Malavasi, Aurelio Cafaro, Mario Falchi, Donatella Valdembri, Giovanni Rezza, Federico Bussolino, Paolo Monini, and Barbara Ensoli. "Hiv Protease Inhibitors Are Potent Anti-Angiogenic Molecules and Promote Regression of Kaposi Sarcoma." *Nat Med* 8, no. 3 (2002): 225-32.

Shangase, L., L. Feller, and E. Blignaut. "Necrotising Ulcerative Gingivitis/Periodontitis as Indicators of Hiv-Infection." *SADJ* 59, no. 3 (2004): 105-8.

Shiels, M. S., S. R. Cole, S. Wegner, H. Armenian, J. S. Chmiel, A. Ganesan, V. C. Marconi, O. Martinez-Maza, J. Martinson, A. Weintrob, L. P. Jacobson, and N. F. Crum-Cianflone. "Effect of Haart on Incident Cancer and Noncancer Aids Events among Male Hiv Seroconverters." *J Acquir Immune Defic Syndr* 48, no. 4 (2008): 485-90.

Shiels, Meredith S., Ruth M. Pfeiffer, H. Irene Hall, Jianmin Li, James J. Goedert, Lindsay M. Morton, Patricia Hartge, and Eric A. Engels. "Proportions of Kaposi Sarcoma, Selected Non-Hodgkin Lymphomas, and Cervical Cancer in the United States Occurring in Persons with Aids, 1980-2007." *JAMA: The Journal of the American Medical Association* 305, no. 14 (2011): 1450-59.

Shroyer, K. R., G. S. Lovelace, M. L. Abarca, R. H. Fennell, M. E. Corkill, W. D. Woodard, and G. H. Davilla. "Detection of Human Papillomavirus DNA by in Situ Hybridization and Polymerase Chain Reaction in Human Papillomavirus Equivocal and Dysplastic Cervical Biopsies." *Hum Pathol* 24, no. 9 (1993): 1012-6.

Skobe, M., L. F. Brown, K. Tognazzi, R. K. Ganju, B. J. Dezube, K. Alitalo, and M. Detmar. "Vascular Endothelial Growth Factor-C (Vegf-C) and Its Receptors Kdr and Flt-4 Are Expressed in Aids-Associated Kaposi's Sarcoma." *J Invest Dermatol* 113, no. 6 (1999): 1047-53.

Sugiyama, Masaru, Ujjal Kumar Bhawal, Tamiko Dohmen, Shigehiro Ono, Miwa Miyauchi, and Takenori Ishikawa. "Detection of Human Papillomavirus-16 and Hpv-18 DNA in Normal, Dysplastic, and Malignant Oral Epithelium." *Oral Surgery, Oral Medicine, Oral Pathology, Oral Radiology & Endodontics* 95, no. 5 (2003): 594-600.

Swift, Patrick S. "The Role of Radiation Therapy in the Management of Hiv-Related Kaposi's Sarcoma." *Hematology/Oncology Clinics of North America* 10, no. 5 (1996): 1069-80.

Taiwo, J. O. "Oral Hygiene Status and Necrotizing Ulcerative Gingivitis in Nigerian Children." *J Periodontol* 64, no. 11 (1993): 1071-4.

Tanabe, Shin-ichi, Charles Bodet, and Daniel Grenier. "Treponema Denticola Lipooligosaccharide Activates Gingival Fibroblasts and Upregulates Inflammatory Mediator Production." *Journal of Cellular Physiology* 216, no. 3 (2008): 727-31.

Tominaga, Kaoru, Hirobumi Morisaki, Yoko Kaneko, Atsushi Fujimoto, Takashi Tanaka, Motoaki Ohtsubo, Momoki Hirai, Hiroto Okayama, Kyoji Ikeda, and Makoto Nakanishi. "Role of Human Cds1 (Chk2) Kinase in DNA Damage Checkpoint and Its Regulation by P53." *Journal of Biological Chemistry* 274, no. 44 (1999): 31463-67.

Trattner, A., E. Hodak, M. David, and M. Sandbank. "The Appearance of Kaposi Sarcoma During Corticosteroid Therapy." *Cancer* 72, no. 5 (1993): 1779-83.

Tukutuku, K., L. Muyembe-Tamfum, K. Kayembe, W. Odio, K. Kandi, and M. Ntumba. "Oral Manifestations of Aids in a Heterosexual Population in a Zaire Hospital." *J Oral Pathol Med* 19, no. 5 (1990): 232-4.

Vaughan Hudson, B., G. Vaughan Hudson, K. A. MacLennan, L. Anderson, and D. C. Linch. "Clinical Stage 1 Non-Hodgkin's Lymphoma: Long-Term Follow-up of Patients Treated by the British National Lymphoma Investigation with Radiotherapy Alone as Initial Therapy." *Br J Cancer* 69, no. 6 (1994): 1088-93.

Vega, Francisco, Pei Lin, and L. Jeffrey Medeiros. "Extranodal Lymphomas of the Head and Neck." *Annals of Diagnostic Pathology* 9, no. 6 (2005): 340-50.

Vogler, W. R., L. G. Malcom, and E. F. Winton. "A Randomized Trial Comparing Ketoconazole and Nystatin Prophylactic Therapy in Neutropenic Patients." *Cancer Invest* 5, no. 4 (1987): 267-73.

Weninger, W., T. A. Partanen, S. Breiteneder-Geleff, C. Mayer, H. Kowalski, M. Mildner, J. Pammer, M. Sturzl, D. Kerjaschki, K. Alitalo, and E. Tschachler. "Expression of Vascular Endothelial Growth Factor Receptor-3 and Podoplanin Suggests a Lymphatic Endothelial Cell Origin of Kaposi's Sarcoma Tumor Cells." *Lab Invest* 79, no. 2 (1999): 243-51.

Williams, C., J. M. Whitehouse, T. A. Lister, and P. F. Wrigley. "Oral Anticandidal Prophylaxis in Patients Undergoing Chemotherapy for Acut- Leukemia." *Med Pediatr Oncol* 3, no. 3 (1977): 275-80.

Worthington, H. V., J. E. Clarkson, and O. B. Eden. "Interventions for Preventing Oral Candidiasis for Patients with Cancer Receiving Treatment." *Cochrane Database Syst Rev*, no. 3 (2002): CD003807.

6

Epidemiology and Treatment of Kaposi's Sarcoma in HIV-1 Infected Individuals in a Poor Resource Setting

Ahmed A.[1] and Muktar H.M.[2]
[1]*Departments of Surgery, HIV Control Programme Ahmadu Bello University Teaching Hospital Zaria*
[2]*Haematology and Blood Transfusion, HIV Control Programme Ahmadu Bello University Teaching Hospital Zaria*
Nigeria

1. Introduction

Kaposi's sarcoma was first described in 1872 by Moritz Kaposi, a Vienna-based Hungarian dermatologist, as a rare multifocal angioproliferative tumour involving blood and lymphatic vessels in elderly men of Jewish origin (Kaposi, 1872). Before the AIDS epidemic three clinico-epidemiological forms with similar histological features have been described. The classic Kaposi's sarcoma (KS) originally described by Kaposi is primarily a skin disease with a chronic indolent course that can sometimes regress spontaneously (Kaposi, 1872). Most of the cases occurred in elderly men of Mediterranean and Jewish origin. The African-endemic KS is seen in the indigenous population of sub-Saharan Africa (Franceschi & Geddes, 1995). It is also seen more commonly among male patients, but differs from the classic form in that it may affect a younger population and is more likely to spread to visceral organs and lymphatics. In addition, it has a variable clinical presentation ranging from a benign disease with few skin lesions to a widely disseminated disease associated with high morbidity and mortality (Franceschi & Geddes, 1995; Taylor et al 1971). Kaposi's sarcoma seen in patients as a result of immunosuppression complicating organ transplantation may have chronic or progressive course and spontaneous remission after discontinuation of immunosuppressive therapy is observed in the majority of patients (Penn, 1979).

The first description of AIDS-associated Kaposi's sarcoma (AAKS) was in 1981, when Friedman-Kien et al (1981) reported some previously healthy young homosexual men with Kaposi's sarcoma involving lymph nodes, viscera, and mucosa as well as skin. This was associated with life-threatening opportunistic infections and a profound defect in cell-mediated immunity. This aggressive and frequently fatal form of Kaposi's sarcoma is the most common cancer in patients with HIV infection (Schwartz, 2004). Before the discovery and widespread use of highly active antiretroviral therapy (HAART) KS was over 20,000 times more common in AIDS patients than the general population (Engels et al 2006). However, several studies showed that HAART reduced the incidence of KS in high income countries (.Franceschi et al, 2008; Pipkin et al, 2011; Simard et al, 2011). The cumulative incidence of Kaposi sarcoma declined from 14.3% during 1980 to 1989, to 6.7% during 1990 to 1995, and to 1.8% during 1996 to 2006 (Simard et al, 2011). In a Swiss HIV cohort study, the overall KS incidence was 33.3 per 1000 person year (py) in 1984–1986 and did not change significantly in the subsequent periods until 1996–1998, when it fell to 5.1 (95% CI, 3.9–6.5) . The incidence further decreased to 1.4 per 1000 py in 1999–2001 and remained constant thereafter (Franceschi et al, 2008). In another recent pan-European multi-centre study, there was a decrease in the incidence rate of KS from 24.7 cases (95% CI 17.2–32.2) per 1000 py in 1994 to 4.7 (95% CI 2.7–6.7) per 1000 py in 1997 and 1.7 (95% CI 0.7–3.4) per 1000 in recent years among HIV-infected individuals (Pipkin et al, 2011). In a report from Sao Paulo Brazil, a low income country, 17% of a cohort of patients on HAART was seropositive for human herpesvirus-8 of which only 2% developed AAKS in 5 years compared to 20% prevalence of AAKS detected in the same region before the HAART era (Yoshioka et al, 2004). In contrast, the incidence of KS has been steadily increasing in parallel with the AIDS epidemic in sub-Saharan Africa (Bassett et al, 1995; Parkin et al, 2008; Sasco et al, 2010). In 2002, of 66,200 estimated KS cases worldwide, 58,800 ware estimated to be in Africa (Parkin et al, 2008). Of these, about 39,500 cases in males and 17,100 cases in females occurred in sub-Saharan Africa compared to 102 males and 17 females in Northern Africa (Parkin et al, 2008). In areas such as Malawi, Uganda and Zimbabwe where Kaposi's sarcoma was common before the AIDS epidemic, the incidence of this cancer has increased by about 20-times and it is now the most common cancer in males and second most common cancer in females (Sasco et al, 2010). In Zimbabwe, the age-adjusted incidence of KS per 100,000 population was 2.3 in men and 0.3 in women before the AIDS epidemic, compared to 48 and 18, respectively, during the AIDS epidemic (Bassett et al, 1995). Recent studies conducted in South Africa and Rwanda found a clear association between HIV infection and KS with odd ratio ranging from 21.9 (95% CI 12.5–38.6) to 47.1 (95% CI 31.9–69.8) (Newton et al, 1995; Stein et al, 2008). Similarly, Newton et al (2001)in a study carried out in Kampala, Uganda found a higher risk of KS among HIV- infected compared to HIV-negative children with an odd ratio of 94.9 (95% CI 28.5–315.3).

Although the course of AAKS is variable most patients would eventually develop progressive and disseminated disease requiring active therapy. The choice of treatment is determined by the stage of KS, its rate of progression, the degree of immune competence and HIV associated diseases. Several therapeutic options are available for AAKS but the optimal therapy is still unclear. Highly active antiretroviral therapy including protease inhibitors may be the first treatment step for indolent slowly progressive disease (Martellotta et al, 2009). Following treatment with HAART, there may be complete remission in patients with good immunological response and limited disease (Martellotta et al, 2009). However, recent studies indicate that there is no significant regression when patients with advanced, symptomatic AAKS are treated with HAART without simultaneous chemotherapy (Krown, 2004; Martin-Carbonero 2004). A wide variety of chemotherapeutic agents, individually and in combination, have been evaluated for the treatment of AAKS. In high income countries, combination of vincristine, doxorubicin and bleomycin (VAB) that was considered the standard chemotherapy regimen for AAKS has been supplanted by liposomal anthracylines due to their higher efficacy and reduced toxicity (Ashish et al 2007; Cooley, 2007). In addition, the angiogenic nature of KS makes it particularly suitable for therapies based on targeted agents such as metalloproteinase inhibitors, angiogenesis inhibitors and tyrosine kinase inhibitors (Koon et al, 2011; Sullivan et al, 2009). In low income countries, the choice of therapeutic agents is limited to the combination of VAB or even more toxic drugs such as therlidomide because liposomal anthracyclines are not available or affordable (Makombe et al, 2009).

1.1 Aetiology and pathogenesis

For a long time, the aetiology and pathogenesis of KS remained unclear. The discovery in 1994 of KS-associated herpes virus (KSHV), also known as human herpes virus-8 (HHV-8), in cells isolated from an AAKS lesion was followed by molecular and epidemiological data confirming an aetiological link between this virus and all clinical forms of KS (Chang et al, 1994; Hengge et al, 2002). Though infection with HHV-8 is not sufficient for tumour development, the virus has developed various mechanisms to manipulate host cell signal transduction, and thereby lead to the activation of numerous pro-growth and anti-apoptotic pathways. HIV-1 transactivation (Tat) protein is a short-term growth factor for KS (Guadalupe et al, 2011; Hassman et al, 2011). Tat protein through the mediation of IFN-γ, b-FGF and other cytokines has the capacity to induce endothelial cell proliferation and facilitate invasion of extracellular matrix (Hassman et al, 2011). In addition, it enhances HHV-8 infectivity for endothelial cells and increases its viral load by reactivating it from latent state (Guadalupe et al, 2011). On the other hand, HHV-8 activates nuclear receptors NF-kappa and NF-AT and this level of activation is synergistically increased by HIV-1 Tat protein (Guadalupe et al, 2011). Thus, infection with HHV-8 is associated with KS the risk for which correlates with HHV-8 viral load. However, for a given HHV-8 titre, the risk is greater in HIV-seropositive, as compared to HIV-seronegative individuals (Casper, 2011). Exceptions have been found in some parts of West Africa, South America and Australia where although the incidence of HHV-8 infection is high only few cases of KS are found (Ablashi et al 1999; Rezza et al, 2001). This indicates that other factors are important in the pathogenesis of KS.

In Nigeria, the incidence of HIV/AIDS was estimated at 4.1 million and is on the downward trend (National Action Committee on AIDS (NACA) 2010). KS has become the most common malignant skin tumour with the disease appearing in areas where it did not exit in the past (Asuquo & Ebughe, 2009; Iregbu & Elegba, 2006). A report from Calabar South Eastern Nigeria showed that KS is the most common malignant skin tumour accounting for 38.0% cases (Asuquo & Ebughe, 2009). Reports from Abuja and Benin both in Nigeria showed KS in 0.8% of newly diagnosed HIV infected patients compared to a prevalence of 0.5% a decade earlier (Akinsete et al, 1998; Iregbu & Elegba, 2006; Onunu et al, 2007). Most of our patients present with extensive and advanced disease that usually required a combination of HAART and chemotherapy. This together with limited therapeutic facilities resulted in poor outcome of treatment (Ahmed et al, 2001; Asuquo & Ebughe, 2009). With improved AIDS awareness and access to HAART more patients are likely to present earlier. Our institution is one of the Federal Government HIV/AIDS designated treatment centre and we see patients from various parts of Nigeria. There is little information on the treatment and outcome of KS in HIV-1infected patients who have been treated with HAART in Africa. The objective of this study was to review the clinical features, treatment and outcome of AIDS -associated Kaposi's sarcoma patients in our institution particularly in the context of increasing use of highly active antiretroviral therapy. We shall also highlight the difficulties in the evaluation and treatment of these patients.

2. Patients and method

This prospective study was carried out at Ahmadu Bello University Teaching Hospital Zaria, the premier referral and teaching hospital in Northern Nigeria. Patients with concurrent diagnosis of HIV infection and Kaposi's sarcoma seen between January 2007 and

December 2010 were included. Only patients 18 years or more were included. Consent was obtained from each patient after counselling and at the time of taking blood sample, tissue specimen or taking photographs of accessible lesions. Permission for the study was also obtained from the hospital ethical committee.

2.1 Patient's evaluation and treatment

Patients were assessed at the time of diagnosis of AAKS and at four to eight weekly intervals during follow-up. At each visit, weight, vital signs and Kaposi's sarcoma symptoms were recorded, and a physical examination was performed. During evaluation efforts were made to discover the probable mode of HIV transmission to the patient. The dimension, number, appearance and sites of involvement of KS lesions were recorded. Lesions causing disfigurement were photographed. Tumour size was defined as the sum of the greatest diameters of each measurable tumour. The Karnofsky score status of the patients was also recorded. The tumour was staged according to AIDS Clinical Trials Group (ACTG) classification using the tumour (T), immune system (I) and systemic illness (S) (Krown et al, 1997). Tumour was defined as T0 if disease was confined to the skin and lymph nodes or oral involvement was confined to the hard palate, or T1 if there was pulmonary or gastrointestinal involvement, tumour associated oedema or ulceration, or extensive oral involvement. Cutaneous KS lesions confined to one anatomical area were classified as local while lesions involving two or more sites as disseminated. Morphologically the lesions were classified as macular, nodular and ulcerative. Tumour response was assessed by comparing lesion characteristics to the baseline tumour evaluations. Treatment responses were assessed according to ACTG criteria. A complete response (CR) was defined as the absence of any detectable residual disease, including tumour-associated oedema, persisting for at least four weeks. Partial response (PR) was defined as ≥50% decrease in the number or size of previously existing evaluable lesions lasting for at least four weeks without the appearance of new lesions or tumour-associated oedema. Stable disease (SD) was defined as any response that did not meet the criteria for progression or PR. Overall response rate was defined as both complete and partial response rates. Progressive disease (PD) was defined as ≥25% increase in the size of previously existing lesions or the appearance of new ones or the development of new or increasing tumour-associated oedema or effusion. Relapse was defined as the development of progressive disease in the presence of a documented CR, or PR.

Screening test for HIV antibodies were performed by parallel testing using Enzyme-linked immunoabsorvent assay (ELISA) with Immunocomb II, HIV-1 and HIV-2 (M/S Orgenics, Israel) and Stat Pak (Trinity Biotech, Wicklow, Ireland). Positive test results from the two different kits were taken as confirmatory evidence of HIV antibodies. The CD4 cell counts were performed using the Dynabeads method (Dynal Biotech LLC, Milwaukee, WI, USA). Patients that presented from 2008 to 2010 were screened with Stat Pak (Trinity Biotech, Wicklow, Ireland) and Bundi HIV-1 and HIV-2 (Bundi International Diagnostics, Abia, Nigeria) and confirmed with Western blot method. Their CD4 count was performed with Partec flow cytometre (Partec GmbH, Munster, Germany). Plasma HIV-1 RNA levels were measured with Roche-Ampiclor HIV-1 monitor test, (version 1.5 (Roche-Ampiclor-Roche Diagnostics, Branchburg, USA). Viral load less than 400 copies/mL was considered undetectable. Diagnosis of Kaposi's sarcoma was based on histological examination of tissue specimens fixed in 10% formalin embedded in paraffin wax and stained with haematoxylin

and eosin. Special stains were employed in selected cases. Serum urea and electrolytes, liver function test and complete blood count with differential and platelet count were done at the time of diagnosis of AAKS and before administration of chemotherapy. Chest radiographs, ECG, abdominal ultrasound, faecal occult blood and gastrointestinal endoscopic examination were performed in appropriate cases.
Our protocol for the treatment of AAKS has been presented previously (Ahmed et al, 2001). Following evaluation, patients were resuscitated and started on HAART which we defined as therapy consisting of at least three antiretroviral drugs in accordance with national guidelines (NACA, 2007). Our protocol recommends that patients with AAKS are started on HAART irrespective of CD4 count. Stable patients that have KPS of ≥40 and adequate bone marrow, renal and hepatic functions were then commenced on specific anti-KS chemotherapy. This consisted of six courses of three weekly cycles of vincristine 1.5mg/m^2, doxorubicin 10mg/m^2 and bleomycin 15mg/m^2 by bolus intravenously. Treatments were delayed for up to two weeks for recovery from grade ≥3 neutropenia, thrombocytopenia or severe diarrhoea. Patients with relapse were treated with same course. Radiotherapy and surgical excision of localised lesions were performed in appropriate cases. Treatment complications and outcome were monitored. Patients were followed-up at four to eight weekly intervals until death or lost to follow-up.

2.2 Statistical analysis

We analysed data using SPSS statistical software (version 17.0, SPSS, Chicago IL). Data were reported as proportions, mean ± standard deviation (SD) or median (range). Categorical variables and proportions were compared by Fisher's exact test while continuous variables were compared by Wilcoxon two-sample test. In patients that responded to treatment, the duration of response was summarised using Kaplan Meier method. Fisher's exact test was used to test for agreement between the occurrence of clinical benefit and the presence of clinical response. Survival was calculated from the day of KS diagnosis until death or the date of last follow-up. Overall survival duration curves and duration of tumour response were plotted according to Kaplan-Meier method. Logistic regression modeling performed to identify independent determinants of survival and tumour response was done using the following clinicopathologic variables: age, sex, presence of comorbid condition, presence of systemic symptoms, KPS, stage of tumour, viral load and CD4 count at presentation. Risk factors were first analysed univariately, and the statistically significant variables were used to construct a multivariate model. Interactions were also analysed to confirm independence. We considered $p \leq 0.05$ to be statistically significant.

3. Results

3.1 Patient's characteristics

During the period of study 7,155 patients with HIV infection were seen of which 98 (1.4%) had associated Kaposi's sarcoma. The number of patients with AAKS increased steadily from 2007 to 2010 (table 1). Their ages ranged from 18 to 54 years (Figure 1), mean of 33.6 ± 3.8 SD. Nine (9.2%) patients were less than 21 years old while 44 (44.9%) were in the third decade. There were 56 males and 42 females, male to female ration of 1.3:1. The male to female ratio decreased from 1.5:1 in 2007 to 1:1 in 2010. Females were younger than males (mean age of 27years vs. males 34; $p < 0.04$). Comorbid conditions were seen in 43 (43.9%)

patients including 20 (20.4%) pulmonary tuberculosis, 17 (17.3%) oral candidiasis, 15(15.3%) hypertension and 2 diabetes mellitus. Duration of symptoms of AAKS ranged from 1 to 13 months, mean 5.7 ±1.2SD. Symptoms were present in 91 (92.9%) patients and included pain (62.2%), swelling of the limbs (figure 2) (52.6%) and cosmetic disability (31.6%). Seven (7.1%) patients had no symptoms of Kaposi's sarcoma and the diagnosis was made during routine clinical evaluation (figure 3) at antiretroviral therapy (ART) clinic. Kaposi's sarcoma was the AIDS defining disease in 64 (65.3%) patients while in the remaining 34 (34.7%) it was diagnosed between 1 and 15 months after the initial diagnosis of AIDS. Sixteen patients had used HAART for 1- 13 months at the time of diagnosis of AAKS. The KPS ranged from 20% to 100%, median of 60%. All the patients were heterosexual although 11 were men having sex with men (MSM). Patients on anti-retroviral therapy at the time of diagnosis had a mean CD4 count of 267± 65SD cell/mm^3. Overall, the mean CD4 count at presentation was 165 cells/mm^3 (range: 26 – 875; 95% CI: 97 - 425). The mean HIV-1 viral load (VL) assessed in 71 patients was 48,593 copies/mL (range: 200- 989,571; 95% CI: 28,593- 76,225).

3.2 Tumour characteristics

The anatomic distribution of AAKS lesions is shown in table 2. All patients had multiple lesions the lower limbs being most frequently involved (45.9%). In 20 (20.4%) patients, tumour was limited to extremities, with fungating and exophytic growth invading and destroying the subcutaneous and surrounding tissues including the underlying bones (Figure 4). Unusual sites including 7 conjunctiva, 9 penile and 12 vulva were also involved. Perineal involvement was more common in females. Visceral lesions included 3 rectal, 5 intestinal and 2 gastric tumours. Tumour size ranged from 2.0 to 58.0cm, mean 29± 15.7SD. The histological type was mixed cellularity in 63 (64.3%) patients and anaplastic in 9 (9.2%). KS stage at presentation was T1, I1, S1 in 47 (48.0%); T1, I1, S0 in 22 (22.4%); T0, I0, S1, in 8 (8.2%) and T0, I0, S0 in 21 (21.4%). Overall, 77 (78.6%) patients had poor prognosis stage comprising 38 (90.5%) females and 39 (69.6%) males (OR= 3.5, 95% CI 1.7–5.6, P < 0.01). Women also had more disseminated cutaneous AAKS lesions involving an increased number of lesions at multiple anatomical sites, compared to more localised lesions in males (OR =3.4, 95% CI = 1.7–5.5, P = 0.001). Despite the differences in age and disease severity between males and females, no gender-specific differences were observed in CD4 counts or plasma HIV-1 viral load. However, when males and females were analysed separately, there were significant correlations between the severity of KS and the degree of immune suppression as measured by CD4 count (χ^2 test, P= 0.001) and between poor disease prognosis and immune suppression (P= 0.001)

Year	HIV infected patients		AIDS associated Kaposi's sarcoma patients		
	No	%	No.	% of HIV patients	Male: Female
2007	1667	23.3	20	1.2	1.5:1
2008	1755	24.5	23	1.3	1.3:1
2009	1837	25.7	25	1.4	1.2:1
2010	1896	26.5	30	1.6	1:1
Total	7155	100	98	1.4	1.3:1

Table 1. Prevalence of HIV infection and AIDS-associated Kaposi's sarcoma

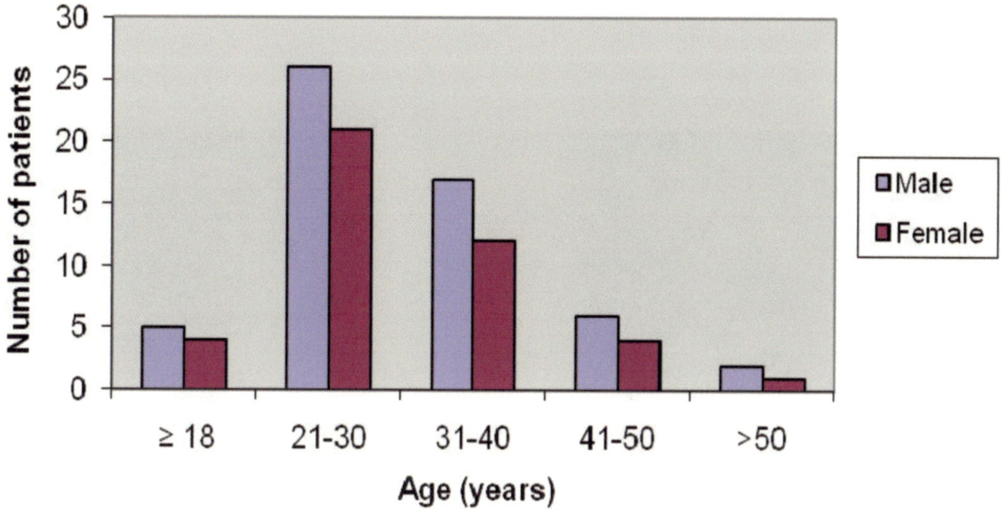

Fig. 1. Age and sex distribution of patients with AIDS-associated Kaposi's sarcoma

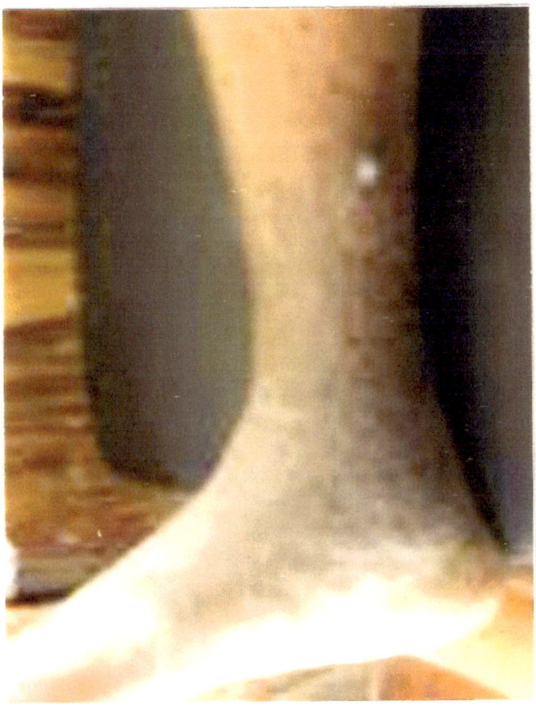

Fig. 2. Nodular Kaposi's sarcoma with swelling of the lower limb

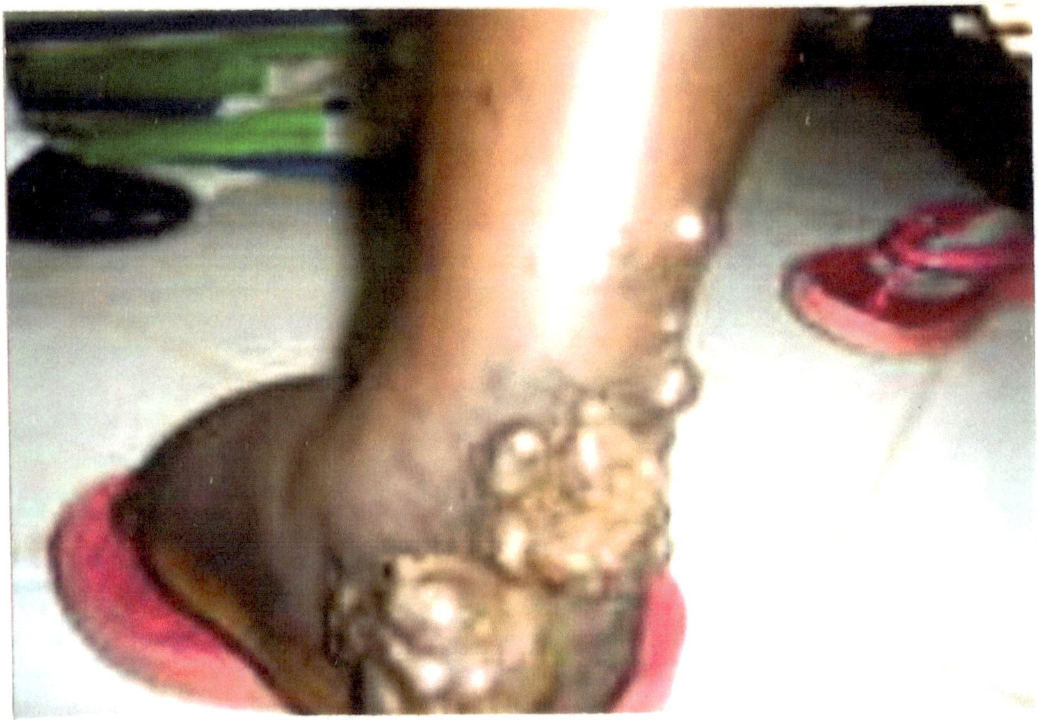

Fig. 3. Asymptomatic Kaposi's sarcoma lesion discovered during routine clinical evaluation

Site	No.	%
Lower limb	45	45.9
Trunk	37	37.8
Lymph node	33	33.7
Perineum	19	19.4
Oropharynx	15	15.3
Upper limb	13	13.3
Visceral	9	9.2
Other	6	6.1

Table 2. Anatomical distribution of AIDS-associated Kaposi's sarcoma lesions

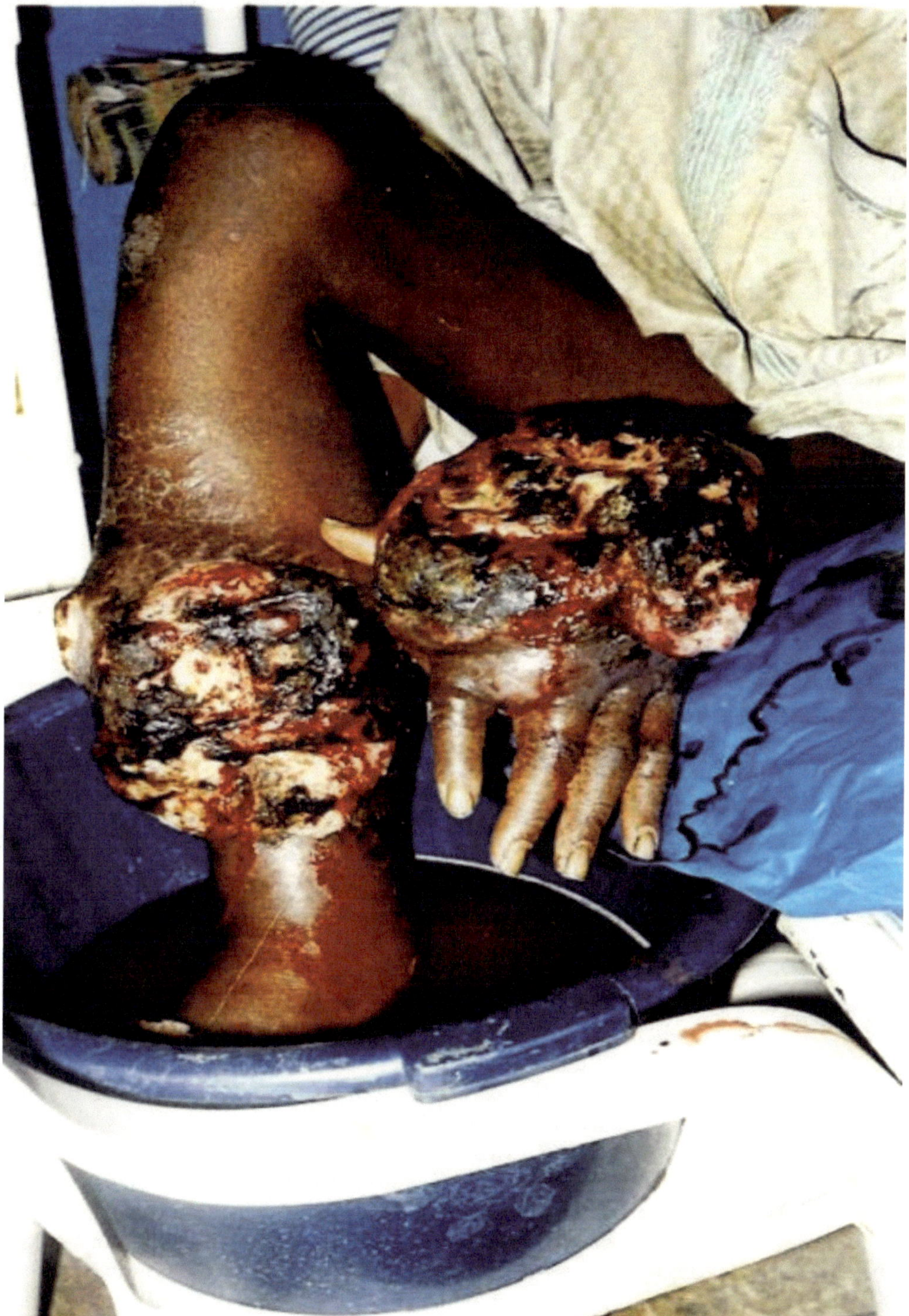

Fig. 4. Fungating Kaposi's sarcoma lesions of upper and lower limbs

Characteristics at presentation	HAART alone n	Mean	(SD)	Standard error of mean	HAART +VAB n	Mean	(SD)	Standard error of mean	P - value
Age (years)	19	32.5	(4.7)	4.21	67	31.8	(7.5)	2.94	0.29
Duration of symptom (months)	19	3.5	(1.7)	0.84	67	3.9	(1.3)	1.25	0.14
Viral load ($x10^3$ copies/mL)	10	503	(128.8)	17.50	41	512	(125.0)	15.9	0.15
CD4 count (cell/uL)	19	162	(56.4)	2.37	67	168	(55.8)	1.45	0.07
Sex									0.75
Male	12				42				
Female	7				25				
ACTG Stage									
Good prognosis	4	(21.1%)			16	(23.9%)			
Poor prognosis	15	(78.9%)			51	(76.1%)			
Time of diagnosis of KS									0.18
At diagnosis of AIDS	12	(63.2%)			43	(64.2%)			
After diagnosis of AIDS	7	(36.8%)			24	(35.8%)			

SD= standard deviation; ACTG = AIDS clinical trials group; KS= Kaposi's sarcoma
HAART= highly active antiretroviral therapy; VAB= combination of Vincristine, Doxorubicin and Bleomycin

Table 3. Characteristics of patients that were treated with HAART alone or HAART and VAB

3.3 Treatment and outcome

Overall, 67 (68.4%) patients were treated with both HAART and VAB of which 53 had completed six cycles. Of the 14 patients that did not complete anti-KS therapy, eight died in the course of treatment after two to five courses, treatment was stopped in two because of severe side effects and four were lost to follow-up (LTF). The median time to start chemotherapy after diagnosis of AAKS was three months (range 1 to 5months). Because of financial constraints, 19 (19.4%) patients had only antiretroviral therapy. The patients that had both HAART and VAB and those that had HAART alone had similar ACTG clinical stage, KPS and CD4 counts (table3). The remaining 12(12.2%) patients had only supportive care because of poor KPS (7) and refusal of consent (5). Two patients had limb amputation, five had excision of localised ulcerated lesions while 17(17.4%) had radiotherapy. Overall, 69 (70.4%) patients had improvement of AAKS symptoms that lasted a median duration of ten months (range 3 months to 4 years). The cumulative tumour response is shown in figure 5.

Fifty four (80.6%) patients treated with HAART and VAB had tumour response compared to 8 (42.1%) of those treated with HAART alone ($p< 0.005$). Patients treated with both HAART and VAB were more likely to have tumour response or stable disease (OR 2.7; CI: 1.8- 3.6) compared to those that had HAART alone (table 4). There was a positive correlation between symptoms control and tumour response (Pearson correlation coefficient, $r = 0.35$ and $r = 0.28$; $p < 0.05$ by two tailed Fisher exact test). While haematotoxicity was the most frequent toxicity in both treatment groups, neutropenia grades three and four was higher in patients treated with both HAART and VAB (22.4%) compared to HAART alone (10.5%)($P < 0.001$). Digestive toxicity was frequently observed in both groups, with a higher rate of diarrhea in the HAART and VAB group. Five patients had peripheral neuropathy while two others had asymptomatic cardiomyopathy. These toxicities delayed chemotherapy by 1-2 weeks in 15 patients.

Patient's response	HAART alone (n=19)	HAART +VAB (n=67)	P -value
Symptom control			0.003
No. (%)	10 (52.6)	59 (88.1)	
Median duration of symptoms control, months (range)	5 (1- 13)	12 (5- 54)	0.001
Overall tumour response	8 (42.1)	54 (80.6)	0.005
Complete response	2 (10.5)	31 (46.3)	0.001
Partial response	6 (31.6)	23 (34.3)	0.075
Median duration of tumour response, months (range)	5 (1-17)	11 (2- 54)	0.001
Median time to relapse, months (range)	3 (2.5-15)	9 (5-26)	0.001
Treatment related complications			
No. (%)	7 (36.8)	38 (56.7)	0.015
Median KPS (range)			
At diagnosis of KS	60 (30-90)	60 (30-90)	
3 months after diagnosis of KS	60 (20-90)	60 (40-90)	0.017
Mortality at 6 months			
No. (%)	6 (31.5)	7 (10.4)	0.005

KS= Kaposi's sarcoma; KPS= Kernofsky performance score
HAART= highly active antiretroviral therapy; VAB= combination of Vincristine, Doxorubicin and Bleomycin

Table 4. Response of patients to treatment with HAART alone or HAART and VAB.

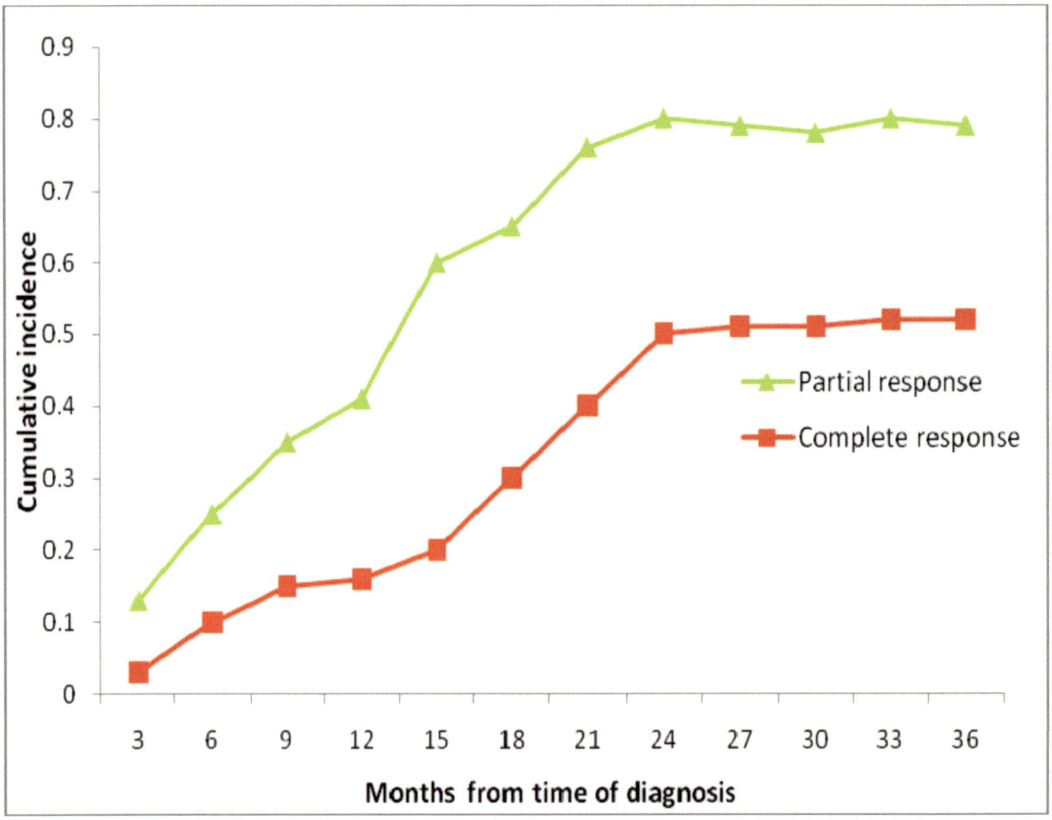

Fig. 5. Cumulative tumour response following treatment of AIDS-associated Kaposi's sarcoma

Overall, median survival was 14 months from the time of diagnosis of AAKS. The median survival was 12 months for patients treated with HAART compared to 18 months for those treated with both HAART and VAB (figure 6). Overall 56 (57.1%) patients had significant improvement in quality of life. Seven (7.1%) patients died during their first admission in the hospital while additional 7 were lost to follow-up. At one year 34 (34.7%) patients had died, comprising of 12 (100%) patients that had only supportive treatment, 9(47.4.0%) of those treated with HAART and 13 (19.4%) treated with HAART and VAB (figure 6). Univariate analysis showed that females, poor ACTG stage, CD4 count <200 cells/mm^3, viral load > 21,000 copies/mL, and not using antiretroviral therapy were significantly associated with poorer survival (table 5). When these factors were subjected to multiple regression analysis, poor ACTG stage (p=0.015), viral load > 21,000 copies/mL (p=0.001), not using antiretroviral (p=0.005) and not using anticancer chemotherapy (p=0.003) were the significant independent factors associated with poorer survival. Patient's follow-up ranged from one month to four years. Fifty two (53.1%) patients were followed-up for one year.

Variable	Number of patients	Death		OR	95% CI	P-value
		No	%			
Sex						
Male	56	21	37.5	1		
Female	42	20	47.6	1.4	1.2 - 2.9	0.049
Age (years)						
1-20	9	4	44.4	1		
21-40	76	32	42.1	1.5	1.4 - 3.5	
41-60	13	5	38.5	1.3	1.1 -2.7	0.175
Time of diagnosis of KS						
After diagnosis of AIDS	34	13	38.2	1		
As AIDS defining disease	64	27	42.2	1.7	1.5 - 4.9	0.075
ACTG stage						
Good prognosis	21	5	23.8	1		
Poor prognosis	77	35	45.5	4.8	3.7 - 12.4	0.005
CD4 count (cells/mm^3)						
>200	40	15	37.5	1		
≤200	58	25	43.1	2.4	1.6 - 3.9	0.016
Viral load (copies/mL)						
0-20,000	11	2	18.2	1		
≥ 21,000	40	19	47.5	2.9	2.7 - 6.5	0.003
Use of HAART						
Yes	86	28	32.5	1		
No	12	12	100.0	5.5	3.9 - 14.6	0.001
Use of VAB						
Yes	67	18	26.8	1		
No	31	22	71.0	3.2	2.1 - 5.7	0.001

OR= odd ratio; CI = confidence interval; ACTG = AIDS clinical trials group; KS= Kaposi's sarcoma
HAART= highly active antiretroviral therapy; VAB= combination of Vincristine, Doxorubicin and Bleomycin

Table 5. Univariate analysis of factors related to mortality in patients with AIDS-associated Kaposi's sarcoma

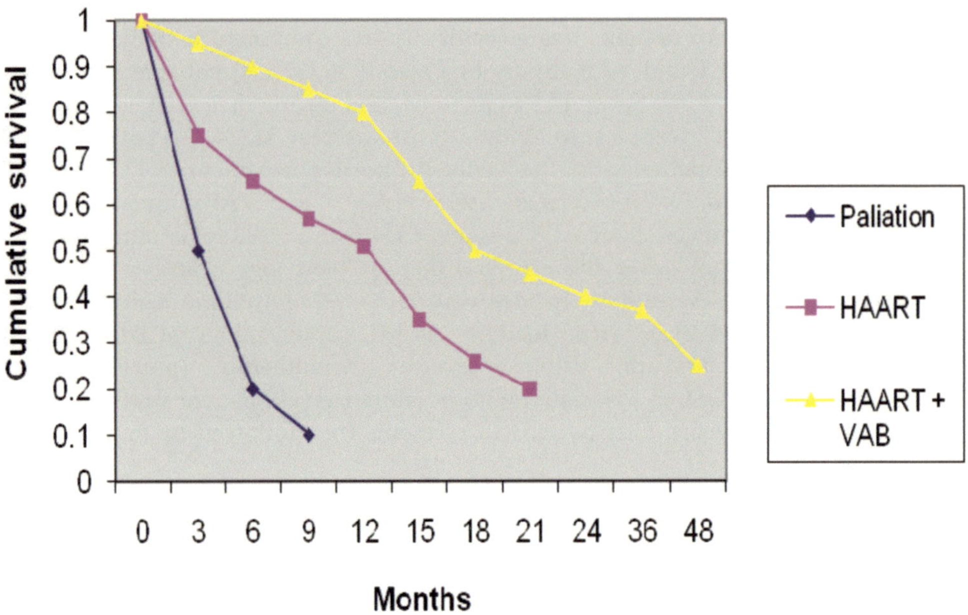

Fig. 6. Cumulative survival following treatment of patients with AIDS-associated Kaposi's sarcoma

4. Discussion

To our knowledge, this is the largest study to date on the treatment and outcome of patients with AIDS-associated Kaposi's sarcoma from Nigeria. The present study identified KS in 1.4% of HIV-1 infected patients. The patients are young with female patients being relatively younger than males. The male to female ratio decreased from 1.5:1 in 2007 to 1:1 four years later. Majority of the patients (78.6%) presented with high tumour burden that was categorised as poor prognosis disease, while 20 (20.4%) had pulmonary tuberculosis. Simultaneous treatment with HAART and combination chemotherapy was carried out on 67(68.4%) patients. This treatment was associated with significant morbidity but was the only chance for control of symptoms and prolonged survival.

In high income countries the incidence of AAKS has decreased significantly from mid 1990s (Franceschi et al, 2008; Pipkin et al, 2011). This reduced AAKS incidence is due to wide spread use of HAART which has the effect of immune reconstitution and direct inhibitory effects on angiogenesis. In addition, there are safer sex practices and other preventive and therapeutic measures against HIV infection. Recently, Phatak et al (2010) from India identified no case of KS among 46 AIDS-associated cancers reviewed over 5 years. In another report from Thailand, the incidence was 0.026 per 100,000 despite high incidence of HIV infection because HHV-8 infection is low at 4.0% (Sriplung & Parkin, 2004). In the present study, there was progressive increase in prevalence of AAKS over the study period (table 1). In a previous report from our institution, 15 AAKS patients were seen from 1991 to 1995 compared to 98 patients seen from 2007 to 2010 in the present study (Ahmed et al, 2001). Overall, the prevalence of AAKS in this study was 1.4% which is lower than 1.6% reported from Jos, Nigeria and 3.4% from South Africa, but higher than 0.8% reported from other centres in Nigeria (Agaba et al, 2009; Iregbu & Elegba, 2006; Chu et al 2010). The high incidence of HHV-8 infection and limited access to HAART and other preventive measures explain in part the reason for increasing incidence of AAKS in sub-Saharan Africa.

Prior to the HIV epidemic KS was a disease of middle-aged men (Penn, 1979; Taylor et al, 1971). The mean age of 33.6 years in the present study is similar to that reported in other studies in our sub-region (Chu et al, 2010; Phipps et al, 2010). The lower age of these patients is probably due to the high risk behaviour and incidence of HIV infection is highest in the age group 20-40 years in sub-Saharan Africa. In addition, our female patients were younger than males. The finding that AAKS occurs at an earlier age in women when compared with men has been reported previously (Mosam et al, 2008; Phipps et al, 2010). In the present study, the proportion of KS patients was highest among women in their mid-20s who heterosexually acquired HIV-1 infection. This indicates that females acquire HIV-1 infection at an earlier age than males. Alternatively, immunosuppression from HIV infection and KS pathogenesis might progress more rapidly in females compared to males. Previous studies have shown that the age-specific distribution pattern for female KS was essentially similar to that previously reported for HIV-1 infection (Jombo et al, 2006). Therefore, the risk of developing AAKS is closely related to the epidemiology of HIV-1 infection in females.

Variable	Category	OR	95% CI	P-value
Sex	Female vs. Male	1.8	1.5- 2.9	0.075
ACTG stage	Poor vs. Good prognosis	5.3	2.2- 17.3	0.015
CD4 count (cells/mm³)	≤ 200 vs. > 200	1.6	1.3- 3.8	0.075
Viral load (copies/mL)	≥ 21,000 vs. < 21,000	3.1	2.6- 9.5	0.001
Use of HAART	No vs. Yes	2.8	2.3- 6.9	0.005
Use of VAB	No vs. Yes	1.9	1.5- 3.8	0.003

OR= odd ratio; CI = confidence interval; ACTG = AIDS clinical trials group;
HAART= highly active antiretroviral therapy; VAB= combination of Vincristine, Doxorubicin and Bleomycin

Table 6. Multiple regression analysis of factors related to mortality in patients with AIDS-associated Kaposi's sarcoma

In Western countries all forms of KS are more common among men than women (Simard et al, 2011; Martellotta et al 2009). This is similar to the findings in Africa before the advent of HIV infection (Sasco et al, 2010; Taylor et al, 1971). Among HIV-infected individuals other than MSM, reported incidence rates of KS are still higher in men in other studies (Kagu et al, 2006; Sissolak & Mayaud, 2005). In a recent study from Brazil 94.4% of 107 AAKS patients were men, giving a male to female ratio of 18:1 (Yoshioka et al, 2004). The observations that a tumorigenic KS cell line could not be established in pregnant immunodeficient mice and that human chorionic gonadotropin (hCG) inhibited KS growth in-vitro suggested a possible biologic basis for the lower KS incidence among women (Lunardi-Iskandar et al, 1995;

Rabkin et al, 1995). However, therapeutic trials with hCG have been inconclusive while studies in women with HIV infection revealed that pregnancy afforded no protection from KS development or dissemination (Rabkin et al, 1995). In our patients, the male to female ratio was 1.3:1 which decreased progressively from 1.5:1 in 2007 to 1:1 four years later. This is similar to 1.4:1 recently reported from South Africa (Chu et al, 2010). A report from Jos Nigeria revealed a reversal of the gender ratio from a male to female ratio of 10:1 about four decades ago to 1:1.4 (Agaba et al, 2009). The reason for the near equivalent distribution of AAKS cases among men and women in recent studies may be a reflection of the high proportion of HIV infected females with >60% of person living with the virus in Africa being women. Additionally, women are more frequently subjected to HIV testing as routine counselling and testing has been applied to perinatal settings, and this may lead to higher number of AAKS cases being identified among women. Finally, unlike in Western countries where MSM constitute a high proportion of AAKS cases, the heterosexual mode of HIV transmission in our patients mean that HHV-8 would be equally distributed among men and women. Therefore, the trend in increasing proportion of female patients with AAKS may continue until when females predominate.

Patients in this study presented with extensive and disseminated disease with 78.6% having poor prognosis stage, a much higher proportion than reported from resource rich countries (Ashish et al, 2007; Krown 2004). Other reports from poor resource countries revealed that poor prognosis disease constitute 60-82% of cases (Agaba et al, 2009; Bassett et al, 1995; Phipps et al 2010). Cutaneous lesions were present in 64.7% of patients in this series followed in order of frequency by lymphadenopathy and visceral lesions. Moderate enlargement of peripheral lymph nodes is not uncommon in HIV infected patients. A biopsy of such nodes would often reveal a focus of KS, a finding that appears to have little clinical consequence (Krown 2004). However, 11 of our patients had massive generalised lympadenopathy in the absence of evidence of KS elsewhere. In sub-Saharan Africa lymphadenopathy is comparatively common and has various causes including tuberculosis, lymphoma, KS and HIV infection. There is a significant overlap in the clinical presentation of these diseases although each requires distinctly different treatment. Histology provides a reliable and cost effective definitive diagnosis since each disease can be distinctively diagnosed under the microscope. However, it has been suggested that co-existing lesions can be missed even in biopsy material if special stains for demonstration of microorganisms are not performed (Pantanowitz et al 2010). Involvement of the gastrointestinal tract (GIT) was seen in only nine of our patients. However, most patients with GIT KS are asymptomatic, and because the lesions are submucosal they are not visualized on contrast-enhanced radiographs (Kibria et al 2010). Previous studies showed that asymptomatic GIT lesions have little clinical consequences hence, endoscopy should be carried out only on symptomatic patients (Kibria et al, 2010; Sissolak & Mayaud, 2005). In our patients, KS involved multiple anatomical regions. The lower limbs were most frequently affected with an associated lymphoedema which may be extensive and disproportionate to the extent of cutaneous disease. This lymphoedema may result from tumour involvement of dermal lymphatics or from the production by KS cells of growth factors that increase vascular permeability (Feller et al, 2008). Additionally, HHV-8-induced exuberant proliferation of endothelial cells may lead to the occlusion of lymphatic vascular lumens leading to lymphoedema (Feller et al, 2008).

In this as in other reports, at the time of diagnosis women had more widespread and advanced AAKS compared to men (Chu et al 2010; Meditz et al, 2007). It is probable that the reason for the increased severity of AAKS in women is not related to virological or immunological differences since both men and women in our study had similar mean VL and mean CD4 counts. This is in agreement with studies from Zimbabwe and South Africa (Meditz et al, 2007; Mosam et al, 2008). Of special interest is a small cohort of 14 patients who were on HAART for 6-13 months at the time of diagnosis of KS. These patients had a median CD4 count of 375 cells/mm^3 and undetectable HIV viral load. They required systemic therapy to control their KS but were more likely to have complete resolution of their tumours and demonstrated a trend towards better survival than patients having KS with lesser CD4 counts and detectable HIV viral loads. In the past, AAKS has been reported in African patients with CD4 counts of >350 cells /mm^3 indicating that severe immunosuppression is not necessary for development of KS (Morgan et al, 2000). Similarly, recent reports from high income countries have identified a group of patients that developed AAKS despite effective and sustained HIV suppression and good immune system function (Crum-Cianflone et al, 2010; Mani et al, 2009; Maurer et al, 2007). This raises questions about the integrity of the immune system and its ability to control certain viruses in patients with long-standing HIV infection. It has been suggested that with the ageing of HIV infected patients those who are co-infected with HHV-8 may develop KS despite good control of HIV infection (Crum-Cianflone et al, 2010). The impacts of AAKS on quality of life are varied. In our patients, extensive oedema of the lower limbs was associated with stiffness and pain that may interfere with walking while ulcerated tumours were infected and foul smelling. Lesions of the face and genitalia also have social and emotional consequences, including isolation because of obvious disfiguring lesions, and depression and anxiety from the constant visible reminder of illness.

The disability and suffering associated with AAKS means that treatment to reduce symptoms and improve quality of life should be carried out promptly and efficiently. HAART is an essential treatment for all AAKS patients (Krown, 2004; Tirelli & Bernardi, 2001). In patients with low tumour burden and slowly progressing disease, histological regression of existing KS lesions has been shown in response to HAART (Martellotta et al, 2009). However, HAART alone can not effectively control all cases of KS and there may be initial tumour progression as part of the immunoreconstitution syndrome (Bower et al, 2005). In addition, it is not possible to state with certainty what proportion of patients with AAKS will benefit from HAART alone, or what are the precise characteristics that can be use to identify such patients. In our patients as in others, HAART is an effective post-chemotherapy maintenance treatment in patients with advanced and extensive disease that has been reduced significantly as a result of conventional chemotherapy (Cooley et al, 2007; Martin-Carbonero, 2004). The effects of HAART on Kaposi's sarcoma are multifactorial and include inhibition of HIV replication, diminished production of HIV-1 transactivating protein Tat, reconstitution of immune response against HHV-8 and possibly direct antiangiogenic activity by inclusion of protease inhibitors (Tirelli & Bernardi, 2001). In the present study, decision to initiate systemic chemotherapy was based on the extent of Kaposi's sarcoma in addition to other considerations such as patient KPS, end organ function, degree of immunosuppression, and other HIV comorbidities.

Our patients were treated with a combination of vincristine, doxorubicin and bleomycin, similar to reports from other low income countries (Chu et al, 2010; Dedicoat et al, 2003). In high income countries liposomal anthracyclines and taxanes are being used for treatment of AAKS due to higher efficacy and reduced toxicity (Ashish et al, 2007; Cooley et al, 2007). In a meta- analysis comparing pegylated doxorubicin (PLD) and VAB among 499 patients, Dedicoat et al (2003) found a better response among the PLD group although there was no survival advantage by either group. However, liposomal anthracyclines are unlikely to be available or affordable in low income countries where the majority of AAKS patients live. In a recent analysis from Brazil, PLD was found to be associated with improved efficacy and less toxicity but in terms of cost effectiveness, the VAB regimen is the most rational treatment option for AAKS patients in poor resource settings (Vanni et al, 2006). Our results showed that six cycles of this regimen could produce a significant and quick response in symptomatic patients with advanced AAKS. Overall response rate of 80.6% in our patients compares favourably to 50% to 88% reported in other studies (Dedicoat et al, 2003; Makombe et al, 2008; Phipps et al, 2010). Differences in response rates are largely attributable to differences in the patient populations evaluated, the lack of strictly defined response criteria and variations in the dosing schedules used. Of the 67 patients that had chemotherapy in this study, 52% had complete resolution of their disease within 36 months of diagnosis. This is similar to observed resolution rates of 44%-60% reported using similar regimen (Bihl et al, 2007; Nasti et al, 2000; Nguyen et al, 2008). However, we found the median time to complete resolution to be 9 months which is considerably longer than 5 months previously reported (Bihl et al, 2007). This is provably because chemotherapy was not immediately started in many of our patients due to financial constraints. In the present study, both HAART and VAB were independently associated with complete resolution of tumour suggesting that even in the HAART era, chemotherapy plays a significant role in the treatment of advanced AAKS patients. In addition, HIV viral load was significantly associated with resolution of KS. This finding is consistent with other reports of AAKS improvement or resolution associated with significant decrease or undetectable HIV viral load (Nguyen et al, 2008). Indeed, it seems that controlling HIV viral load is essential for clinical improvement, disease resolution of KS, and perhaps decreased risk of relapse. In this as in other studies there was no association between CD4 T-cell count and KS response, suggesting that suppression of HIV replication plays a more vital role in the resolution of KS than immune reconstitution (Mosam et al, 2008; Iregbu & Elegba, 2006). In our patients, there was positive correlation between tumour response and clinical response, and the response was maintained for a significant period of time after discontinuation of chemotherapy. Clinical response was associated with improved quality of life as evidenced by control of fungating and foul smelling ulcers and improvement of pain, cosmetic appearance and KPS. In the present study, median survival was 18 months following chemotherapy compared to 12 months following HAART alone. Both VAB and HAART are independently associated with improved survival, similar to the Multicenter AIDS Cohort Study which demonstrated an 81% reduced risk of death for KS patients treated with HAART (Tam et al, 2002). Whilst CD4 count <200 cells/mm^3 was associated with mortality on univariate analysis, it was not on multivariate analysis. This may be due to the effects of advanced KS disease (T1 and S1 stages) whose effects were stronger than CD4 count.

The toxicities observed following chemotherapy in our patients are similar to those reported in other studies using same regimen and are well tolerated (Dedicoat et al, 2003; Guadalupe et al, 2011). In the absence of haemopoetic growth factors, cytotoxic chemotherapy was used cautiously in our patients to minimise the risk of bone marrow suppression that may lead to infectious complications. Bacterial infections which resulted from severe neutropenia secondary to chemotherapy were observed in three of our patients. Doxorubicin causes significant bone marrow suppression which is at its nadir on day 14 after administration. This bone marrow suppression recovers slowly over 7-10 days but in an HIV infected individual the magnitude and duration of the bone marrow suppression may be longer, hence the need to wait for three weeks to allow the bone marrow to recover before the next cycle of chemotherapy is given. The selection of therapy for KS must take into account the potential benefit and adverse effects of treatment, interactions with other medications, and potential impact on underlying immunosuppression.

When dealing with localised bulky or cosmetically disturbing lesions, radiotherapy is the most effective local therapy. In this as in other reports, irradiated lesions regress with treatment, but regrowth, after 6 months is common (Bih et al, 2007; Nguyen et al, 2008). In addition to providing effective palliation, radiotherapy is associated with minimal side effects. Although surgery is effective in excision of localised isolated lesions, heroic surgery is unjustified. Our study has several limitations. Among the patients that died, other risk factors for mortality such as tuberculosis were not independently considered hence the actual death due to KS were not isolated. In addition, some of our patients were lost to follow-up and a previous study indicates that about 40% of these patients were actually dead (Brinkhof et al, 2009). Similarly, because many patients lost to follow-up were treated with VAB, the beneficial effects of chemotherapy may be underestimated. Finally, follow-up of patients was difficult and inconsistent hence, it was not possible to monitor the timing of treatment outcome accurately.

5. Conclusion

In conclusion KS is not uncommon in patients with HIV-1 infection. The patients present with extensive and advanced disease that requires systemic treatment. All AAKS patients should receive HAART. In low income countries like ours, chemotherapy consisting of a combination of vincristine, doxorubicin and bleomycin should be given simultaneously with HAART to patients that can physiologically withstand such therapy. The usual number of cycles for effective therapy is six cycles. However, chemotherapy may continue for 1-2 cycles beyond complete remission to maximise the chance of attacking all microscopic KS cells. Following successful treatment chemotherapy can be restarted for recurrent tumour. If KS continues to grow in the presence of effective HAART regimen, chemotherapy with VAB should be stopped and alternative treatment modalities should be instituted if possible, or else palliative KS management should be started. Palliative care for KS may include adequate pain relief, reduction of the size of tumours with radiotherapy and reduction of the offensive smell of ulcerated lesions with appropriate dressing argent. Prevention and treatment of other opportunistic infections is necessary as uncontrolled infections may stimulate KS progression probably due to production of angiogenic cytokines. Using this approach we achieved quick and prolonged tumour response in addition to improved quality of life as evidenced by symptoms control and improved cosmetic appearance and KPS. High satisfaction and reduced toxicities as well as availability, affordability and ease of administration of the drugs led to good patient's compliance. This approach is recommended for treating AAKS patients in a poor resource setting. It is necessary to identify KS patients early in the disease when treatment is likely to provide significant benefits in terms of reducing the bulk of disease and improving long-term survival. However, early access to highly active antiretroviral therapy constitutes the best hope for the control of this stigmatizing and lethal disease in sub-Saharan Africa. With improvement in the access to antiretroviral therapy in sub-Saharan Africa, it is necessary to designed studies that investigate the effects of cheaper and more widely available chemotherapeutic argents for the treatment of AIDS-associated Kaposi's sarcoma among patients on highly active antiretroviral therapy.

6. Acknowledgement

We sincerely appreciate the cooperation of the patients and their relations that were included in this study. We are also very grateful to all physicians and other personnel that participated in the management of these patients.

7. References

Ablashi D, Chatlynne L, Cooper H, et al. (1999) Seroprevalence of human herpesvirus-8 (HHV-8) in countries of Southeast Asia compared to the USA, the Caribbean and Africa. *Br J Cancer*. 81:893-897.

Agaba PA, Sule HM, Ojoh RO, Hassan Z, Apena L, Mu'azu MA. (2009). Presentation and survival of patients with AIDS-related Kaposi's sarcoma in Jos, Nigeria. *Int J STD AIDS* 20: 410–413

Ahmed A, Isa MS, Habeeb AG, Kalayi GD, Muhammad I, Eagler LJ. (2001) Influence of HIV infection on presentation of Kaposi's sarcoma. *Trop Doct* 31:42-45

Akinsete I, Akanmu AS, Okany CC. (1998) Spectrum of clinical diseases in HIV-infected adults at the Lagos University Teaching Hospital: a five-year experience (1992–96). *Afr J Med Sci* 28: 147–151

Ashish U, Keith M S, Donald WN. (2007) Pegylated liposomal doxorubicin in the treatment of AIDS-related Kaposi's sarcoma. *Int J Nanomedicine*. 2: 345–352.

Asuquo ME, Ebughe G. (2009). Cutaneous cancers in Calabar, Southern Nigeria. *Dermatol Online J* 15: 11-13

Bassett MT, Chokunonga E, Mauchaza B, et al. (1995) Cancer in the African population of Harare, Zimbabwe, 1990–1992. *Int J Cancer* 63: 29–36.

Bihl F, Mosam A, Henry LN, et al. (2007) Kaposi's sarcoma-associated herpes virus-specific immune reconstitution and antiviral effect of combined HAART/chemotherapy in HIV clade C-infected individuals with Kaposi's sarcoma. *AIDS*. 21:1245–1252

Bower M, Nelson M, Young AM, et al. (2005) Immune reconstitution inflammatory syndrome associated with Kaposi's sarcoma. *J Clin Oncol*. 23: 5224–5228.

Brinkhof MW, Pujades-Rodriguez M, Egger M. (2009) Mortality of patients lost to follow-up in antiretroviral treatment programmes in resource-limited settings: systematic review and meta-analysis. *PLoS One*. 4:e5790

Casper C. (2011). The increasing burden of HIV-associated malignancies in resource-limited regions. *Annual Rev Med*. 62:157-170.

Chang Y, Cesarman E, Pessin MS, Lee F, Culpepper J, Knowles DM. (1994). Identification of herpesvirus-like DNA sequences in AIDS-associated Kaposi's sarcoma. *Science* 266:1865-1869.

Chu KM, Mahlangeni G2, Swannet S, Ford NP, Boulle A, Cutsem GV. (2010) AIDS-associated Kaposi's sarcoma is linked to advanced disease and high mortality in a primary care HIV program in South Africa. *J Int AIDS Soc* 13:23 doi:10.1186/1758-2652-13-23

Cooley T, Henry D, Tonda M, Sun S, O'Connell M, Rackoff W. (2007) A Randomized, Double-Blind Study of Pegylated Liposomal Doxorubicin for the Treatment of AIDS-Related Kaposi's sarcoma. *Oncologist* 12;114-123

Crum-Cianflone NF, Hullsiek KH, Ganesan A, Weintrob A, Okulicz JF, Agan BK. (2010) Is Kaposi's sarcoma occurring at higher CD4 cell counts over the course of the HIV epidemic? *AIDS.* 24:2881-2883

Dedicoat M, Vaithilingum M, Newton RR. (2003) Treatment of Kaposi's sarcoma in HIV-1 infected individuals with emphasis on resource poor settings. *Cochrane Database of Systematic Reviews.* Issue 3. Art. No.: CD003256. DOI: 10.1002/14651858.CD003256.

Engels EA, Pfeiffer RM, Goedert JJ, et al. (2006) Trends in cancer risk among people with AIDS in the United States 1980-2002. *AIDS* 20: 1645–1654

Feller L, Masipa JN, Wood NH, Raubenheimer EJ, Lemmer J. (2008) The prognostic significance of facial lymphoedema in HIV-seropositive subjects with Kaposi sarcoma. *AIDS Research and Therapy* 5:2 doi:10.1186/1742-6405-5-2

Franceschi S, Dal Maso L, Rickenbach M. et al (2008) Kaposi sarcoma incidence in the Swiss HIV Cohort Study before and after highly active antiretroviral therapy. *Br J Cancer* 99: 800–804

Franceschi S, Geddes M. (1995). Epidemiology of classic Kaposi's sarcoma, with special reference to Mediterranean population. *Tumori* 81: 308–314

Friedman-Kien A, Laubenstein L, Marmor M et al. (1981) Kaposi's sarcoma and pneumocystic pneumonia among homosexual men: New York and California. *Morbidity and Mortality Weekly Report* 30, 305–308.

Guadalupe M, Pollock BH, Westbrook S, et al. (2011) Risk factors influencing antibody responses to Kaposi's sarcoma-associated herpesvirus latent and lytic antigens in patients under antiretroviral therapy. *J Acquir Immune Defic Syndr.* 56:83-90.

Hassman LM, Ellison TJ, Kedes DH. (2011) KSHV infects a subset of human tonsillar B cells, driving proliferation and plasmablast differentiation. *J Clin Invest.* 121:752-768.

Hengge UR, Ruzicka T, Tyring SK, Stuschke M, Roggendorf M, Schwartz RA. (2002) Update on Kaposi's sarcoma and other HHV8 associated diseases. Part 1: epidemiology, environmental predispositions, clinical manifestations, and therapy. *Lancet Infect Dis* 2: 281–292

Iregbu KC, Elegba OY. (2006) Prevalence of Kaposi's sarcoma among adult HIV-seropositive patients seen in a designated HIV treatment and care centre in Abuja, Nigeria. *J Int Assoc Physicians AIDS Care.* 5: 115-118.

Jombo GTA, Egah DZ, Banwat EB. (2006). Human immunodeficiency virus in a rural community of plateau state: Effcetive control measures still a nightmare. *Nig J Med.* 15:49-51

Kagu M B, Nggada H A, Garandawa H I, Askira B H, Durosinmi M A (2006) AIDS-associated Kaposi's sarcoma in Northeastern Nigeria. *Singapore Med J* 47: 1069-1074

Kaposi M. (1872). Idiopathic multiple pigmented lesions of the skin. *Arch Dermatol Syph* 4: 265–273

Kibria R, Siraj U, Barde C (2010) Kaposi's sarcoma of the stomach and duodenum in human immunodeficiency virus infection. *Dig Endosc.* 22:241-242.

Koon HB, Fingleton B, Lee JY, et al (2011) Phase II AIDS Malignancy Consortium trial of topical halofuginone in AIDS-related Kaposi sarcoma. *J Acquir Immune Defic Syndr.* 56: 64-68

Krown SE. (2004). Highly active antiretroviral therapy in AIDS-associated Kaposi's sarcoma: Implications for the design of therapeutic trials in patients with advanced, symptomatic Kaposi's sarcoma. *J Clin Oncol* 22: 399–402.

Krown SE, Testa MA, Huang J. (1997). AIDS-related Kaposi's sarcoma: prospective validation of the AIDS Clinical Trials Group staging classification. AIDS Clinical Trials Group Oncology Committee. *J Clin Oncol* 15:3085-3092.

Lunardi-Iskandar Y, Bryant JL, Zeman RA, et al. (1995). Tumorigenesis and metastasis of neoplastic Kaposi's sarcoma cell line in immunodeficient mice blocked by a human pregnancy hormone. *Nature* 375:64-68.

Makombe SD, Harries AD, Kwong-Leung Yu J, et al. (2008). Outcomes of patients with Kaposi's sarcoma who start antiretroviral therapy under routine programme conditions in Malawi. *Trop Doct* 38: 5–7

Mani D, Neil N, Israel R, Aboulafia DM. (2009). A retrospective analysis of AIDS-associated Kaposi's sarcoma in patients with undetectable HIV viral loads and CD4 counts greater than 300 cells/mm^3. *J Int Assoc Physicians AIDS Care* 8:279-285

Martellotta F, Berretta M, Vaccher E, Schioppa O, Zanet E, Tirelli U. (2009). AIDS-related Kaposi's sarcoma: state of the art and therapeutic strategies. *Curr HIV Res.* 7: 634-638.

Martin-Carbonero L, Barrios A, Saballs P et al. (2004). Pegylated liposomal doxorubicin plus highly active antiretroviral therapy versus highly active antiretroviral therapy alone in HIV patients with Kaposi's sarcoma. AIDS 18: 1737–1740.

Maurer T, Ponte M, Leslie K. (2007). HIV-associated Kaposi's sarcoma with a high CD4 count and a low viral load. *NEJM* 357:1352-1353

Meditz AL, Borok M, MaWhinney S, Gudza I, Ndemera B, Gwanzura L. (2007). Gender Differences in AIDS-Associated Kaposi Sarcoma in Harare, Zimbabwe. *J Acquir Immune Defic Syndr* 44:306–308

Morgan D, Malamba SS, Orem J, Mayanja B, Okongo M, Whitworth JA. (2000). Survival by AIDS defining condition in rural Uganda. *Sex Transm Infect* 76:193–197

Mosam A, Hurkchand HP, Cassol E, Page T, Cassol S, Bodasing U. (2008). Characteristics of HIV-1-associated Kaposi's sarcoma among women and men in South Africa. *Int J STD AIDS* 19:400-405

Nasti G, Errante D, Talamini R, et al. (2000). Vinorelbine is an effective and safe drug for AIDS-related Kaposi's sarcoma: results of a phase II study. *J Clin Oncol.* 18:1550-1557.

National Guidelines for HIV and AIDS treatment and care in Adolescents and Adults, Department of Public Health Federal Ministry of Health Abuja, Nigeria in Collaboration with The National Action Committee on AIDS. 2007.

Newton R, Grulich A, Beral V, et al. (1995). Cancer and HIV infection in Rwanda. *Lancet* 345: 1378–1379.

Newton R, Ziegler J, Beral V, et al. (2001). A case control study of human immunodeficiency virus infection and cancer in adults and children residing in Kampala, Uganda. *Int J Cancer* 92: 622–627.

Nguyen HQ, Amalia S M, Kitahata MM, Rompaey SE, Wald A, Casper C. (2008). Persistent Kaposi sarcoma in the era of HAART: characterizing the predictors of clinical response. *AIDS.* 22: 937–945.

Onunu AN, Okoduwa C, Eze EU, Adeyekun AA, Kubeyinje EP, Schwartz RA. (2007). Kaposi's sarcoma in Nigeria. *Int J Dermatol.* 46, 264 -267

Pantanowitz L, Kuperman M, Goulart RA. (2010). Clinical history of HIV infection may be misleading in cytopathology. *Cytojournal.* 7: 7. doi: 10.4103/1742-6413.64375

Parkin DM, Sitas F, Chirenje M, Stein L, Abratt R, Wabinga H. (2008). Cancer in Indigenous Africans—burden, distribution, and trends. *Lancet Oncol* 9:683-692

Penn I. (1979). Kaposi's sarcoma in organ transplant recipients: report of 20 cases. *Transplantation* 27, 8–11.

Phatak UA, Joshi R, Badakh DK, Gosavi VS, Phatak JU, Jagdale RV. (2010). AIDS-associated cancers: an emerging challenge. *J Assoc Physicians India.* 58:159-162.

Phipps W, Sewankambo F, Nguyen H, et al (2010). Gender differences in clinical presentation and outcomes of epidemic Kaposi Sarcoma in Uganda. *PLoS ONE* 5: e13936. doi:10.1371/journal.pone.0013936

Pipkin S, Scheer S, Okeigwe I, Schwarcz S, Harris DH, Hessol NA. (2011). The effect of HAART and calendar period on Kaposi's sarcoma and non-Hodgkin lymphoma: results of a match between an AIDS and cancer registry. *AIDS* 25: 463-471.

Rabkin CS, Chibwe G, Muyunda K, Musaba E. (1995). Kaposi's sarcoma in pregnant women. *Nature* 377:21-22

Rezza G., Danaya R.T., Wagner T.M., et al. (2001). Human herpesvirus-8 and other viral infections, Papua New Guinea. *Em Infect Dis* 7: 893-895.

Sasco AJ, Jaquet A, Boidin E, et al. (2010). The Challenge of AIDS-related malignancies in sub-Saharan Africa. *PLoS ONE* 5: e8621. doi:10.1371/journal.pone.0008621

Schwartz AA. (2004). Kaposi's sarcoma: an update. *J Surg Oncol* 87:146-151.

Simard EP, Pfeiffer RM, Engels EA. (2011). Cumulative incidence of cancer among individuals with acquired immunodeficiency syndrome in the United States. *Cancer.* 117:1089-1096

Sissolak G, Mayaud P. (2005). AIDS-related Kaposi's sarcoma: epidemiological, diagnostic, treatment and control aspects in sub-Saharan Africa. *Trop Med Int Health* 10:981–992

Sriplung H, Parkin DM. (2004). Trends in the incidence of Acquired Immunodeficiency Syndrome–related malignancies in Thailand. *Cancer.* 101:2660-2666

Stein L, Urban MI, O'Connell D, et al. (2008). The spectrum of human immunodeficiency virus-associated cancers in a South African black population: results from a case-control study, 1995–2004. *Int J Cancer* 122: 2260–2265.

Sullivan RJ, Pantanowitz L, Dezube BJ. (2009). Targeted therapy in Kaposi sarcoma. *Bio Drugs.* 23: 69–75.

Tam HK, Zhang ZF, Jacobson LP, Margolick JB, Chmiel JS, Rinaldo C. (2002). Effect of highly active antiretroviral therapy on survival among HIV-infected men with Kaposi sarcoma or non-Hodgkin lymphoma. *Int J Cancer* 98:916-922.

Taylor JF, Templeton AC, Vogel CL et al. (1971). Kaposi's sarcoma in Uganda: a clinicopathological study. *Int J Cancer.* 8, 122–135.

The National AIDS and STD Control Programme, Department of Public Health Federal Ministry of Health Abuja, Nigeria in Collaboration with The National Action Committee on AIDS Sentinel report. 2010.

Tirelli U, Bernardi D. (2001). Impact of HAART on the clinical management of AIDS-related cancers. *Euro J Cancer 37: 1320–1324*

Vanni T, Fonseca BAL, Polanczyk CA. (2006). Cost-Effectiveness Analysis Comparing Chemotherapy Regimens in the Treatment of AIDS-Related Kaposi's Sarcoma in Brazil. *HIV Clin Trials* 7:194–202

Yoshioka MC, Alchorne MDA, Porro AM, Tomimori-Yamashita J. (2004). Epidemiology of Kaposi's sarcoma in patients with acquired immunodeficiency syndrome in Sao Paolo, Brazil. *Int J Dermatol* 43:643–647

7

Thiourea Derivatives: A Promising Class Against HIV/TB Co-Infection

Marcus Vinicius Nora de Souza[1,2], Marcelle de Lima Ferreira Bispo[1,2], Raoni Schroeder Borges Gonçalves[1,2] and Carlos Roland Kaiser[2]

[1]*Fundação Oswaldo Cruz (Fiocruz)- Instituto de Tecnologia em Fármacos – Farmanguinhos*

[2]*Programa de Pós-Graduação em Química, Instituto de Química, Universidade Federal de Rio de Janeiro, Brazil*

1. Introduction

Nowadays, the Human Immunodeficiency Virus (HIV), which is the causative agent of Acquired Immune Deficiency Syndrome (AIDS), represents a serious public health problem. According to the World Health Organization (WHO), in 2009 there were 33.3 million people living with HIV worldwide, and more particularly in sub-Saharan Africa, where the overwhelming majority (67%) of cases appear. Furthermore, 2.6 million people have been recently infected with the virus in 2009, when HIV/AIDS was estimated to have caused 1.8 million deaths (United Nations Program on HIV/AIDS [UNAIDS], 2010).

Due to the impairment of their immune system, HIV bearers are more susceptible to opportunistic infections, such as Tuberculosis (TB), which is a leading cause of HIV-related deaths worldwide. The risk for TB is 20-37-fold greater among HIV-infected individuals, depending on the status of the HIV epidemic. According to WHO, one-third of people living with HIV are infected with TB, and there was an estimate of 1.4 million new TB cases per year among said population. Moreover, one in four TB deaths occurs in HIV-positive patients, while TB was responsible for 23% of AIDS-related deaths (WHO, 2010a).

This situation becomes especially alarming in view of the number of challenges in the control and management of TB in HIV-infected individuals, such as the difficulties to conclude a TB diagnosis, as well as the complexity involved in the treatment of HIV infection-related TB. Due to their great relevance to the subject matter of this work, the above factors will be emphasized in the next section.

2. Challenges in the management of HIV infection-related TB

2.1 Diagnosis of TB in HIV-infected individuals

Within the context of lung diseases, there are some aspects that may constitute a bar to the diagnosis of TB (Box **1**): HIV-infected patients are minimally symptomatic or asymptomatic, as they present few or less specific classic symptoms of TB (productive cough, chest pain, fever, night sweats, weight loss, hemoptysis); patients with low $CD4^+$ T lymphocyte counts have atypical chest radiograph findings, with lower prevalence of cavitary disease, while the findings could be normal in up to 22% of HIV-infected individuals; the main method used worldwide for TB detection, namely the microscopic examination of Ziehl-Neelsen-stained sputum smears, has low sensitivity among HIV-infected individuals, as they develop acid-faster smear negative diseases with higher frequency than HIV-uninfected people (Sterling et al., 2010).

Furthermore, HIV-infected individuals present more often the subclinical form of TB, said factor leading to a delay in the diagnosis and treatment. Another difficulty for the TB diagnosis in HIV-infected individuals is the increased risk (10-20% in HIV-uninfected individuals, compared to 40-80% in HIV-infected persons) to develop extrapulmonary TB, whose most prevalent forms are pleural effusion, lymphadenopathy, pericardial disease, miliary disease, meningitis and disseminated TB (Chaisson et al., 1987).

Box 1. Usual difficulties involved in the diagnosis of TB in HIV-infected individuals

- Minimally symptomatic or asymptomatic patients;
- Atypical chest radiograph findings;
- Acute prevalence of acid--fast smear negative disease ;
- High frequency of subclinical TB form;
- Increased risk of development of extrapulmonary TB.

2.2 TB treatment in HIV bearers

In addition to diagnostic difficulties, the treatment of HIV infection-related TB also presents several challenges, such as duration and frequency, determining the precise moment to start antiretroviral therapy (ART), management of drug interactions, as well as several side effects from therapy.

As regards the duration of TB therapy, WHO recommends a 6-month rifampicin-based treatment (2HRZE/4HR, Table **1**), applying to both HIV-infected and uninfected individuals. Nevertheless, Perriens and collaborators showed that, after providing a 12-month therapy with 2HRZE/4HR, the recurrence rate at the 18th month shall be lower than those observed at the standard regime (Perriens et al., 1995). Furthermore, another study performed by Fitzgerald et al indicated that the administration of isoniazid for 1 year upon termination of the therapy under standard regime reduces the recurrence of TB only among HIV-infected patients (Fitzgerald et al., 2000). It is worthy to mention that, in both studies, patients had no access to antiretroviral therapy, which contributes to extend the beneficial effects from TB treatment, without presenting the risks that are inherent to the combination of TB-HIV drugs.

Phase	Duration (months)	Dosing Frequency	Drugs
Intensive	2	Daily	HRZE
Continuous	4	Daily or three times per week[a]	HR

[a] For the continuation phase, the optimal dosing frequency may be also daily; should the administration of such a dosage be impossible, three times per week is a suitable alternative.
H = isoniazid, R= rifampicin, Z = pyrazinamide, E= ethambutol

Table 1. TB treatment for HIV bearers, as recommended by WHO.

Providing another relevant instruction on TB treatment in HIV-infected patients, WHO also recommends a daily TB therapy within, at least, the intensive phase (WHO, 2010b). Such orientation is based on a recent study, which showed that the incidence of relapse and failure among HIV-positive TB patients who were treated with intermittent TB therapy throughout treatment was 2–3 times higher, in comparison with patients who received a daily intensive therapy (Kahn et al., 2010). Moreover, another study indicated that, among HIV-positive patients, the risk of acquired resistance to rifampicin is higher when failing a three times weekly short-course intermittent regime (Kahn et al., 2010).
In relation to HIV treatment (Box **2**), WHO recommends that the first-line ART regime should comprise a combination of two nucleoside reverse transcriptase inhibitors (NRTIs) and one non-nucleoside reverse transcriptase inhibitor (NNRTI), as said drugs are effective, available at low costs in the market, and present generic and fixed-dose combinations (FDCs). Therefore, protease inhibitors (PIs) should be kept for second-line regimes (WHO, 2010b).

Box 2. Combined regime for both HIV and TB treatment.

- First-line regime: **2NRTIs + 1NNRTI**
  - [AZT or TDF] and [3TC or FTC] plus [EFV or NVP];
  - ART regime containing EFV is preferred, since interactions with anti-TB drugs are minimal;
  - EFV should not be administrated to women during the first trimester pregnancy, due to its teratogenic effects .
- **In cases of EFV intolerance, of HIV resistant to EFV, or contraindications to an EFV-based regime:** [AZT + 3TC + NVP] or TDF + [3TC or FTC] + NVP or the triple NRTI regime [AZT + 3TC + ABC] or [AZT + 3TC + TDF]
- **ART regime containing a boosted protease inhibitor** (PIs)
  - If available, a rifabutin-based TB treatment should be preferable.
  - Hepatitis among healthy adults is recurrent.

AZT= zidovudine, TDF= tenofovir, 3TC= lamivudine, FTC= emtricitabine, EFV= efavirenz , NVP= nevirapine.

2.3 Optimal timing to start the ART treatment

A critical issue among HIV-infected individuals diagnosed with TB is to determine the precise moment to initiate ART. Although ART improves the survival of HIV-positive patients, including those with TB, the optimal deadline from the onset of TB to start such a treatment is a matter that still requires further clarification. According to WHO, the TB treatment should be initiated in all HIV bearers showing active TB disease, regardless of their $CD4^{+}$ lymphocyte count. TB treatment should be started first, and, then, followed by ART as soon as possible, and preferably within the first weeks from the beginning of the TB treatment (WHO, 2010b). However, the concomitant treatment of both diseases results in several disadvantages, whose examples are listed and discussed at the Table **2**.
In spite of a number of clinical trials intended to determine the optimal timing for ART administration in bearers of HIV infection-related TB, the question still requires further studies (Piggot & Karakousis, 2011). Among the above referred works, Abdool Karim and collaborators have been performing the Starting Antiviral Therapy at Three Points in TB (SAPIT), which is an open-label, randomized and controlled trial conducted in Durban,

South Africa, with 642 HIV-positive patients with a CD4 count <500/mm^3 and with smear-positive TB (Abdool et al., 2010). The preliminary findings of SAPIT showed a decreased mortality rate among individuals who had started ART during anti-TB regime, in comparison with those who initiated ART only upon completion of the anti-TB therapy.

Disadvantage	Comments
High pill burden	More than 10 pills daily; discourage treatment adherence.
Overlapping of adverse effects	Hepatotoxicity promoted by H, R and Z and also by PI and NNRTI; increased risk of hepatitis C virus infection (Velasco et al., 2009). Gastrointestinal upset and rash are common in both therapies Peripheral neuropathy promoted by H, didanosine and stavudine
Immune reconstitution inflammatory syndrome (IRIS)	Although ART triggers the regeneration of immune cells, the immune system unexpectedly produces an overwhelming inflammatory response that unmasks or worsens the co-infection symptoms (TB is the most common among them); The risk of IRIS is the main ground to initiate TB treatment prior to ART, whenever it is possible. Its frequent symptoms comprise fever, swollen lymphonodes, skin lesions and rashes, changes in breathing, pneumonia, hepatitis, abscesses and eye inflammation. They often appear within 2-6 weeks from the beginning of HIV therapy (Antonelli et al., 2010).
Drug-drug interactions	**See Table 3**

Table 2. Disadvantages from the concomitant treatment of TB and HIV.

Following these conclusions, another study performed by Blanc and collaborators provided strong evidences for an early start of ART administration (Blanc et al., 2010). The Cambodian Early versus Late Introduction of Antiretrovirals (CAMELIA) was an open label, prospective, randomized controlled trial, registering HIV-positive patients with a CD4 count <200/mm^3 and smear-positive TB living in Cambodia. This study demonstrated that the group treated with ART within 2 weeks from the beginning of the TB therapy showed a relevant decline of 34% at the mortality rate, when compared with patients who received ART only 8 weeks after the initiation of TB treatment. In both studies, an increased incidence of IRIS was observed in patients who were early treated with ART. Nevertheless, the data shown by the SPIT trial, namely a lack of mortality or changes in antiretroviral regime attributable to IRIS, also corroborate the early ART initiation in HIV infection-related TB patients.

2.4 Management of drug-drug interactions between antiretroviral and anti-TB agents

The most delicate kind of interactions involves the concomitant use of rifamycins (among which the most usual are rifampicin and rifabutin), NNRTIs and PIs, given that these last two classes of antiretroviral drugs are essentially metabolized through cytochrome P450 (CYP) 3A4 enzymes, whose expression is induced by rifamycins. Consequently, the plasma concentration and exposure of NNRTIs and PIs are significantly reduced, when they are concomitantly administrated with rifamycins (Burman et al., 2001). Furthermore, rifampicin improves the activity of the efflux multidrug transporter P-glicoprotein, which promotes the elimination of PIs (Kim et al., 1998; Schuetz et al., 1996). Due to the reduction of NNRTIs and PIs at the plasma concentration, as a result from the simultaneous administration of rifamycins, the HIV treatment can fail, thus giving rise to the emergence of drug resistance.

The Table **3** below summarizes the most relevant interactions between rifamycins and antiretroviral agents (Centers for Disease Control and Prevention [CDC], 2007).

Antiretroviral agent	Effects on pharmacokinetics parameters and comments	
	Rifampicin	Rifabutin
NNRTIs		
EFV	EFV AUC↓ by 22%	Rifabutin AUC↓ by 38% **Increase Rifabutin dose to 450-600mg (daily or intermittent)**
NVP	NVP AUC↓ 37-58% and Cmin↓ 68% with 200mg 2x/day dose	NVP and Rifabutin AUC are not significantly changed
DLV	DLV AUC↓ 95% **Simultaneous use of such drugs should be avoided.**	DLV AUC↓ 95% Rifabutin AUC↑100% **Simultaneous use of such drugs should be avoided.**
PIs		
Ritonavir	Ritonavir AUC*↓ by 35% **Monitor for antiretroviral activity of ritonavir**	
Fos-Amprenavir	**Simultaneous use of such drugs should be avoided.**	**Rifabutin dose ↓ to 150mg/day or 300mg 3x/week**
Atazanavir	Atazanavir AUC↓ by >95% **Simultaneous use of such drugs should be avoided.**	Rifabutin AUC ↑ by 250% **Rifabutin dose ↓ to 150mg every other day or 3x/week**
Indinavir	Indinavir AUC↓ by 89% **Simultaneous use of such drugs should be avoided.**	Rifabutin AUC ↑ by 34% **Rifabutin dose ↓ to 150mg/day or 300mg 3x/week**
Nelfinavir	Nelfinavir AUC↓ by 82% Simultaneous use of such drugs should be avoided.	Rifabutin AUC ↑ by 207% **Rifabutin dose ↓ to 150mg/day or 300mg 3x/week**
Saquinavir	Saquinavir AUC↓ by 84% **Simultaneous use of such drugs should be avoided.**	
Saquinavir + Ritonavir	**Caution. The use of this combination could cause hepatitis.**	
Lopinavir + Ritonavir	**Caution. The use of this combination could cause hepatitis.**	Rifabutin AUC ↑ by 303% **Rifabutin dose ↓ to 150mg every other day or 3x/week**
Fusion Inhibitors		
Enfuvritide	No interaction. No dose adjustment.	No interaction. No dose adjustment.
CCR5 receptor antagonists		
Maraviroc	Maraviroc Cmin↓ by 78% **Increase Maraviroc to 600mg twice-daily**	**Change Maraviroc dose to 300mg twice daily and rifabutin to 300mg daily**
Integrase Inhibitors		
Raltegravir	Raltegravir concentratios ↓ by 40-61%	Rifabutin trough ↓ by 20% Raltegravir AUC is not affected **Change Rifabutin dose to 300mg daily and Raltegravir to 400mg twice daily**

*AUC= area under the plasma concentration time curve; estimated bioavailability.

Table 3. Management of interactions among anti-TB and anti-HIV drugs.

3. Thiourea derivatives: A promising class against HIV/TB co-infection

Due to such a number of complications that may possibly arise in the course of treatment of HIV-related TB, as described above, the development of new drugs against HIV and TB should be mandatory. Said medications should produce relevant effects, such as the improvement of patient well-being by means of the reduction of pill burden, as well as by the careful management of the overlapping toxicity resulting from the treatment of TB and HIV infections. Therefore, an alternative could be the development of drugs that might be able to simultaneously act in the treatment of both diseases. In this context, thiourea derivatives appear as a promising class of compounds. For instance, the tetrahydroimidazobenzodiazepinthiones (TIBO) derivative **9-Cl-TIBO** and the phenylethylthiazolylthiourea (PETT) derivatives **LY73497** and **trovirdine (TRV)** play a significant role in the inhibition of HIV reverse transcriptase (Fig. 1). On the other hand, the compound **isoxyl (ISO**, thiocarlide), another thiourea derivative, is known by its strong anti-TB activity (Fig. 1). By the way, although used as part of the TB clinical treatment since the 1960's, it may be pointed out that the relevance of **ISO** emerged from recent researches, and particularly from studies in the field of new treatments against MDR-TB. Therefore, the main purpose of this chapter is to highlight the importance of thioureas for the TB-HIV drug discovery, and to proceed with a review of data from recent literature, by focusing the most relevant contributions to the development of new prototypes containing this promising scaffold.

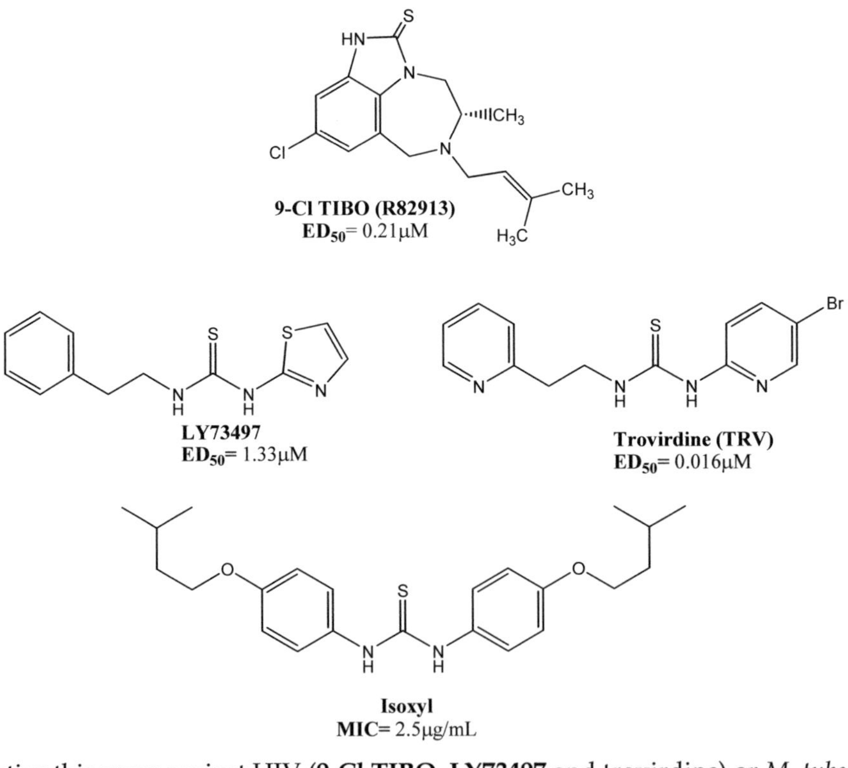

Fig. 1. Active thioureas against HIV (**9-Cl TIBO, LY73497** and trovirdine) or *M. tuberculosis* (**ISO**).

3.1 Thiourea derivatives showing a potential activity against HIV

3.1.1 TIBO derivatives

TIBO and HEPT [1-(2-hydroxyethoxymethyl)-6-(phenylthio)thymine] derivatives, yet discovered independently from each other, can be reputed a landmark in the history of the antiretroviral therapy. These compounds were the first congeners from a new category of anti-HIV drugs, currently known as NNRTIs (De Clercq, 2004). At the beginning of the 1990s, the only drug that had been approved for AIDS treatment was AZT, so that patients had to live at imminent risk to develop resistant mutant virus. Therefore, it becomes quite clear that the identification of a different class of antiretroviral drugs brought new perspectives in the treatment of AIDS.
The development of TIBO derivatives started from a screening program from the library of Janssen Research Foundation, working with 600 compounds that were selected due to their failure in producing effects on the standard pharmacological assays, and to their low toxicity in rodents as well (De Clercq, 2004). Upon evaluation of the biological activity of these compounds against HIV-1/$HTLV_{IIIB}$ in MT-4 cells, researchers identified the tetrahydro-benzodiazepine derivative **R14458** (Fig. 2), which presented a moderate anti-HIV-1 activity (IC_{50}= 62μM) (Pauwels et al., 1990). Using this substance as a lead compound, they started a program aiming at the improvement of its anti-HIV properties. Thereafter, several analogues were synthesized, thus allowing the performance of an extensive structure-activity relationship (SAR) study of this class of compounds.

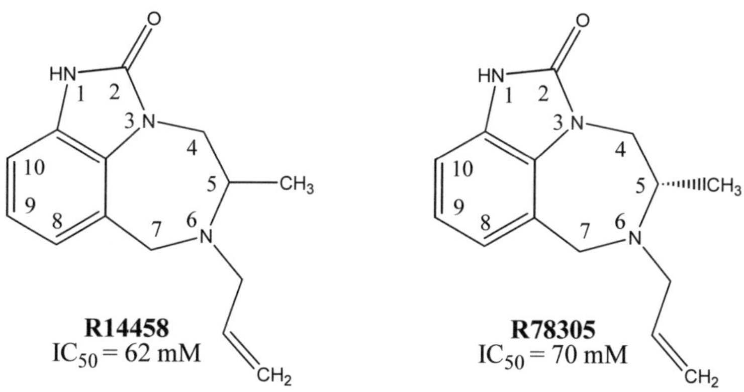

R14458 IC_{50} = 62 mM

R78305 IC_{50} = 70 mM

Fig. 2. Structure of TIBO derivatives **R4458** and **R78305**.

3.1.1.1 SAR of TIBO derivatives

Considering that the compound **R14458** is a racemic mixture, the authors initially investigated the role of stereochemistry in the biological activity of this substance. Although the two optical isomers were synthesized and tested against HIV-1, only the enantiomer **R78305** (Fig. 2) with *S* configuration was found to be active, showing that this configuration is required for the anti-HIV-1 properties of TIBOs (Pauwels et al., 1990). The subsequent studies aimed at the evaluation of systematic alterations in the structure of the lead compound, and its scaffold was independently modified in four different portions: the substituent bonded to the 6-positon nitrogen of the diazepine ring (Kukla et al., 1991a), the 5-ring urea portion (Kukla et., 1991b), the 7-membered ring portion (Breslin et al., 1995) and the substituent of the aromatic ring (Ho et al., 1995). The results obtained in these studies are described in the next sections.

3.1.1.1.1 Modifications in the substituent bonded to the 6-position nitrogen of the diazepine ring

Initially, it was verified that the presence of bulky groups attached to this position was mandatory to trigger anti-HIV-1 activity, since compounds containing hydrogen, ethyl or a linear propargyl substituent were inactive. The strongest activities were observed whenever an unsaturated allyl group was attached to the 6-positon nitrogen, such as in the lead compound, and it was verified that the substitution at the 2-position of this group led to more active compounds. The improvement degree of said activity varied in accordance with the following sequence: ethyl > methyl = vinyl = bromo > H. On the other hand, all compounds containing 2-propyl, phenyl, benzyl or fused cyclohexenyl were inactive. Substitutions at the 3-positon of the allyl group were also verified, and the dimethyl substituted compound showed the highest degree of activity found in these series. Introduction of bulky groups at this position usually led to completely inactive compounds. In view of the above results, an optimum size to the substituent for both 2- and 3-positions is required, since the substance loses its activity, as the length of the side chain increases or decreases. Moreover, the groups attached to the nitrogen which led to inactive compounds were the following: acetylene, alkyl groups containing heteroatom, and methylene attached to functional groups such as, nitrile, ketone, ester, alcohol, ether or a heteroaromatic pyrrole or imidazole (Kukla et al., 1991a).

3.1.1.1.2 Modification in the 5-ring urea portion

This portion of the tricyclic TIBO structures underwent several modifications, among which we can mention the replacement of carbonyl carbon by: nitrogen, sulfur dioxide or deletion of the carbonyl oxygen yielding, that are, respectively, a triazine, a sulfonamide and an imidazole. However, in the most part of trials, these modifications gave rise to inactive compounds. The most promising result was found by the replacement of the urea group by a thiourea, yielding a compound around one hundred times more active than the original prototype. The ring expansion, by insertion of a methylene or another carbonyl, led to a loss of anti-HIV-1 activity, and it was also verified that methylation of 1-positon nitrogen also gave rise to an inactive compound, probably in view of the need of NH to form hydrogen bonding (Kukla et., 1991b).

3.1.1.1.3 Modifications at the 7-membered ring portion

The demethylation of carbon in 5-position or introduction of bulky groups at this position yielded inactive or less active compounds, thus demonstrating that the size of the methyl group is optimum for the biological activity. The C-4 position showed a greater tolerance for larger groups, and the analogues presented a good anti-HIV-1 activity. The 7-position also underwent replacements, whereby high levels of activity were once more achieved. However, among the modifications performed at the 7-membered ring, none of them led to the discovery of compounds showing a better HIV inhibitory activity than the simplest 5-mono-methyl-substituted analogue (Breslin et al., 1995).

3.1.1.1.4 Evaluation of substituent effect on the aromatic ring

In order to evaluate the substituent effect on the aromatic ring, researchers used both urea and thiourea derivatives, and maintained the optimal conditions described by previous works, such as the attachment of a methyl group to the 5-position, and bonding of a dimethylallyl group to nitrogen at the 6-positon (except in case of compounds presenting synthetic problems, where scientists had to use a cyclopropylmethyl, also able to lead to high levels of activity). The best results were found for 8-substituted analogues, which, in comparison to the lead compound, showed much higher potency, so that halogens reached the highest level of activities in the substituent group. Iodine was the only exception to the above conclusions, probably due to its larger volume. Compounds containing a methoxy or an acetylene group bounded at 8-positon displayed similar activities, when compared to the parent unsubstituted compound. Although the substitution of 8-methoxy group by 8-thiomethyl may have led to an improvement in the biological activity, the replacement of methoxy by the ethoxy group, which is larger, resulted in a decrease in anti-HIV activity. Amino, aminoacetyl, dimethylamino and nitro analogues remained inactive. Furthermore, the substitutions at 9-positon led to the formation of compounds, whose activities are similar to those of the parent unsubstituted compound, while 10-substituted compounds were found to be less active. The replacement of the aromatic ring by a heteroaromatic ring was also evaluated, but the derivatives were inactive (Ho et al., 1995).

3.1.1.1.5 Clinical trial with 9-Cl-TIBO (R82913)

Extensive SAR studies with TIBO derivatives allowed the identification of substances with similar or better activities than other known antiretroviral drugs, such as AZT, dideoxycytidine (ddC) and Dideoxyinosine (ddI). Among these substances, thiourea **9-Cl TIBO (R82913)** (Fig. 1) was selected for a phase I clinical trial. This study evaluated 22 patients, within the age group between 27-59 years old, who showed HIV infection in an advanced stage (Pialoux et al., 1991). The drug was administrated by daily intravenous injection through a peripheral or a central venous catheter. **R82913** had to be injected in a dose of 120-200mg, in order to reach the concentration observed *in vitro* (20-40ng/mL), which is required for the protection against HIV cytopathic effects. The measured half-life was of 3 days, and the pharmacokinetic profile of the substance was neither influenced by an increase of the dose, nor by its long-term administration. In spite of its side effects, which usually comprised phlebitis, drowsiness and fatigue, a general absence of toxicity could be attributed to **R82913**.

3.1.2 PETT derivatives

3.1.2.1 Discovery of PETT series and preliminary SAR studies

Phenethylthiazolylthiourea (PETT) analogues integrate the powerful class of NNRTIs, first described by researchers from Lilly laboratories in the second half of the 1990's (Ahgren et al., 1995). These compounds were discovered in an attempt to indentify the minimal structural elements that might be necessary for the development of the thiourea derivative **9-Cl TIBO** biological activity (Fig. 1). The researchers disconnected some bonds from the rigid tricyclic nucleus of this substance, thus producing simpler structures. The potential pharmacophores produced after the systematically disconnections were used to search similar structures in the organic compound database of Lilly Research Laboratories. The study disclosed approximately 250 substances, whose activity against HIV was duly evaluated. The *N*-(2-phenethyl)-*N'*-(2-thiazolyl)thiourea, **LY73497** (Fig. 3), was identified as the lead compound, and used in subsequent SAR studies (Bell et al., 1995).
SAR studies were performed by dividing **LY73497** into four portions and proceeding with an aleatory variation of each of them (Fig. 3) (Bell et al., 1995). Initially, the authors

modified the quadrant 1 of phenyl ring, introducing different substituents, or replacing it by other aromatic heterocycles. They observed that *meta* and *ortho* substitutions generally triggers better activities, when compared with the *para* one. As regards the electronic nature of *ortho* substituents, both small electron-donating and small electron-withdrawing groups presented good activities, and, among said elements, the preferred groups are the following: fluoro, chloro, azido and methoxy. A combination of alkoxy and halogen substitution resulted in compounds with improved activity. Although the introduction of an ethoxy group in *meta* position may have led to a good activity, the use of bulky alkoxy groups, such as propoxy and isopropoxy, seems to have been responsible for a reduction in the activities. Among the substances containing a heterocycle in replacement of the phenyl ring, the best activity was observed for the 2-pyridyl compound. Changes at the nitrogen atom for the 3- and 4-position induced a decrease in the activity.

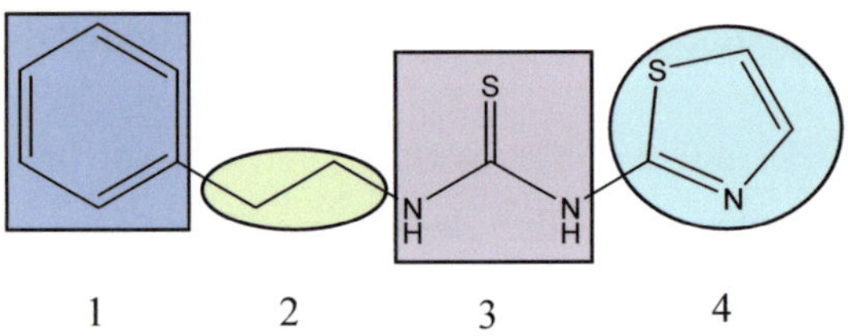

LY73497

Fig. 3. SAR studies with PETTs derivatives.

The modifications in quadrant 2 were characterized by changes in the length of the alkyl linker. The main conclusion was the identification of an ethyl linker as optimal to the activities. It was also noted that the introduction of a methyl group in the benzylic position of ethylene linker enhanced the activity, while a methyl group in the phenethyl position led to its reduction.

The variations in quadrant 3 demonstrated the crucial role played by thiourea moiety at the anti-HIV activity of these compounds. In fact, the replacement of thiourea by urea resulted in an inactive compound and other isosters, such as cyanoguanidine derivatives, which appeared to be less potent. The methyl substitution at the nitrogen adjacent to the thiazole ring leads to a less active compound, while methyl substitution on the nitrogen adjacent to the phenethyl side chain provided compound with no activity at all. This result is attributed to presence of an internal hydrogen bond between the hydrogen bonded to nitrogen adjacent to the phenethyl side chain and the nitrogen of the thiazole nucleus in **LY73497**.

As regards quadrant 4, it was observed that a heterocycle in this position is determinant to reach a good activity. In general, substituted thiazoles were highly active, excepting the 4-carboxythiazolyl compound, whose lack of activity indicated that the allosteric site of the enzyme does not accept a polar group. When thiazole nucleus was replaced by another heterocyle, the 2-pyridyl analog showed the highest level of activity.

During a second phase of SAR studies, the authors combined the optimal substituents in quadrants 1-4, and observed that these parameters are additive, able to give rise to compounds with optimal activity. Among them, the compound **LY300046**, currently known as **trovirdine (TRV;** Fig. 1**)**, was selected for further pharmacological examinations, since the hydrochloride salt of this compound showed acceptable blood levels, when orally administrated in rats (Ahgren et al., 1995).

TRV displayed a comparable or a better ED_{50} than other known antiretroviral drugs, such as **9-Cl TIBO**, L697661, NVP, AZT, ddI and ddC, being capable of inhibiting the replication of HIV-1 in MT-4 cell culture, as well as the replication of various clinical HIV-1 isolates in MT-2 cells and PBL human cells. However, this substance showed no action against HIV-2. When it was tested against resistant isolates containing mutations in Ile-100, Cys-181, and Ile-100–H-188 reverse transcriptase (RT), the trials disclosed a cross resistance between trovirdine and other non-nucleoside compounds. Nevertheless, within the group of said non-nucleoside derivatives, trovirdine was found to present the highest level of activity against these mutants.

In the enzymatic assay with wild-type and mutant RT enzymes, **TRV** was also more active than the non-nucleosides **9-Cl TIBO**, L697661 and nevirapine, showing a lower IC_{50}.

After **TRV** oral administration in rats (20mg/kg), a peak concentration in plasma of 3.5μg/mL was observed at 0.5h. The overall half-life was of 1 h, and the area under the concentration-time curve was 6.9μg/h/mL. The peak concentration in brain was 2.9μg/g, and the area under the concentration-time curve was 5.9μg/h/mL. This result shows that **TRV** crosses the blood-brain barrier, which is a desirable property of anti-retroviral agents, due to the risk of HIV-associated encephalopathy in contaminated patients (Ahgren et al., 1995).

Despite the promising outcomes related to the use of **TRV** as NNRTI, the clinical trials focused on this compound were suspended. Anyway, this substance is still considered a standard lead compound for the development of new PETT analogues, as it encouraged the course of an extensive serie of SAR studies based on modern approaches, such as crystallographic techniques and molecular modeling. These works will be discussed in the next section.

3.1.2.2 Rational design of new PETT analogues

This study was initiated when Vig and collaborators (Vig et al., 1998) proposed to synthesize series of novel PETT derivatives based on the structure of the non-nucleoside inhibitor (NNI) binding pocket of HIV-1 reverse transcriptase (RT). This composite binding pocket was built by superimposing nine individual crystal structures of RT-NNI complexes (Sudbeck et al., 1998). After having conducted docking studies with **TRV**, they verified the existence of multiple sites, which can be used for incorporation of larger functional groups, mainly surrounding the pyridyl ring, the ethyl linker and near the 5-bromo position. Hence, they proposed that a better use of these spaces by strategically designed functional groups could lead to a high-affinity binding and to the discovery of more potent anti-HIV agents. In view of the above, they decided to study the effects of introduction of several substituents in different positions of the phenyl ring, such as methoxy group, fluorine atom or chlorine atom (Table **4**).

These results disclosed by a preliminary SAR study attest to the potency of PETT derivatives phenyl ring substitutions on various positions (Fig. 4). After analyzing the composite NNI binding pocket, the authors identified three promising PETT derivatives with *ortho*-F **(HI-240)**, *ortho*-Cl (**HI-253**) and *metha*-F (**HI-241**) substituents on the phenyl ring, which showed potent anti-HIV activity (IC_{50} [p24] values of < 1nM), selectivity indexes (SI) of > 100,000, and were recognized to be more active than AZT or **TRV**. Among them, **HI-240** has been chosen as the lead compound, as it presented the highest level of activity against wide-type HIV RT. This finding could be grounded on the examination of a composite binding pocket model, showing that Wing 2 region is predominantly hydrophobic, except at the area nearby *ortho* positions on both sides of the phenyl ring, which would be compatible with polar groups, such as, for instance, halogen atoms.

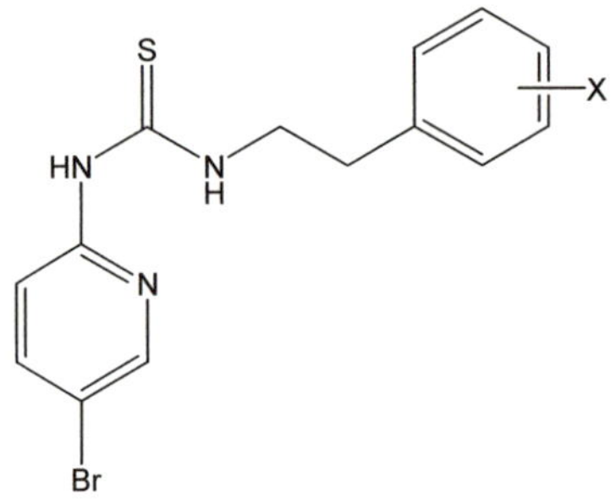

Compound	X	IC_{50} rRT (μM)[a]	IC_{50} p24 (μM)[b]	SI[c]
HI-237	*o*-OMe	1.0	0.01	>1 x 10^4
HI-240	*o*-F	0.6	<0.001	>1 x 10^5
HI-253	*o*-Cl	0.7	<0.001	>1 x 10^5
HI-239	*m*-OMe	0.4	0.003	>3 x 10^4
HI-241	*m*-F	0.7	<0.001	>1 x 10^5
HI-254	*m*-Cl	3.1	N.D.	N.D.
1	*p*-OMe	0.9	0.015	>6 x 10^3
HI-242	*p*-F	6.4	N.D.	N.D.
HI-255	*p*-Cl	2.5	N.D.	N.D.
TRV	----	0.8	0.007	>1 x 10^4
AZT	----	>100	0.004	7 x 10^3

[a] Purified recombinant HIV RT assay.

[b] IC_{50} p24 values represent the inhibition of HIV-1 replication in relation to the virus control, as measured by p24 EIA.

[c] SI (selectivity index) = IC_{50}[MTA]/ IC_{50}[p24]. IC_{50}[MTA] values were >100μM.

Table 4. IC_{50} and SI values for series of PETT derivatives.

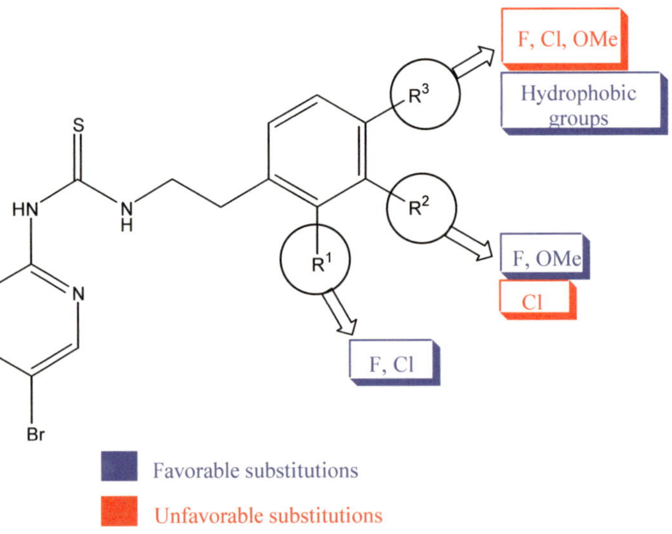

Fig. 4. Preliminary SAR of PETT derivatives.

The authors postulated that the lead compound **HI-240** would be effective against HIV RT mutants (Mao et al., 1999). This hypothesis was confirmed, since **HI-240** is three times more potent than **TRV** against the multiple-drug-resistant of HIV RT, thus emphasizing the relevance of a polar ring substituent, which could provide more favorable interactions with binding site residues (Table **5**).
During this SAR study, Mao and collaborators (Mao et al., 1999) rationally designed a novel PETT analogue (**HI-236**), by using the computer model of NNI binding pocket. This derivative was designed through the optimization of van der Waals contact with the binding pocket, mainly at Wing 2 region, that presents unrecognized spacious regions surrounding the phenyl ring. This strategy would improve the potency against wild-type RT, and also against Wing 2 mutants of RT. In view of the above, the authors proposed the synthesis of **HI-236**, whose 2,5-dimethoxy-substituted phenyl ring allows favorable contacts with Wing 2 region, and also decreases the unoccupied volume surrounding phenyl ring of **HI-240** by 25 $Å^3$. Therefore, **HI-236** showed a potent anti-HIV activity ($IC_{50} <$ 0.001μM), which is lower than IC_{50} values for AZT (0.004 μM). This substance was not cytotoxic, and its calculated selectivity index was > 10^5.
Furthermore, **HI-236** was found to be highly effective against multidrug-resistant HIV-1 strain RT-MDR, whose multiple mutations involve several RT residues (Table **5**). These results are consistent with the prediction according to which **HI-236** would be more active than **HI-240**.

Compounds	**IC_{50} p24**	**IC_{50} RT-MDR[a]**	**IC_{50} A17[b]**	**IC_{50} A17 variant[b]**
HI-236	<0.001	0.005	0.1	11
HI-240	<0.001	0.005	0.2	41
DLV	0.009	0.4	50	>100
NVP	0.034	5	>100	>100
TRV	0.007	0.02	N.D.	N.D.
AZT	0.004	0.15	0.006	0.004

[a] V106A mutation
[b] Genotypic NNRTI-resistant HIV-strains (A17 and A17 variant) carrying clinically relevant mutations Y181C and K103N + Y181C, respectively.

Table 5. Inhibitory activity of **HI-236** and **HI-240** on p24 production in peripheral blood mononuclear cells infected with HIV strains HIV_{IIIB}, RT-MDR, A17 and A17 variant.

In another work, Mao and collaborators (Mao et al, 1998) proposed the synthesis of new PETT analogues through replacement of the planar pyridyl ring of TVR by a non-planar ring, such as a piperidinyl (**HI-172**) or piperazinyl ring (**HI-258**). This modification was based on the presence of unrecognized spacious regions surrounding the pyridyl ring of **TRV** (molecular volume (MV)= 160$Å^3$), which could be better filled than the spacious Wing 2 region of the butterfly-shaped NNI binding pocket. In comparison with the MV of **TRV**, **HI-172** and **HI-258** presented larger MVs (calculated in 276 and 272$Å^3$ respectively), being thus predicted to better fit into the potentially usable space of the binding site.
Furthermore, these heterocyclic rings are conformationally more flexible than the pyridyl ring, such a factor being likely to contribute to fit an uncompromising binding pocket in a more efficient way. Table **6** shows that both compounds were more potent than **TRV**, and that they inhibited HIV replication at nanomolar concentrations, without showing cytotoxicity. These findings indicate that, when compared to **TRV** analogues, double substitutions at axial or equatorial positions on these heterocyclic rings could lead to PETT derivatives with a broader range of curvatures, and that they would also better fit to Wing 2 region.

Compound	IC50 p24	IC50 [MTA]*	SI
HI-172	<0.001	>100	>1 x 105
HI-258	0.002	>100	>5 x 104
TRV	0.007	>100	>1 x 104
AZT	0.006	50	8 x 103

* MTA= Methyl tetrazolium assay

Table 6. IC_{50} and SI values for series of PETT derivatives.

Following their continuous program aiming at the development of new potent PETTs, Uckun and collaborators (Uckun et al., 1999a) decided to replace the pyridyl ring of **TRV** by an aciclyc cyclohexenyl, adamantly or *cis*-myrtanyl ring. Such a proposal of modifications was due to the fact that these chosen groups would fit well with Wing 2 region of the NNI binding pocket. Given the existence of a region compatible with polar atoms at Wing 1, the authors also suggested the replacement of bromine atom by chlorine or trifluoromethyl group (Table **7**). After a biological evaluation, they observed that the replacement of the pyridyl ring of **TRV** by the adamantly **(HI-504)** or *cis*-myrtanyl **(HI-444)** rings resulted in a complete loss of RT inhibitory function. In another important finding, bromine **(HI-346)** / chlorine **(HI-445)** atoms were found to reach the best biological result, thanks to their capacity of making more hydrophobic contacts at the binding pocket, when compared to trifluoromethyl group **(HI-347)**. Moreover, the lead compounds **HI-346** and **HI-445** showed a significant activity against the multidrug resistant (MDR) strain, without presenting cytotoxicity, when administrated at effective concentrations (Table **7**).

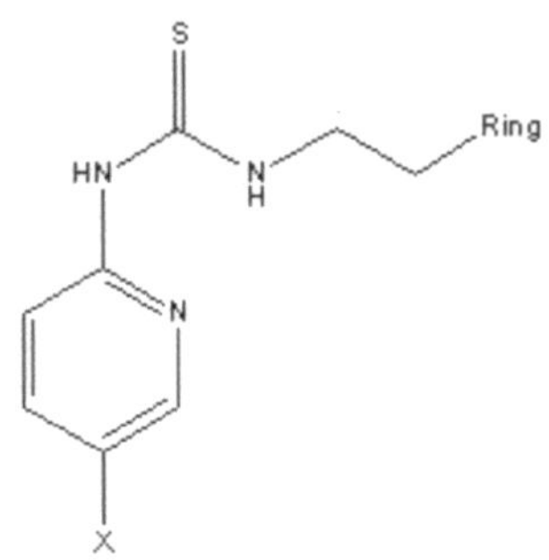

Compound	Ring	X	CC_{50} MTA (μM)	IC_{50} (μM) p24	RT-MDR	A17	A17 variant
HI-346	Cyclo-hexenyl	Br	>100	0.003	0.020	N.D.	18.7
HI-445	Cyclo-hexenyl	Br	>100	0.003	0.001	0.068	30
HI-347	Cyclo-hexenyl	Cl	>100	0.079	0.038	0.300	>100
HI-504	Adamantyl*	CF_3	N.D.[a]	N.D.[a]	N.D.[a]	N.D.[a]	N.D.[a]
HI-444	Myrtanyl*	Br	N.D.[a]	N.D.[a]	N.D.[a]	N.D.[a]	N.D.[a]
TRV	Pyridyl	Br	>100	0.007	0.020	0.500	>100
AZT	-----	----	>100	0.004	0.2	0.006	0.004

* methylene group, instead of ethyl linker
[a] N.D.= not determined, because IC_{50} rRT (μM) > 100

Table 7. CC_{50} and IC_{50} values for series of PETT derivatives.

Uckun and collaborators (Uckun et al., 1999b) carried on performing their PETT derivatives SAR study, and decided to promote new replacements of the pyridyl ring of **TRV** with eight different heterocyclic substituents, including heterocyclic amines, heteroaromatic rings furan and thiophene, as well as aromatic acetal piperonyl. After evaluation of HIV-RT inhibitory activity, the authors concluded that these proposed modifications were critical for the biological activity of said series of compounds, as only the thiophene-substituted derivative **HI-443** inhibited recombinant RT *in vitro* in more than 90% (Table **8**).

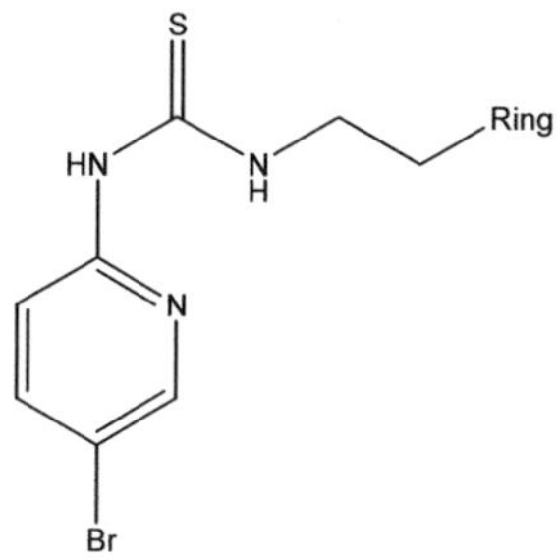

Compound	Ring	IC_{50} rRT (μM)	IC_{90} rRT (μM)
HI-443	Thiophene	0.8	15.0
HI-230	Pyrrolidine	4.9	>100
HI-436	Imidazole	>100	>100
HI-442	Indole	0.9	>100
HI-206	1-methyl-pyrrolidine	>100	>100
HI-276	Morpholine	>100	>100
HI-257	Piperonyl*	0.7	>100
HI-503	Furan*	1.2	>100
TRV	Pyridine	0.6	12.0

* Methylene linker group, instead of an ethyl linker.

Table 8. RT inhibitory activity of PETT derivatives, expressed as IC_{50} and IC_{90} values.

After proceeding with docking studies, it was observed that the thiophene group of **HI-443** occupies the same Wing 2 region of the NNI binding pocket of RT as **TRV**, although with a smaller molecular volume. Moreover, the geometry of hydrogen bond between 2′-NH atom and the amide carbonyl or TR residue 101 deviates from the optimum geometry that authors had observed in relation to **TRV** and other PETT derivatives, such as **HI-172** (Table **6**). Said remarks could justify the lower inhibitory activity of **HI-443** against $HTLV_{IIIB}$ RT, in comparison with **TRV** (Table **9**). Surprisingly, when **HI-443** was assayed against NNI-resistant and MDR-HIV strains, it showed excellent results (Table **9**). This finding is in perfect accordance with the docking analysis, as this latter revealed that thiophene group is located very close to the Y181 residue. Therefore, in the Y181C mutant strains, the sulfur atom from its thiophene group may be more compatible with the sulfur-containing cysteine 181 residue than the pyridyl group of **TRV**.

Compound	CC_{50} MTA (μM)	IC_{50} (μM)			
		p24	RT-MDR	A17	A17 variant
HI-443	>100	0.030	0.004	0.048	3.3
HI-172	>100	<0.001	>100	>100	>100
HI-240	>100	<0.001	0.005	0.200	41
TRV	>100	0.007	0.020	0.500	>100
AZT	>100	0.004	0.2	0.006	0.004

Table 9. Anti-HIV activity of PETT derivatives.

In their next work, Venkatachalam and collaborators (Venkatachalam et al., 2001) designed, synthesized and evaluated 13 aromatic/heterocyclic thiazolyl thiourea compounds, since thiazolyl group was expected to favorably bind to Wing 1 region of the binding pocket of HIV-1 RT (Table **10**).

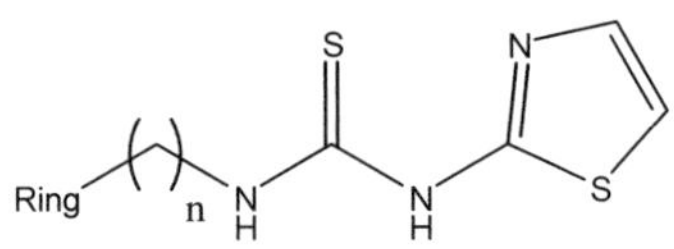

2-14

Compound	n	Ring	IC_{50} (μM)			CC_{50} (μM)	SI
			HTL_{VIIIB}	A17	A17 variant		
2	Et	2-Thiophene	<0.001	>100	N.D.	71	71,000
3	Et	2-Cyclo-hexenyl	0.007	0.9	>100	4	571
4	Et	1-phenoxy	<0.001	4.4	>100	>100	>100,000
5	Et	4-methyl-phenyl	0.07	3.9	>100	>100	1459
6	Me	1-Adamantyl	<0.001	0.6	1.3	40	40,000
7	Pr	2-Furan	<0.001	2.0	0.6	>100	>100,000
8	Et	1-Imidazole	<0.001	>100	>100	35	35,000
9	Et	3-indole	<0.001	2.2	3.7	28	28,000
10	Et	1-pyperidine	>100	N.D.	N.D.	N.D.	N.D.
11	Et	4-hydroxy-phenyl	>100	N.D.	N.D.	N.D.	N.D.
12	Et	2-pyridine	1	N.D.	N.D.	100	100
13	Pr	1-pyrrolidinone	9	N.D.	N.D.	18	2
14	2-Bu	Phenyl	0.009	2.1	1.5	10	1111
NVP	----	----	0.034	>100	>100	N.D.	N.D.
DLV	----	----	0.009	50	>100	N.D.	N.D.

Table 10. Anti-HIV activity of thiazolyl thiourea derivatives.

Among 13 compounds, six lead ones were detected (**2**, **4** and **6-9**). They were 9-34 times more active than the standard NNRTI nevirapine and delavirdine. The compounds **2-9** and **14** were also tested against NNRTI-resistant strains A17 with Y181C mutation and A17 variant with a Y181C plus K103N mutations in RT. The most promising compounds were **6**, **7**, **9** and **14**, as they were effective against both NNRTI-resistant HIV-1 isolates and showed much greater potency against both wild-type and NNRTI-resistant HIV-1 than nevirapine and delavirdine. Among these compounds, the most promising was the **7**, due to its minimal cytotoxic effects on PBMC, as well as to its selectivity index > 100,000.

Subsequently, Venkatachalam and collaborators (Venkatachalam et al., 2000) proposed to study the influence of stereochemistry of Halopyridyl and Thiazolidyl thiourea compounds on their potency as NNRTI. For this purpose, they synthesized and measured anti-HIV activity of *R* and *S* stereoisomers of two cyclohexyl methyl haloperidyl thiourea compounds (**HI-509** and **HI-510**), of two α-methyl benzylhalopyridyl thiourea compounds (**HI-511** and **HI-512**) and of one cyclohexyl ethyl thiazolyl thiourea compound (**HI-513**) (Table **11**).

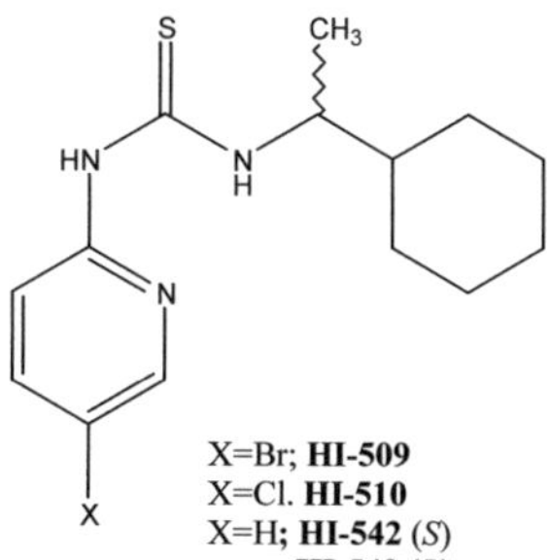

X=Br; **HI-509**
X=Cl. **HI-510**
X=H; **HI-542** (*S*)
HI-543 (*R*)

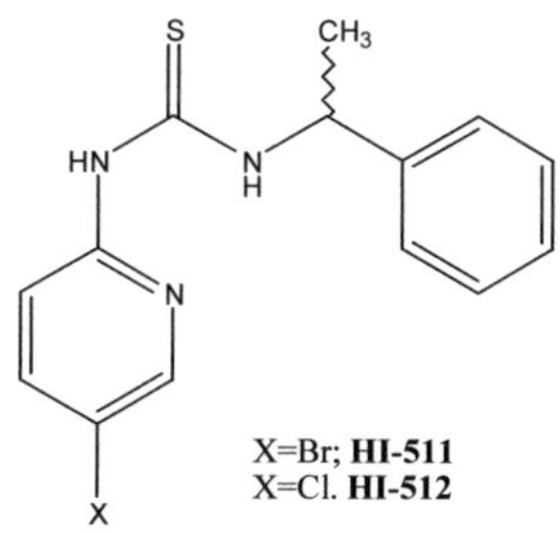

X=Br; **HI-511**
X=Cl. **HI-512**

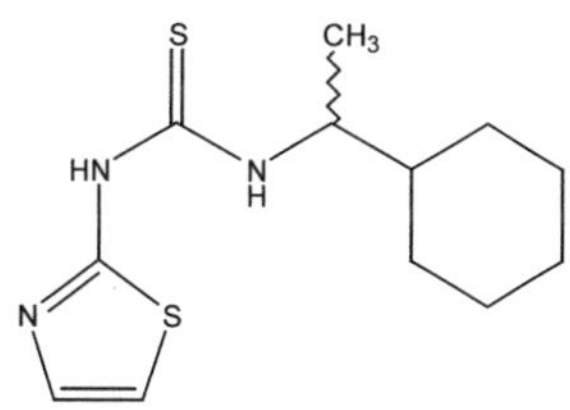

HI-513

Compound	IC$_{50}$ (μM)				
	rRT	**HTLV$_{IIIB}$**	**RT-MDR**	**A17**	**A17 variant**
HI-509(*R*)	1.2	0.001	0.2	0.4	10.0
HI-509(*S*)	>100	>1	N.D.	N.D.	N.D.
HI-510(*R*)	1.4	0.025	0.06	0.07	8.2
HI-510(*S*)	>100	>1	N.D.	N.D.	N.D.
HI-511(*R*)	1.6	0.01	0.005	0.01	2.7
HI-511(*S*)	>100	>1	N.D.	N.D.	N.D.
HI-512(*R*)	1.2	0.010	0.010	0.2	10.2
HI-512(*S*)	>100	>1	N.D.	N.D.	N.D.
HI-513(*R*)	13.0	0.001	5.6	0.9	5.8
HI-513 (*S*)	>100	>1	N.D.	N.D.	N.D.
HI-542 (*S*)	>100	>1	N.D.	N.D.	N.D.
HI-543 (*R*)	>100	>1	N.D.	N.D.	N.D.
TRV	0.8	0.007	0.02	0.5	>100

Table 11. Effects of stereochemistry on anti-HIV activity of thiourea compounds.

The results showed that *R* stereoisomers of all five compounds inhibited the recombinant RT *in vitro* with IC_{50} values that were 100-fold lower. Each one of these five compounds was also active against NNI-resistant HIV-1 strains. Among them, **HI-511(*R*)** (see Table **11**) presented a potent antiviral activity against NNI-resistant and multidrug resistant strains of HIV-1.

Molecular modeling studies indicated that the *R* steroisomer [**HI-509(*R*)**] would fit the target NNI binding pocket on HIV-RT much better than its enantiomer [**HI-509(*S*)**]. Due to the presence of unfavorable steric interactions with the NNI binding pocket residues near the Y181 side chain, **HI-509(*S*)** adopts an energetically unfavorable eclipsed conformation, which reflects in its higher IC_{50} value. These assumptions could also apply in favor of **HI-510(*R*)**. As a relevant data concerning this study, it is worthy to mention that the methyl group on chiral carbon of **HI-509(*R*)** and **HI-510(*R*)** probably promotes the strong binding to the NNI binding pocket via van der Waals with residue V179.

The substitution of the pyridyl ring of **HI-509(*R*)** and **HI-510(*R*)** by a thiazolyl ring (compound **HI-513(*R*)**) resulted in 10-fold higher IC_{50} values in cell free RT inhibition assays, as the unsubstituted thiazole could be better accommodated by the binding site than the unsubstituted pyridine (in combination with the bulky cyclohexylethyl group) as a whole molecule. Nevertheless, halogen substitution on pyridine adds a considerable number of favorable interactions at Wing 1 region, which improves the final interaction score for the substituted pyridine thiourea compounds.

While studying the effect of stereochemistry on anti-HIV activity of chiral thiourea compounds, Venkatachalam and collaborators (Venkatachalam et al., 2004) synthesized two new series of PETT compounds: β-methyl phenylethyl thiourea (β-MPT), and α-methyl benzyl thioureas (α-MBT) (Fig. 5).

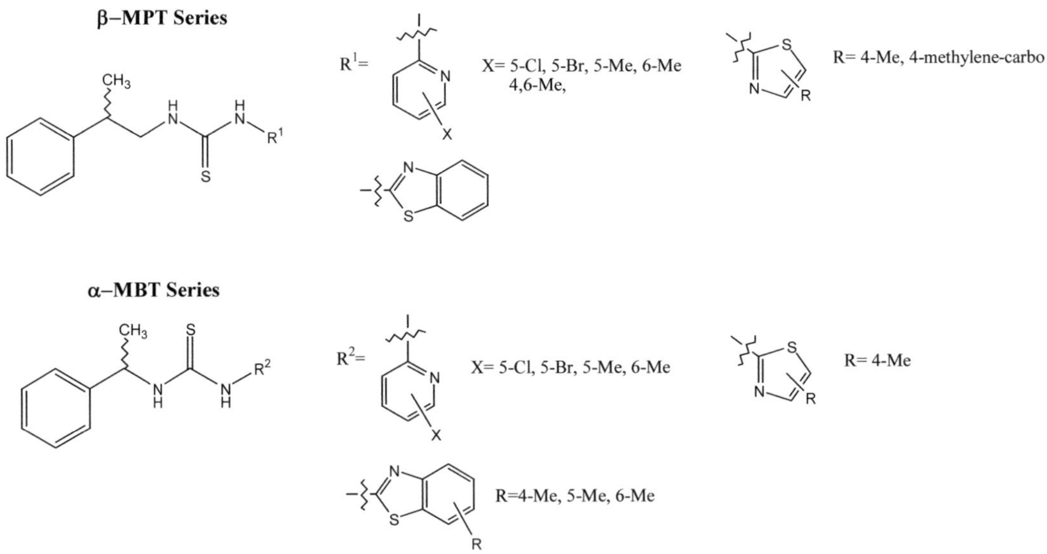

Fig. 5. β-MPT and α-MBT series.

These derivatives were evaluated against HIV-1 strain $HTLV_{IIIB}$, and also against NNRTI-resistant strains. Upon analysis of these results, the authors expressed critical positions regarding SAR of this class of compounds (Fig. 6).

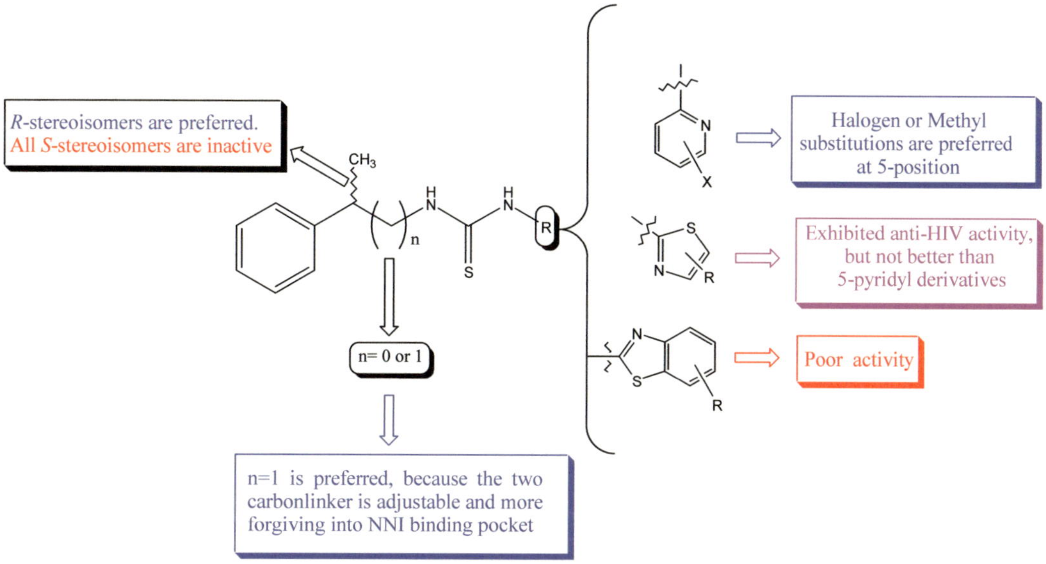

Fig. 6. Complementary SAR study of chiral thiourea compounds.

Among all synthesized compounds, the derivative **15** (Table **12**), namely the *R* isomer 5-chloropyridyl (β-MPT Series), was 380-fold more active than nevirapine, 2-fold more active than trovirdine and 190-fold more potent against A17 than delavirdine. The compound **15** was also >200-fold more potent against A17V than nevirapine, trovirdine or delavirdine. In view of these results, the authors postulated that β-MPT compounds may be useful candidates to further development as anti-HIV agents, especially due to their remarkable activity against mutant strains of HIV-1.

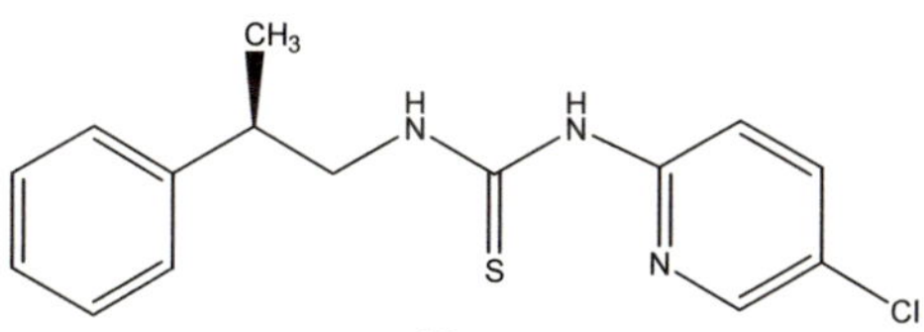

15

Compound	**IC_{50} (μM)**				
	rRT	**$HTLV_{IIIB}$**	**RT-MDR**	**A17**	**A17 variant**
15	0.1	<0.001	0.02	0.3	0.5
TRV	0.8	0.007	0.02	0.5	>100

Table 12. Anti-HIV activity of thiourea derivative 15.

Besides the modifications on the pyridyl ring, Sahlberg and collaborators (Sahlberg et al., 1998) decided to investigate the replacement of thiourea by urea moiety in PETT derivatives. Furthermore, they have prepared compounds with an ethyl linker (Series **I**) and other conformationally restricted cyclopropyl analogues (Series **II**, Table **13)**.

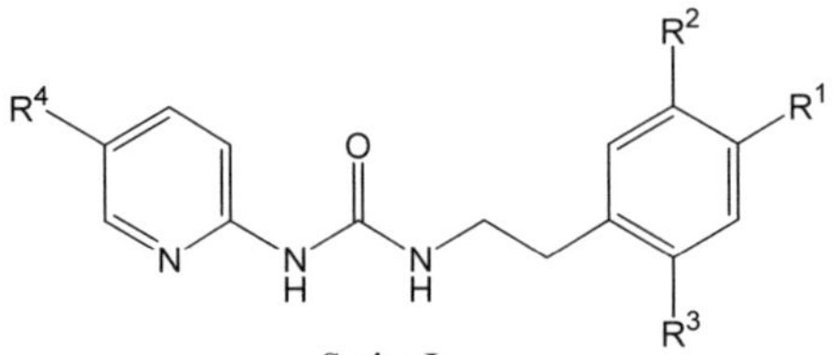

Series **I**
16-21

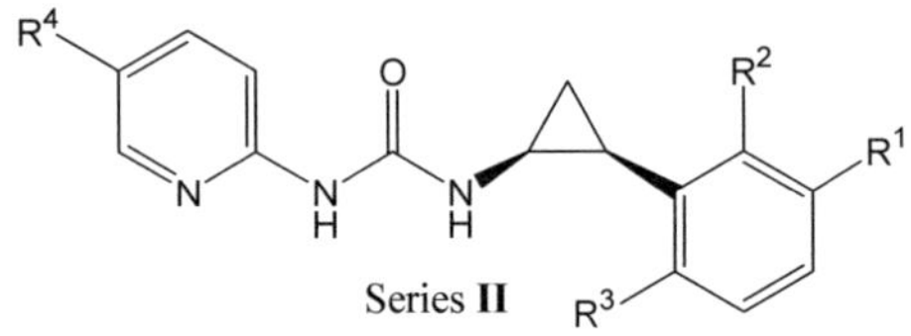

Series **II**
22-28

Compound	R^1	R^2	R^3	R^4	ED_{50} (μM)[a]			
					wt	wt[b]	T181C	L100I
16	H	F	F	Cl	0.03	0.85	>32	32
17	NMe_2	F	F	Br	0.5	N.D.	>25	>25
18	OMe	F	OMe	Cl	0.011	0.09	3	17
19	OEt	F	OMe	Cl	0.13	N.D.	>27	14
20	COMe	F	OMe	Cl	0.2	N.D.	>27	>27
21	OEt	Cl	F	Br	0.07	N.D.	8	15
22	H	F	F	Cl	0.006	0.01	N.D.	N.D.
23	OEt	Cl	F	Cl	0.016	0.06	N.D.	0.1
24	OEt	Cl	F	CN	0.01	0.02	0.53	0.27
25	OEt	F	F	Cl	0.008	0.03	0.27	0.75
26	OMe	F	OMe	Cl	0.012	0.1	2.7	1.6
27	OEt	F	Cl	Cl	0.008	N.D.	0.1	0.1
28	OEt	F	Br	Br	0.025	0.8	N.D.	N.D.
TRV	----	----	----	----	0.02	5	>5	0.8

[a] The cell culture assay used MT4 cells infected with HIV-1_{IIIB}.
[b] The assay contains 15% human AB serum.

Table 13. Inhibition of HIV-1 by urea-PETT compounds.

Cyclopropyl compounds use to be more potent than the ethyl linked ones, especially on mutants (Table **13**). The authors hypothesized that, in comparison with the most restricted cyclopropyl analogues, the most flexible ethyl derivatives might present inconvenient in adopting conformations that fit in the mutant enzymes.
When compared with thiourea analogues, urea derivatives are less active (Fig. 7), although these compounds might have better toxicological and pharmacokinetic properties. In addition, it was verified later that, in cell culture and in the presence of added human serum, urea-PETT compounds keep their antiviral activity in standards that are much higher than those shown by the respective thiourea compounds.

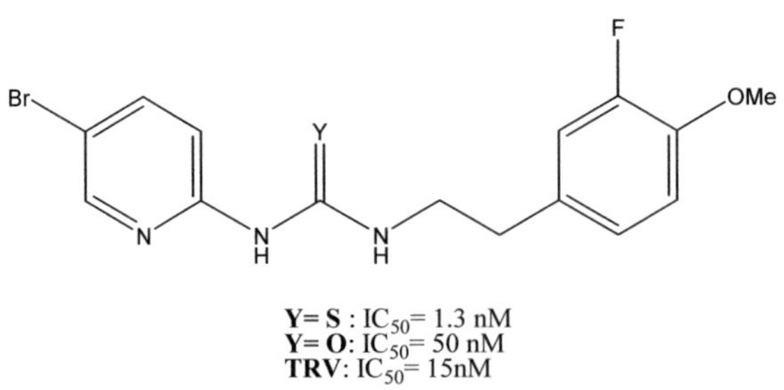

Fig. 7. Anti-HIV activities of thiourea and urea derivatives.

Following this study, Högberg and collaborators (Högberg et al., 2000) have proposed several bioisosteric substitutions of both thiourea and urea moieties of PETT compounds by sulfamide, cyanoguanidine and guanidine groups (Series **III**, Fig.8). Furthermore, they have promoted the replacement of the phenetyl group by benzophenethyl group, in an attempt to evaluate the influence of said modifications on the antiviral activities of this class of compounds (Series **IV**, Fig.8).

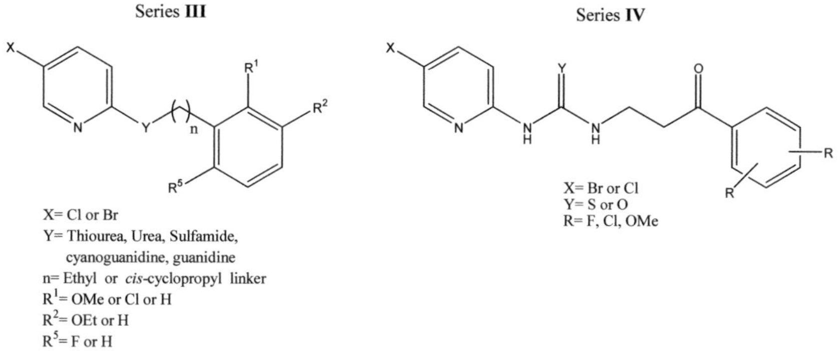

Fig. 8. Structures of two series of PETT analogues, obtained through bioisosteric modifications.

The biological results showed that thiourea and urea moieties play an essential role in the optimal activity of PETT compounds, as all the proposed bioisosteric replacements lead to a reduction (compounds with guanidine group) or to the complete loss of activity (sulfamide and cianoguanidine derivatives). Moreover, the benzoylethyl derivatives were reasonably potent inhibitors of wild-type HIV-1 RT and HIV-1 virus in cell culture. However, these derivatives were less active than the phenethyl compounds (see compound **39**, Table **14**).

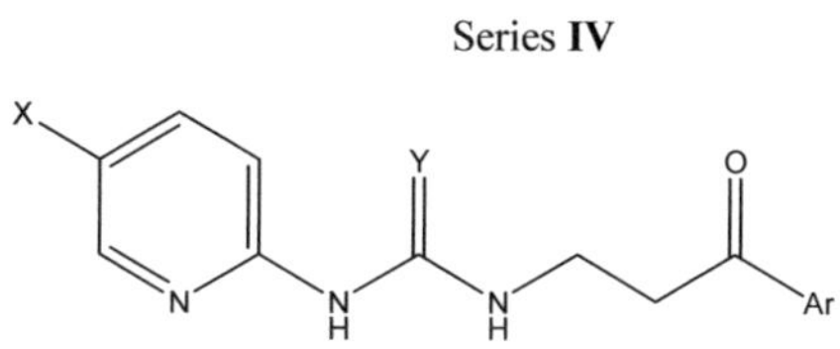

Compound	Ar	Y	X	IC_{50} HIV-1 RT (μM)[a]	ED_{50} (μM)[b]
29	phenyl	S	Br	<0.027	0.036
30	2-F- phenyl	S	Br	0.004	0.009
31	2-Cl- phenyl	S	Br	0.010	0.100
32	2-OMe- phenyl	S	Br	0.003	0.076
33	2-F- phenyl	O	Br	0.054	0.201
34	3-OMe- phenyl	S	Br	0.080	0.911
35	4-F- phenyl	S	Br	0.047	0.300
36	2,5-F- phenyl	S	Br	<0.025	0.067
37	2,6-F- phenyl	S	Br	0.006	0.028
38	2,6-F- phenyl	S	Cl	0.003	0.050
39	2,6-F- phenyl*	S	Br	0.001	0.010

[a] HIV-1 RT assay which used (poly)rC.(oligo)dG as the templae/primer.
[b] Anti-HIV activity assay, using MT4 cells (human T cell line) infected with HIV-1_{IIIB}
*Phenylethyl, instead of benzoylethyl linker.

Table 14. IC_{50} and ED_{50} values for Series **IV**.

3.1.2.3 PETT derivatives as anti-HIV microbicides

D´Cruz and collaborators started to develop a vaginal microbicidal contraceptive, which was potentially able to prevent HIV transmission. Thus, they decided to evaluate two potent anti-HIV PETT derivatives (**HI-240** and **HI-236**, Table **5**), that had been previously identified by Venkatachalam and collaborators (Vig et al, 1998; Mao et al., 1998), in an attempt to verify a possible dual-function, namely its anti-HIV and spermicidal activity. After proceeding with the analysis of the results, they observed that only the derivative **HI-240** showed a spermicidal activity, although the underlying mechanism involved in such a function remains unknown. Moreover, **HI-240** inhibited the sperm motility, in a concentration-and time-dependent way (D´Cruz & Venkatachalam et al., 1999).
Subsequently, the authors investigated the cytotoxic characteristics and selectivity of this compound, and, then, compared their results to nonoxynol-9 (**N-9**), which is the most widely used vaginal spermicide. This substance immobilizes sperm, as a result from a detergent-type action on the sperm plasma membrane. Due to its membrane-disruptive properties, a continued use of **N-9** has been shown to be likely to damage the cervicovaginal epithelium, causing an acute tissue inflammatory response, and thus enhancing the probability of HIV infection by heterosexual transmission. When compared with **N-9, HI-240** was selectively spermicidal, without detergent-type toxicity against membrane of the female genital tract, which may present significant clinical advantages. Another important feature of **HI-240** may still be pointed out, namely the possibility for spermicidal NNI to remain stable as protonated species, even within the acidic environment of the vagina, due to the presence of pyridine ring, containing a basic nitrogen atom. Furthermore, the vaginal concentrations of this substance required for dual-action anti-HIV and spermicidal activity are well below the systemic concentrations achieved by the oral dosages that are generally prescribed for NNIs.
In view of these promising results, D´Cruz and collaborators (D´Cruz et al., 2000) decided to evaluate other 31 PETT derivatives for anti-HIV and sperm inhibitory activity (SIA) (Fig.9).

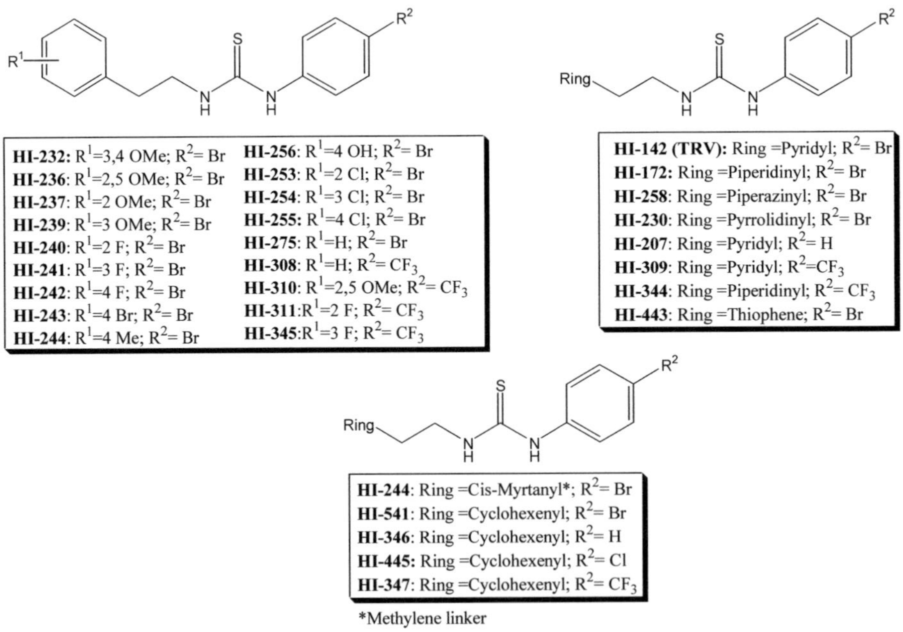

Fig. 9. Structures of thiourea derivatives, evaluated as spermicidal microbicides.

Among all these substances, they identified several dual-function of thiourea compounds, such as the phenyl ring-containing derivatives **HI-240** (2-fluoro), **HI-253** (2-chloro) and **HI-255** (4-chloro) and the cyclohexenyl ring-containing derivatives **HI-346** and **HI-445**, which were identified as potential lead compounds for the development of clinically useful dual-function anti-HIV spermicides (Table **15**). In this study, the authors also demonstrated that, at a spermicidal concentration, the dual-function thiourea derivatives were selectively spermicidal, without cytotoxic effects against human vaginal, ectocervical and endocervical epithelial cells .

Compound	**IC_{50} (μM)**		**EC_{50} (μM) SIA**
	p24	**rRT**	
HI-240	<0.001	0.60	147 ± 18
HI-253	<0.001	0.70	70 ± 8
HI-255	0.001	2.50	160 ± 16
HI-346	0.003	0.6	42 ± 9
HI-445	0.003	0.5	57 ± 5
HI-142 (TRV)	0.007	0.8	>500

Table 15. Effect of PETT derivatives on p24 antigen production in HIV-infected PBMC, as well as enzymatic activity of HIV-1 RT and human sperm mobility.

Considering that the most promising dual-function microbicides PETTs were **HI-346** and **HI-445**, which are cyclohexenyl ring-containing derivatives, D´Cruz and collaborators decided to investigate other cyclohexenyl thiourea (CHET) compounds, in order to examine the way how heterocyclic rings and their functionalization affect the anti-HIV and SIA potency of these substances (D´Cruz et al., 2002a). Furthermore, some urea compounds were also evaluated, in an attempt to determine the role of thiourea moiety in the biological activity of these series (Table **16**).

In view of the data obtained, the authors concluded that, among the thiazolyl-ring containing CHET compounds, only the 4-methyl-substituted derivative (**42**) showed a significant anti-HIV activity. As a matter of fact, compounds containing benzothiazole-ring generally present poor anti-HIV activities. Among the compounds containing *N*-pyridyl nucleus, the functionalization at 5-position with bromine, chlorine and methyl groups led to a potent anti-HIV activity of CHET compounds. The thiourea moiety was essential to trigger said anti-HIV activity, as its replacement by urea group either abolished (**44**) or reduced (**45**) the biological activity.

Among 15 derivative compounds that were evaluated for spermicidal potential, 12 showed an improvement of spermicidal function, when analyzed at micromolar concentrations. The authors observed that compounds with methyl group at 4- or 6-postion were non-spermicidal, even at concentrations >500μM. The pyridyl-ring containing CHET compounds with bromine or chlorine attached to 5-position showed an excellent SIA activity, in addition to their remarkable anti-HIV activity. Interestingly, the urea compounds, although having retained SIA, presented a poor anti-HIV activity, . Another curious data arises from the comparison between the values of $T_{1/2}$ relating to thiourea and urea compounds, showing that urea analogues immobilized sperm 38-fold faster than thiourea derivatives.

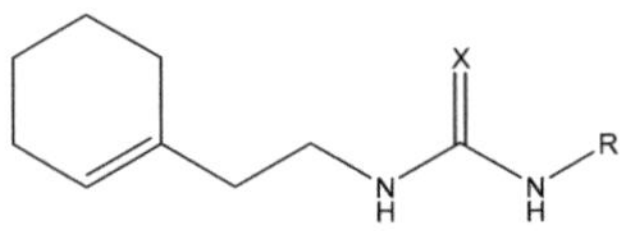

Compound	X	R	HIV		Sperm	
			IC50 [rRT] (μM)	IC50 [p24] (μM)	EC50 [SIA] (μM)	T1/2* (min)
40	S	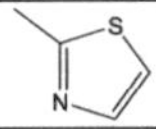	>100	0.03	80 ± 3	1.0 ± 0.2
41	S	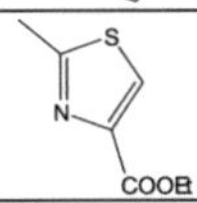	>100	N.D.	132 ± 22	77 ± 3
42	S	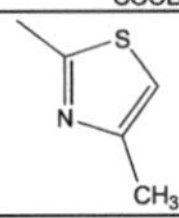	3.0	0.008	>500	>180
43	S	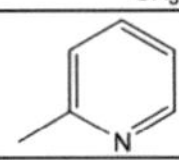	22.2	0.03	144 ± 18	37 ± 5
HI-346	S	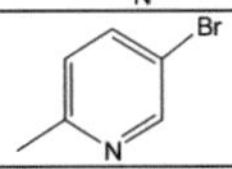	0.6	0.003	45 ± 9	65 ± 6
44	O	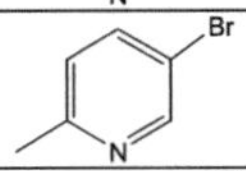	>100	N.D.	100 ± 4	1.5 ± 0.1
HI-445	S	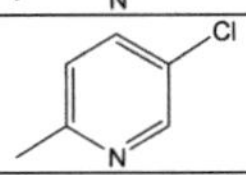	0.5	0.003	60 ± 5	34 ± 2
45	O	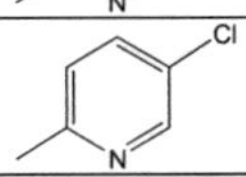	12.3	N.D.	113 ± 9	0.9 ± 0.1
46	S	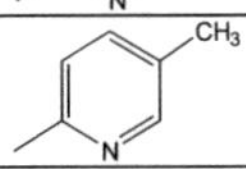	1.2	0.005	96 ± 7	34 ± 2
47	S	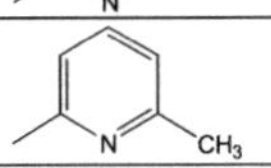	5.6	0.017	>500	>180
48	S	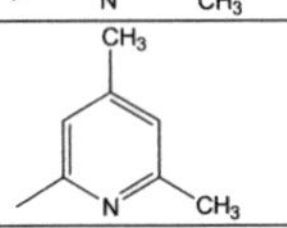	>100	N.D.	45 ± 7	80 ± 2
49	S	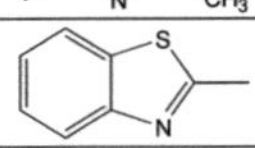	2.0	0.02	149 ±16	70 ± 6
50	S	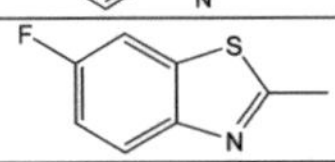	>100	N.D.	194 ± 20	63 ± 2
51	S	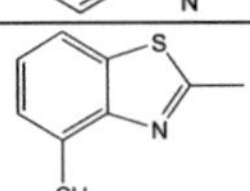	>100	N.D.	>500	>180
52	S	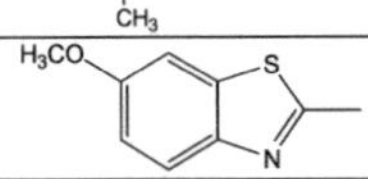	>100	N.D.	261 ± 12	>180

* Time required for 50% sperm mobility loss.

Table 16. Anti-HIV and sperm immobilization activity of a serie of PETT derivatives.

Furthermore, the lead compounds **HI-346** and **HI-445** were evaluated in their activity against NNI-resistant strains (RT-MDR, A17 variant), and were found to be more effective than **TRV**, delavirdine and nevirapine. These findings established the dual-function compounds **HI-346** and **HI-445** as potent NNI of drug-sensitive, as well as multidrug-resistant strains of HIV-1.

Due to the fact that the compound **HI-346** is a broad-spectrum anti-HIV agent with SIA, and also to the characteristic of its urea analogue **44** as an extremely rapid spermicidal, the authors decided to evaluate the *in vivo* fertilizing ability of sperm exposed to the lead dual-function CHET compound **HI-346,** either alone or in combination with its structural analogue (compound **44)**, in the rabbit model. They observed that the conception was completely inhibited after insemination with semen treated with compound **44,** or **HI-346** plus **44**.

As to the cytotoxic profile, CHET-NNIs showed high selectivity indexes against these genital tract epithelial cells *in vitro*. Moreover, in rabbits, the lead thiourea/urea compounds are not harmful to vaginal mucosa, in spite of their potent spermicidal properties, when added either to human or to rabbit semen.

These results indicated that the extremely rapid SIA of the urea analogue, as well as the broad-spectrum anti-HIV activity of spermicidal CHET-NNIs, together with their lack of mucosal toxicity and the remarkable ability to reduce *in vivo* fertility, appear as features that are particularly attractive to encourage the clinical development of a dual-function spermicidal microbicide (D´Cruz et al., 2002a).

The next step performed by D´Cruz and collaborators was the investigation on subchronic intravaginal toxicity of **HI-346** in mice. Thus, **HI-346** was formulated via lipophilic gel-microemulsion for intravaginal use as a potential dual-function microbicide. In order to evaluate the potential toxicity of short-term intravaginal exposure to **HI-346**, groups of 15 female B6C3F1 and CD-1 mice underwent an intravaginal exposure to a gel-microemulsion containing 0, 0.5, 1.0, or 2.0% **HI-346**, 5 days per week, for 13 consecutive weeks. Subsequently, the authors concluded that repetitive intravaginal administration of **HI-346** to yield effective spermicidal and antiviral concentrations is not expected to lead to local, systemic, or reproductive toxicity (D´Cruz et al., 2002b).

In another study, D´Cruz and collaborators decided to evaluate the PETT derivative **HI-236** as microbicide, as, in accordance with a previous work, this compound had already presented a broad-spectrum of anti-HIV activity (Mao et al., 1999). In view of the above the authors demonstrated that **HI-236** showed a high-selectivity index against both human vaginal and cervical epithelial cells, without affecting the human sperm functions. Furthermore, **HI-236** was able to prevent the HIV systemic infection via vaginal route. Therefore, **HI-236** presented a clinical utility as non-spermicidal microbicide to curb the transmission of HIV via semen: (a) in sexually active women, to allow pregnancy, while protecting both mother and her fetus or infant from HIV-1 and (b) as a prophylactic antiviral agent for HIV-1 serodiscordant couples, or for use before assisted reproductive technology procedures (D´Cruz & Uckun, 2005).

3.2 Thiourea derivatives with potential activity against TB

3.2.1 Isoxyl

The thiocarbanilide Isoxyl (**ISO**, thiocarlide, 4,4′-diisoamythio-carbanilide) (Fig.1) was synthesized in 1953 by Buu-Hoi an Xuong. In this work, the authors described the antimicobacterial activity of several thioureas, among which some are more active than **ISO;** however, this substance was chosen for subsequent assays, due to its better absorption, and also to its good tolerance even at the highest therapeutic doses (König, 1970). Pharmacological data demonstrated that, upon this drug ingestion, the human serum presented fluctuating levels of **ISO,** that exceeded its minimum inhibitory concentration (Tousek, 1970). Besides, given its remarkable characteristics, this substance has been used at the clinical treatment of TB since the 1960's. **ISO** was employed both: in monotherapy and in combined therapy, such as: ISO-isoniazid (I), ISO-streptomycin (S), ISO-I-S and ISO-*para*-aminosalicylic acid (PAS). These studies reached good results (some of which are shown at Table **17**), especially in patients with pulmonary TB resistant to isoniazid, streptomycin and PAS, as well as in patients with hyper allergic reactions against others drugs or hepatitis as a result from I (Tousek, 1970; Urbancik, 1970). However, when compared with other combinatory regimes, such as I-PAS and S-PAS, the results achieved with **ISO** appeared to be quite mediocre, thus culminating with the introduction of more powerful antituberculosis drugs, such as ethambutol, and with the consequent discontinuation of **ISO** administration. Nevertheless, in view of the worldwide dissemination of MDR-TB and XDR-TB (World Health Organization, 2010a), a re-evaluation of drugs which were formerly deemed to be effective against TB is a promising strategy for the development of new treatments, so that, in this context, **ISO** may be considered as a strong candidate.

Combination	**Months of therapy**	**Negative on culture (%)[a]**
ISO (6 g)	1.5 - 4.5	47
ISO - I (6 g/600 mg)	4	89
ISO - I (6 g/10 mg/Kg)	6	75
ISO - I (6 g/5 mg/Kg)	6	63
ISO - S - I (4 g/1 g/200 mg)	6	83
ISO - PAS (6 g/12 g)	6	50

[a]percentage of patients who had presented negative cultures.

Table 17. Examples of results achieved in clinical trials with ISO (Tousek, 1970)

In a recent report, Phetsuksiri and collaborators (Phetsuksiri et al., 1999) evaluated the minimal inhibitory concentration (MIC) of **ISO** against various clinical isolates of susceptible and MDR-TB strains (Table **18**). The growing of all tested strains was inhibited at low concentrations, with a MIC ranging between 1-10μg/mL, which are smaller than the maximum serum levels observed in humans for **ISO** (10-13.2μg/mL) (König, 1970). The authors also verified the effect of **ISO** on viable *M. tuberculosis in vitro* bone marrow macrophage assay, where this substance showed an ability to inhibit bacterial growth inside the macrophage, as well as a bactericidal activity, by reducing the initial inoculum of virulent *M. tuberculosis*. Another interesting result from this assay disclosed that **ISO** showed no acute level of toxicity for mouse macrophages.

Together with the early studies performed with **ISO** in the 1960s, the recent results corroborate the capacity of this substance to be used as an anti-TB drug, particularly in the development of new regimes to MDR and XDR-TB treatment. Such a characteristic is a direct result from **ISO** mechanism of action, which considerably differs from those presented by other known anti-TB drugs.

Strain Designation	Drug Resistance	MIC (µg/mL)
CSU 15	I	5.0
CSU 21	I, R, E, S, Rfb	5.0
CSU 22	I, R, E, S, Kan, Cap, AMK	10.0
CSU 31	I, R, E	10.0
CSU 32	I, R, E, Cyc, ETH, Z	10.0
CSU 37	--	5.0
CSU 39	I, R, S, Kan, AMK, ETH	10.0
CSU 44	I, R, E, S, Kan, Z	10.0
W 670	I, R, E, S, Kan	5.0
W 3432	I, R, E, S, Kan, AMK, ETH, Cip	5.0
BB	--	1.0
LL	I, R, S, Kan, AMK, Z	1.0

kanamycin (Kan), cycloserine (Cyc), rifabutin (Rfb), ethionamide (ETH), amikacin (AMK), capreomycin (Cap).

Table 18. Minimal inhibitory concentration of **ISO** against susceptible and MDR-TB strains.

3.2.2 Mechanism of action

Similarly to what happens with Isoniazid, a substance used in the first line treatment of TB, and with ethionamide, a second line drug, **ISO** strongly inhibits the synthesis of mycolic acids. However, **ISO** can also inhibit shorter chain fatty acid synthesis, thus producing an effect that had never been observed in other drugs showing antimycobacterial properties (Phetsuksiri et al., 2003).

ISO interferes in the fatty acid metabolism, through inhibition of the Δ9 desaturase DesA3. This mechanism leads to the inhibition of the of oleic acid synthesis, which is the most abundant unsaturated fatty acid in *Mycobacterium* spp. and a constituent of mycobacterial membrane phospholipids. Due to the vital functions of oleic acid, the inhibition of its synthesis leads to cell death. Another membrane phospholipid constituent which is indirectly affected during this pathway is the tuberculostearic acid, given that this substance is synthesized through direct methylation of oleic acid by S-adenosylmethionine.

ISO inhibitory mechanism in mycolic acids synthesis has not been described. Nevertheless, it was already demonstrated that there is no relationship between oleic acid and mycolic acids synthesis inhibition (Phetsuksiri et al., 2003).

Another relevant aspect involved in the **ISO** mechanism of action concerns the fact that its activation by the flavin-containing monooxygenase EthA is mandatory to trigger an activity against *M. tuberculosis* (Korduláková, 2007). Based on the LC/MS analyses of the compounds formed after **ISO** treatment with the partially purified recombinant EthA (compounds **53**, **55** and **57**, Fig. 10), the following activation pathway was proposed: Initially, oxidation reactions with sulfur atom lead to the formation of intermediary **54**, which undergoes an elimination reaction, yielding the formimidamide **55**. Further reactions lead to the formation of carbodiimide **56**, which can be hydrolyzed, yielding the urea derivative **57** (Fig. 10). The data obtained from previous studies with ETH and thiacetazone could suggest that **ISO** would be a prodrug, activated by oxidations reactions catalyzed by EthA, and that carbodiimide **56** would appear as its active form. However, the real function of this process and its role in the inhibition of oleic acid and/or mycolic acids synthesis are not well understood. Besides, it is worthy to consider that EthA could only serve to retain **ISO** or its metabolites inside the bacterial cell.

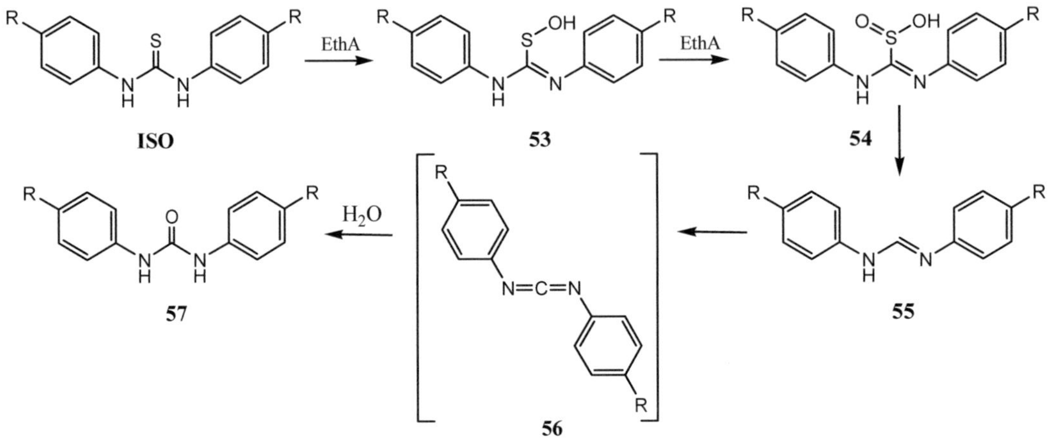

Fig. 10. Proposed pathway for **ISO** activation by EthA.

3.2.3 ISO analogues

In spite of the interesting results shown by the prior clinical trials with **ISO** , this substance was found to present some pharmacokinetic disadvantages, which limited its clinical use as an antimycobacterial agent (Wang & Hickey, 2010). In view of the above, and in an attempt to overcome this kind of inconvenient, several **ISO** derivatives have been synthesized throughout the last years, as may be illustrated by the following examples.

Phetsuksiri and collaborators described the antimycobacterial evaluation of series of **ISO** analogues (Phetsuksiri et al., 1999). These compounds were prepared through random substitutions in the side chains attached to the thiourea nucleus, which it is required for animycobacterial activity (Phetsuksiri et al., 2003; Kordulákovà, 2007). This strategy led to the formation of a pool of new **ISO** derivatives, which present variations both in the symmetric and asymmetric side chains with alkyl, alkoxy or sulfur fuctional groups substituted in *para* and *para´* positions (Table **19**).

Said results show that the most part of derivatives presented a similar or a better activity (MIC <0.1 to 2.5μg/mL), when compared to **ISO** (MIC= 2.0μg/mL). Among some relevant aspects concerning SAR, it may be noted that the replacement of oxygen **(58-60)** by sulfur **(62-64)** in the side chain provides a considerable improvement in the antimycobacterial activity. Moreover, the introduction of a long alkyl chain plus an ester group leads to the formation of inactive compounds **(67,68)**. Bulky groups, such as *t*-butyl, attached to *para* and *para´* position of phenyl ring, also gave rise to an inactive derivative **(65)**. These results suggest that chemical modifications on thiourea nucleus basis could lead to the constitution of an inhibitor, that would be even more powerful against *M. tuberculosis*.

In another study, Bhowruth and collaborators (Bhowruth et al., 2006) synthesized and evaluated series of symmetrical and unsymmetrical **ISO** analogues against *M. tuberculosis* (Table **20**). Several compounds disclosed by this study present similar or better activities than **ISO** (MIC <0.1 to 1.56μg/mL). It is worthy to mention that the introduction of an aliphatic C_4 chain to either or both R^1 and R^2-positions increased the potency of the inhibitor **(76-79, 81)**. Among them, the derivatives **78** and **79** were the most active, with a significant 10-fold increase in potency against *M. tuberculosis,* when compared to **ISO**.

Compound	Structure	MIC_{99} (μg/mL)*
58	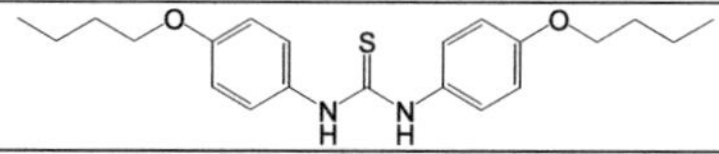	0.1-0.5
59	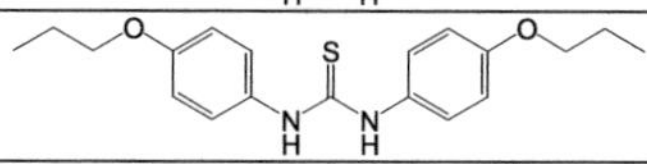	0.1-0.5
60	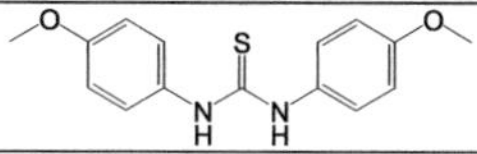	1.0
61	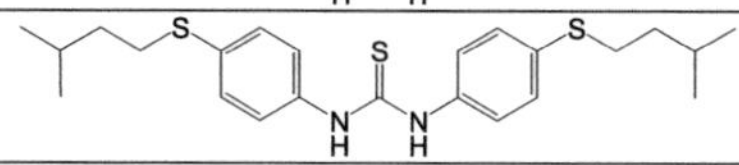	2.5
62	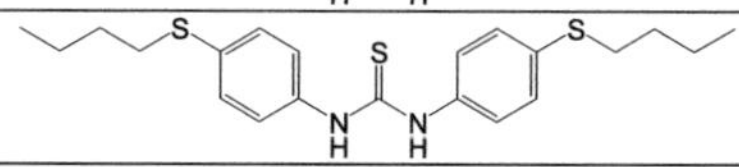	<0.1
63	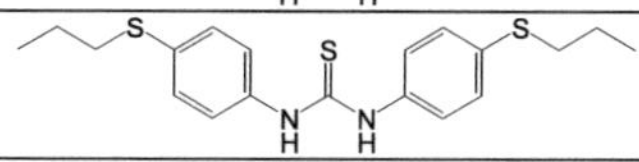	<0.1
64	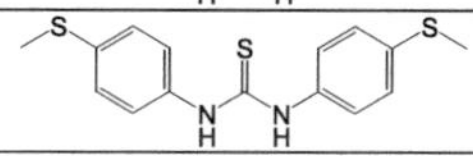	0.5
65	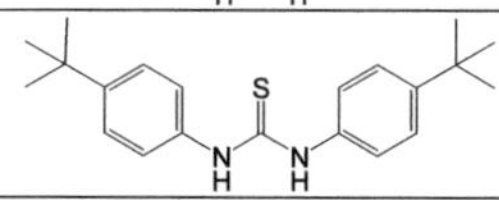	>20.0
66	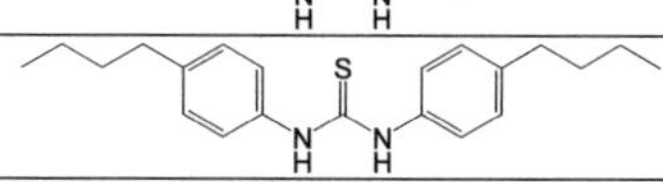	0.1-0.5
67	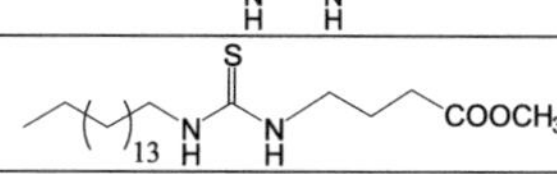	>20.0
68	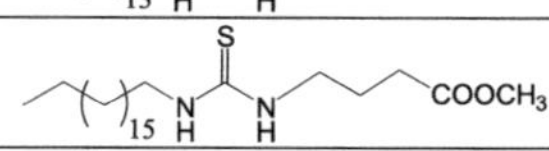	>20.0
69	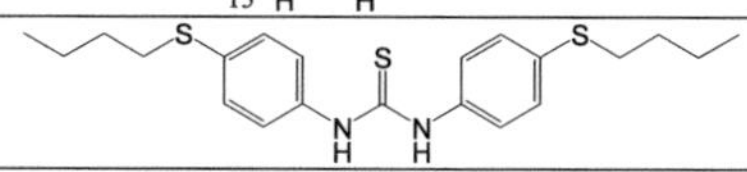	N.D.
70	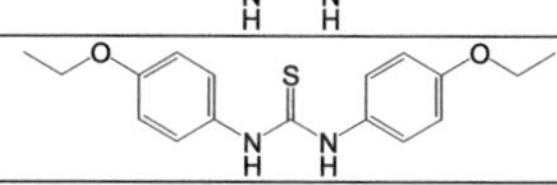	1.0
71	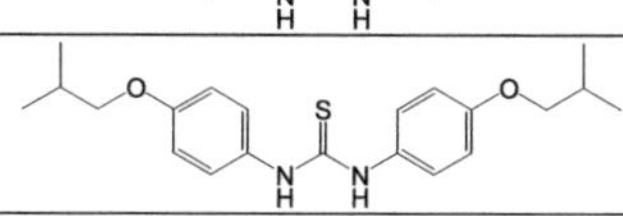	0.5
72	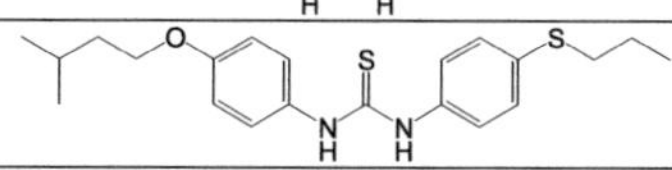	0.1
73	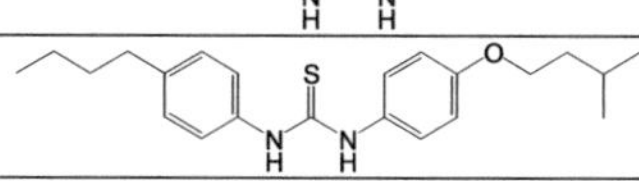	0.5
74	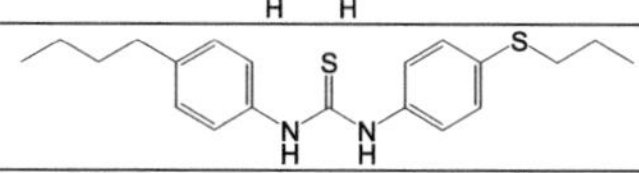	0.5
ISO	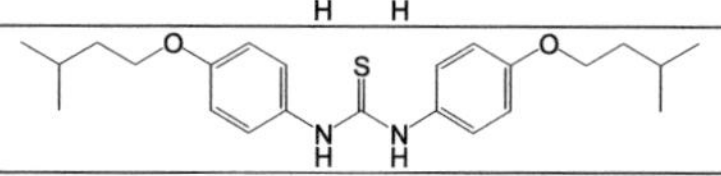	2.0

* MIC_{99} is defined as the lowest concentration of compound that reduced 99% of the number of *M. tuberculosis* colonies on the plates, in comparison with those at the control plate free of compound.

Table 19. **ISO** analogues prepared by Phetsuksiri and collaborators, as well as their respective MIC values.

Compound	Structure	MIC$_{99}$ (μg/mL)*
75	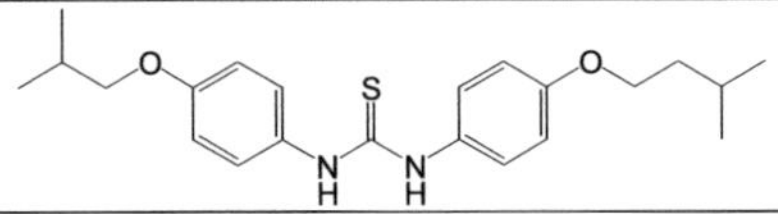	0.9
76	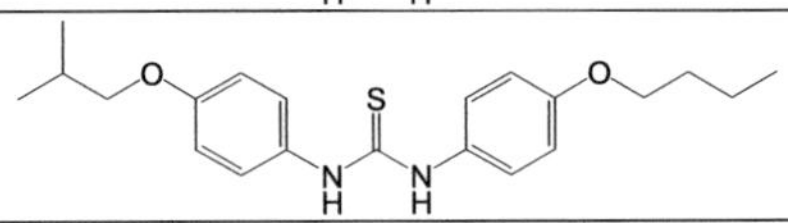	0.6
77	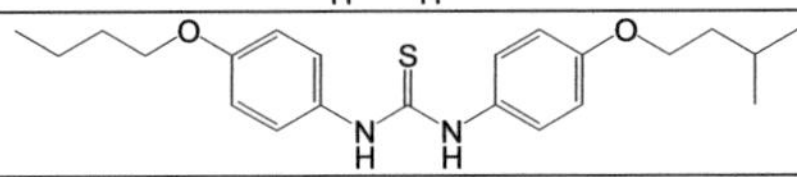	0.4
78	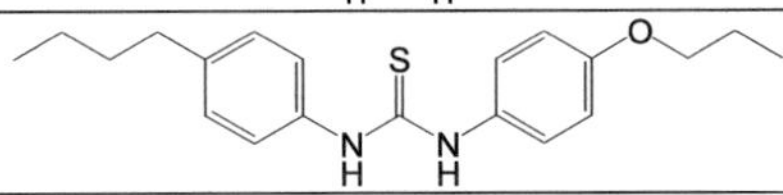	<0.1
79	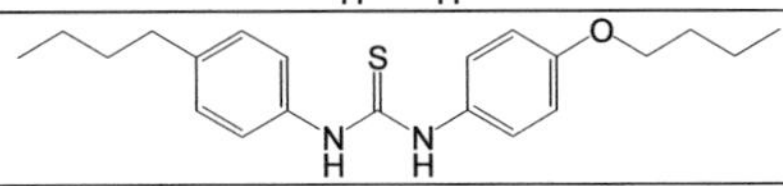	0.7
80	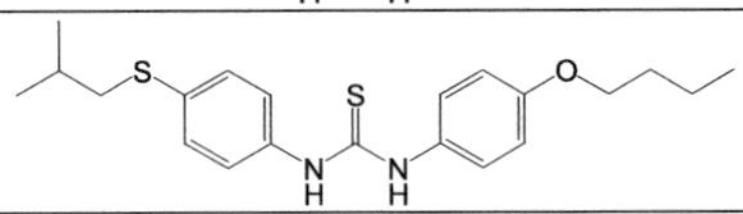	>6.25
81	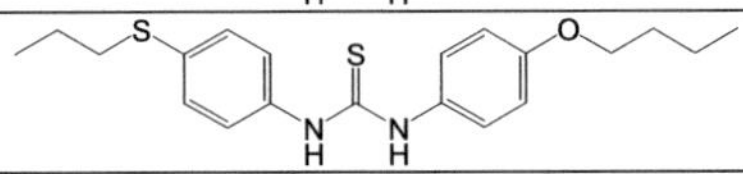	0.2
82	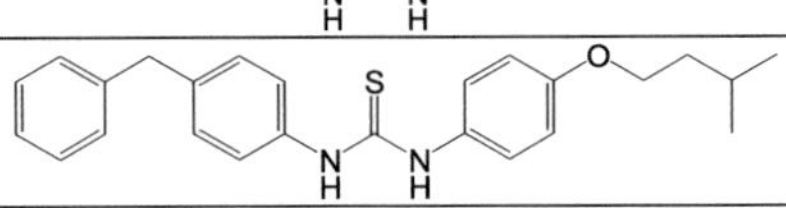	0.2
83	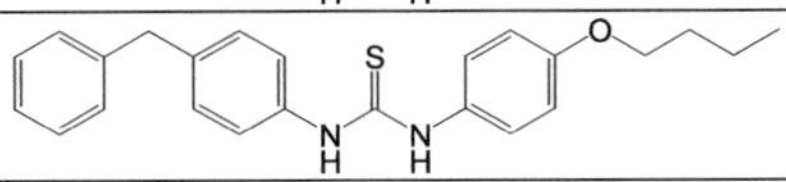	0.39
84	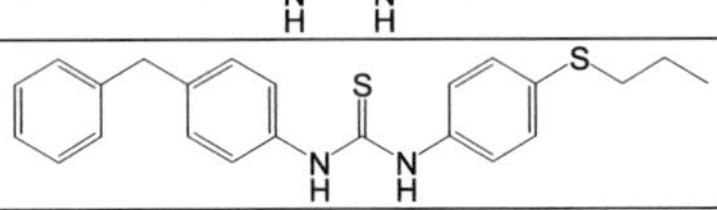	1.56
85	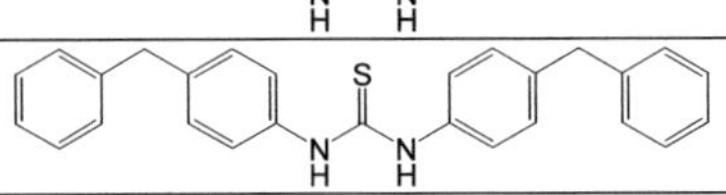	3.13
86	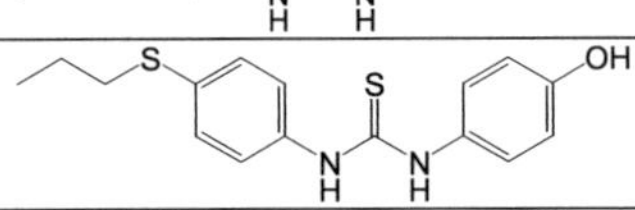	0.39
87	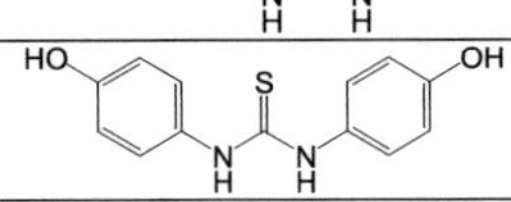	5.0
ISO	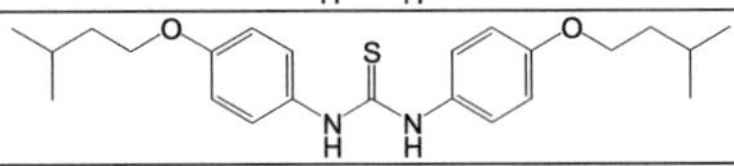	2.0

Table 20. Structures and antimycobacterial activity of ISO derivatives.

Liav and collaborators investigated the effect of replacement of one of the isoamyloxyphenyl **ISO** moieties by a carbohydrate (Liav et al., 2008a). Said modification aimed at the production of **ISO** analogues with better hydrophilic properties, which could be useful to mitigate the inconvenient represented by the poor bioavailability of this drug (Fig.11). Among these compounds, only the arabinfuranosyl derivative **90** has a MIC value of 2.5μg/mL, which is almost more potent than **ISO**.

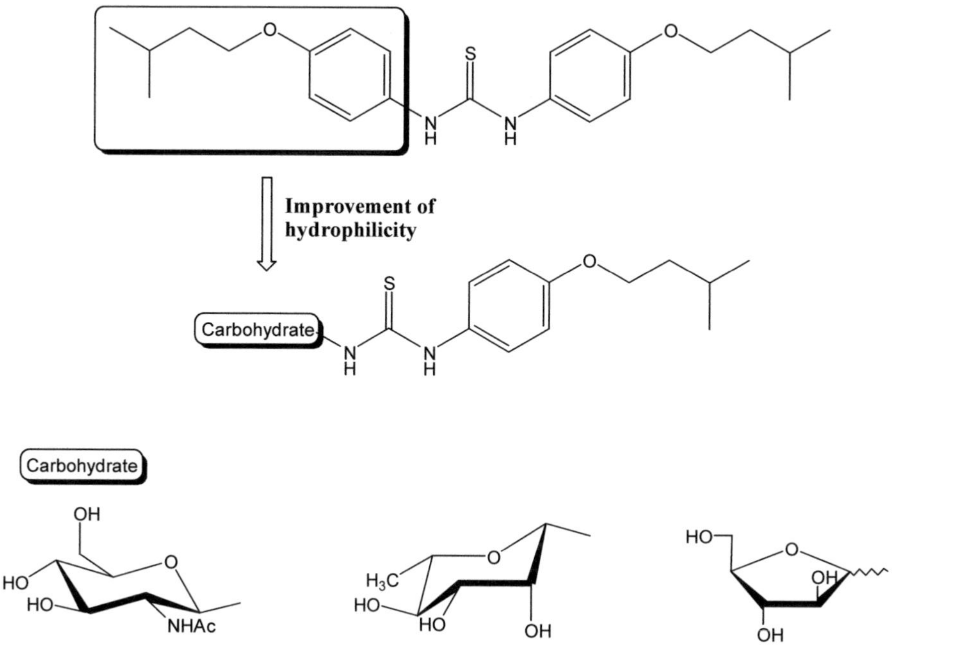

88 MIC= 50-100μg/mL | **89** MIC=8μg/mL | **90** MIC=2.5μg/mL

Fig. 11. **ISO** derivatives containing carbohydrates moieties.

This promising result encouraged Liav and collaborators (Liav et al., 2008b) to synthesize and evaluate the D-aldopentofuranosyl derivatives (**90-93**, Fig.12). Arabino analogue (**90**) was re-tested, and found to be more potent than **ISO**, while the ribo analogue (**91**) presented a MIC value in the same range of **ISO**. The D-xylo analogue (**92**) was rather less active, and the D-lyxo product (**93**) only acted at a concentration of 50μg/mL. These results could suggest that the products are very sensitive to stereochemical configuration, thus indicating that the carbohydrate group does not only add the required hydrophilicity to the molecule, being also responsible for adding specificity to it.

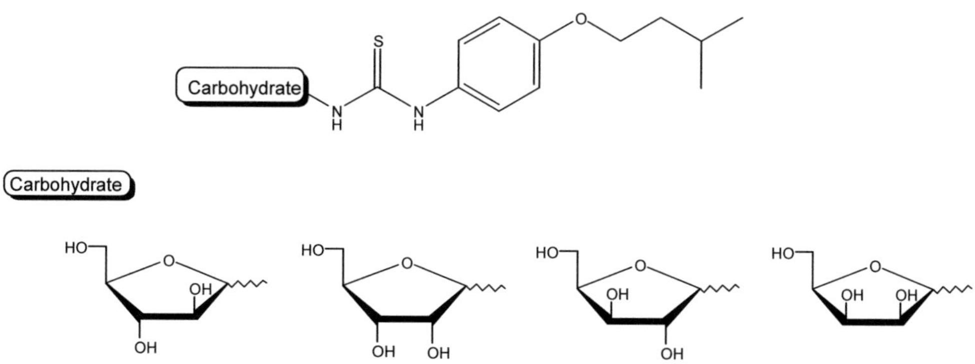

90 MIC=1.56-3.12μg/mL | **91** MIC=3.12-6.25μg/mL | **92** MIC=6.25-12.5μg/mL | **93** MIC=50μg/mL

Fig. 12. Other **ISO** derivatives containing carbohydrates moieties.

4. Conclusion

Thiourea is a very important functional group for anti-HIV and anti-TB drug discovery, and, as seen above, literature has already described the promising biological activities of several derivatives. In the context of AIDS drug discovery, this scaffold is found in two remarkably important classes of compounds, namely among PETT and TIBO derivatives. The PETT compound **TRV** has been exploited as an excellent lead compound, whose several derivatives have been described. TIBO derivatives were essential for the development of NNRTI, a class of antiretroviral agents that currently present a relevant role in AIDS treatment. In parallel, as refers to TB drug discovery, **ISO** was found to present promising activities against resistant strains, especially due to its unique mechanism of action. In view of said data, the development of substances containing thiourea moiety and showing a potential activity against both diseases could be considered an important research field, which should be particularly orientated towards the improvement of therapeutic options for HIV-TB co-infected patients.

5. References

Abdool, K. S. S., Naidoo, K., Grobler, A. et al. (2010). Timing of initiation of antiretroviral drugs during tuberculosis therapy. *The New England Journal of Medicine*, vol. 362, no. 8, pp. 697–706, ISSN 0028-4793.

Ahgren, C., Backro, K., Bell, F.W. et al. (1995). The PETT Series, a New Class of Potent Nonnunleoside Inhibitors of Human Immunodeficiency Virus Type 1 Reverse Transcriptase. *Antimicrobial Agents and Chemotherapy*, vol. 39, No.6, pp.1329-1335, ISSN 0066-4804.

Antonelli, L.R.V., Mahnke, Y., Hodge, J.N. et al. (2010). Elevated frequencies of highly activated CD4+ T cells in HIV+ patients developing immune reconstitution inflammatory syndrome. *Blood*, vol. 116, No.19, pp. 3818-3827,ISSN 0006-4971.

Bell, F.W., Cantrell, A.S., Högberg, M. et al. (1995). Phenethylthiazolethiourea (PETT) Compounds, a New Class of HIV-1 Reverse Transcriptase Inhibitors. 1. Synthesis and Basic Structure-Activity Relationship Studies of PETT Analogs. *Journal of Medicinal Chemistry*, vol. 38, pp.4929-4936, ISSN 0022-2623.

Bhowruth, V., Brown, A.K., Reynolds, R.C. et al. (2006). Symmetrical and unsymmetrical analogues of isoxyl; active agents against Mycobacterium tuberculosis. *Bioorganic & Medicinal Chemistry Letters*, vol.16, No.18, pp. 4743–4747, ISSN 0960-894X.

Blanc, F. X., Sok, T. & Laureillard, D. Significant enhancement in survival with early (2 weeks) vs. late (8 weeks) initiation of highly active antiretroviral treatment (HAART) in severely immunosuppressed HIV-infected adults with newly diagnosed tuberculosis, *Proceedings of the 18th International AIDS Society Conference*, Vienna, Austria, July, 2010.

Breslin, H.J., Kukla, M.J., Ludovici, D.W. et al. (1995). Synthesis and Anti-HIV-1 Activity of 4,5,6,7-Tetrahydro-5-methylimidazo[4,5,1-*jk*][1,4]benzodiazepine-2(1*H*)-one (TIBO) Derivatives 3. *Journal of Medicinal Chemistry*, vol. 38, pp.771-793, ISSN 0022-2623.

Burman, W.J. & Jones, B.E. (2001). Treatment of HIV-related tuberculosis in the era of effective antiretroviral therapy. *American Journal of Respiratory and Critical Care Medicine*, vol.164, No.1, (January 2001), pp. 7–12, ISSN 1073-449X.

Buu-Hoi, N.P., Xuong, N.D. (1953). The Thiourea Type of Tuberculostatic Compounds and Their Mechanism of Action. *Comptes Rendus Chimie*, vol. 237, pp.498-500, ISSN 1631-0748.

Centers for Disease Control and Prevention. (2007). Managing Drug Interactions in the Treatment of HIV-Related Tuberculosis, In: *Centers for Disease Control and Prevention*, 29.01.2011, Available from: <http://www.cdc.gov/tb/TB_HIV_Drugs/default.htm>

Chaisson, R.E., Schechter, G.F., Theuer, C.P. et al. (1987). Tuberculosis in patients with the acquired immunodeficiency syndrome: clinical features, response to therapy, and survival. *American Review of Respiratory Disease*, vol.136, pp.570–574, ISSN 0003-0805.

D'Cruz, O.J. & Uckun. F.M. (1999). Novel derivatives of phenethyl-5-bromopyridylthiourea and dihydroalkoxybenzyloxopyrimidine are dual-function spermicides with potent anti-human immunodeficiency virus activity. *Biology of reproduction*, vol.60, No.6, pp. 1419–1428, ISSN 0006-3363.

D'Cruz, O.J., Venkatachalam, T. K. & Uckun. F.M. (2000). Novel thiourea compounds as dual-function microbicides. *Biology of reproduction*, vol.63, No.1, pp. 196–205, ISSN 0006-3363.

D'Cruz, O.J., Venkatachalam, T. K. Mao, C. et al. (2002a). Structural requirements for potent anti-human immunodeficiency virus (HIV) and sperm-immobilizing activities of cyclohexenyl thiourea and urea non-nucleoside inhibitors of HIV-1 reverse transcriptase. *Biology of reproduction*, vol.67, No.6, pp. 1959–1974, ISSN 0006-3363.

D'Cruz, O.J., Waurzyniak, B. & Uckun. F.M. (2002b). A 13-week subchronic intravaginal toxicity study of the novel broad-spectrum anti-HIV and spermicidal agent, *N*-[2-(1-cyclohexenyl)ethyl]-*N* -[2-(5-bromopyridyl)]-thiourea (PHI-346) in Mice. *Toxicologic Pathology*, vol.30, No.6, pp. 687–695, ISSN 0192-6233.

D'Cruz, O.J. & Uckun. F.M. (2005). Discovery of 2,5-dimethoxy-substituted 5-bromopyridyl thiourea (PHI-236) as a potent broad-spectrum anti-human immunodeficiency virus microbicide. *Molecular Human Reproduction*, Vol.11, No.10, pp. 767–777, ISSN 1360-9947.

De Clercq, E. (2004). Non-Nucleoside Reverse Transcriptase Inhibitors (NNRTIs): Past, Present, and Future. *Chemistry & Biodiversity*, vol. 1, pp.44-64, ISSN 1612-1872.

Fitzgerald, D.W., Desvarieux, M., Severe, P. et al. (2000). Effect of post-treatment isoniazid on prevention of recurrent tuberculosis in HIV-1-infected individuals: a randomized trial. *The Lancet*, vol.356, No.9240, (October 2000), pp.1470–1474, ISSN 0140-6736.

Ho, W., Kukla, M.J., Breslin, H.J. et al. (1995). Synthesis and Anti-HIV-1 Activity of 4,5,6,7-Tetrahydro-5-methylimidazo[4,5,1-*jk*][1,4]benzodiazepine-2(1*H*)-one (TIBO) Derivatives 4. *Journal of Medicinal Chemistry*, vol. 38, pp.794-802, ISSN 0022-2623.

Högberg, M., Engelhardt, P., Vrang, L. et al. (2000). Bioisosteric modification of PETT-HIV-1 RT-inhibitors: synthesis and biological evaluation.*Bioorganic & Medicinal Chemistry Letters*, vol.10, No.3, pp. 265-268, ISSN 0960-894X.

Khan, F.A., Minion, J., Pai, M. et al. (2010).Treatment of active tuberculosis in HIV-coinfected patients: a systematic review and meta-analysis. *Clinical Infectious Diseases*, vol. 50, No.9, pp.1288–1299, ISSN 1058-4838

Kim, R.B., Fromm, M.F., Wandel, C. et al. (1998). The drug transporter Pglycoprotein limits oral absorption and brain entry of HIV-1 protease inhibitors. *Journal of Clinical Investigation*, vol.101, No.2, pp.289–294, ISSN 0021-9738.

König, A. (1970). Discussion on Isoxyl. *Antibiotica et Chemotherapia*, vol. 16, pp.187-202, ISSN 0376-0227.

Korduláková, J., Janin, Y.L., Liav, A. et al. (2007). Isoxyl Activation is Required for Bacteriostatic Activity against *Mycobacterium tuberculosis*. *Antimicrobial Agents and Chemotherapy*, vol. 51, No.11, pp.3824-3829, ISSN 0066-4804.

Kukla, M.J., Breslin, H.J., Pauwels, R. et al. (1991a). Synthesis and Anti-HIV-1 Activity of 4,5,6,7-Tetrahydro-5-methylimidazo[4,5,1-*jk*][1,4]benzodiazepine-2(1*H*)-one (TIBO) Derivatives. *Journal of Medicinal Chemistry*, vol. 34, pp.746-751, ISSN 0022-2623.

Kukla, M.J., Breslin, H.J., Diamond, C.J. et al. (1991b). Synthesis and Anti-HIV-1 Activity of 4,5,6,7-Tetrahydro-5-methylimidazo[4,5,1-*jk*][1,4]benzodiazepine-2(1*H*)-one (TIBO) Derivatives 2. *Journal of Medicinal Chemistry*, vol. 34, pp.3187-3197, ISSN 0022-2623.

Liav, A., Angala, S.K. & Brennan, P.J. (2008a). N-Glycosyl-N0-[p-(isoamyloxy)phenyl]-thiourea Derivatives: Potential Anti-TB Therapeutic Agents. *Synthetic Communications*, vol.38, No.8, pp. 1176–1183, ISSN 0039-7911.

Liav, A., Angala, S.K., Brennan, P.J. et al. (2008b). N-D-Aldopentofuranosyl-N´-[*p*-(isoamyloxy)phenyl]-thiourea derivatives: Potential anti-TB therapeutic agents. *Bioorganic & Medicinal Chemistry Letters*, vol.18, No.8, pp. 2649–2651, ISSN 0960-894X.

Mao, C., Vig, R., Venkatachalam, T. K. et al. (1998). Structure-based design of N-[2-(1-piperidinylethyl)]-N´-[2-(5-bromopyridyl)]-thiourea and N-[2-(1-piperazinylethyl)]-N´-[2-(5-bromopyridyl)]-thiourea a potent non-nucleoside inhibitors of HIV-1 reverse transcriptase. *Bioorganic & Medicinal Chemistry Letters*, vol.8, No.16, pp. 2213-2218, ISSN 0960-894X.

Mao, C., Sudbeck, E.A., Venkatachalam, T. K. et al. (1999). Rational design of N-[2-(2,5-dimethoxyphenylethyl)]-N´-[2-(5-bromopyridyl)]-thiourea (HI-236) as a potent non-nucleoside inhibitor of drug-resistant human immunodeficiency virus. *Bioorganic & Medicinal Chemistry Letters*, vol.9, No.11, pp. 1593-1598, ISSN 0960-894X.

Pauwels, R., Andries, K., Desmyter, J. et al. (1990). Potent and Selective Inhibition of HIV-1 replication *in vitro* by a Novel Series of TIBO Derivatives. *Nature*, vol. 343, pp.470-474, ISSN 0028-0836.

Perriens, J.H., St Louis, M,E., Mukadi, Y.B. et al. (1995). Pulmonary tuberculosis in HIV-infected patients in Zaire: a controlled trial of treatment for either 6 or 12 months. *The New England Journal of Medicine*, vol.332, No.12, (March 1995), pp.779–784, ISSN 0028-4793.

Phetsuksiri, B., Baulard, A.R., Cooper, A.M. et al. (1999). Antimycobacterial activities of isoxyl and new derivatives through the inhibition of mycolic acid synthesis. *Antimicrobial Agents and Chemotherapy*, vol.43, No.5, (May 1999), p. 1042–1051, ISSN 0066-4804.

Phetsuksiri, B., Jackson, M., Sherman, H. et al. (2003). Unique Mechanism of Action of the Thiourea Drug Isoxyl on *Mycobacterium tuberculosis*. *The Journal of Biological Chemistry*, vol. 278, No.52, pp.53123-53130, ISSN 0021-9258.

Pialoux, G., Youle, M., Dupont, B. et al. (1991). Pharmacokinetics of R 82913 in Patients with AIDS or AIDS-related Complex. *The Lancet*, vol. 338, pp.140-143, ISSN 0140-6736.

Piggott, D.A. & Karakousis, P.C. (2011). Timing of Antiretroviral Therapy for HIV in the Setting of TB Treatment. *Clinical and Developmental Immunology*, Vol.2011, pp.1-10, ISSN 1740-2522.

Sahlberg, C., Norren, R., Engelhardt, P. et al. (1998). Synthesis and anti-HIV activities of urea-PETT analogs belonging to a new class of potent nonnucleoside HIV-1 reverse transcriptase inhibitors. *Bioorganic & Medicinal Chemistry Letters*, vol.8, No.12, pp. 1511-1516, ISSN 0960-894X.

Schuetz, E.G., Schinke, A. H., Relling, M.V.,et al. (1996). P-glycoprotein: a major determinant of rifampicin–inducible expression of cytochrome P4503A in mice and humans. *Proceedings of the National Academy of Sciences*, vol.93, No.9, pp. 4001–4005, ISSN 0027-8424.

Sterling, T.R., Pham, P.A. & Chaisson, R.E. (2010). HIV Infection–Related Tuberculosis: Clinical Manifestations and Treatment. *Clinical Infectious Diseases*, vol.50, No.S3, pp.S223–S230, ISSN 1058-4838.

Sudbeck, E.A., Mao, C., Vig, R. et al. (1998). Structure-based design of novel dihydroalkoxybenzyloxopyrimidine derivatives as potent nonnucleoside inhibitors of the human immunodeficiency virus reverse transcriptase. *Antimicrobial Agents and Chemotherapy*, Vol. 42, No. 12, (December 1998), pp. 3225–3233, ISSN 0066-4804.

Tousek, J. (1970). On the Clinical Effectiveness of Isoxyl. *Antibiotica et Chemotherapia*, vol. 16, pp.149-155, ISSN 0376-0227.

Uckun, F.M., Mao, C., Pendergrass, S. et al. (1999a). N-[2-(1-cyclohexenyl)ethyl)]-N´-[2-(5-bromopyridyl)]-thiourea and N`-[2-(1-cyclohexenyl)ethyl)]-N´-[2-(5-chloropyridyl)]-thiourea as potent inhibitors of multidrug-resistant human immunodeficiency virus-1. *Bioorganic & Medicinal Chemistry Letters*, vol.9, No.18, pp. 2721-2726, ISSN 0960-894X.

Uckun, F.M., Pendergrass, S., Maher, D. et al. (1999b). N´-[2-(2-thiophene)ethyl)]-N´-[2-(5-bromopyridyl)]-thiourea a potent inhibitor of NNI-resistant and multidrug-resistant human immunodeficiency virus-1.*Bioorganic & Medicinal Chemistry Letters*, vol.9, No.24, pp. 3411-3416, ISSN 0960-894X.

United Nations Programme on HIV/AIDS. (2010). *Global report: UNAIDS report on the global AIDS epidemic 2010*, WHO press, ISBN 978-92-9173-871-7, Geneva, Switzerland.

Urbancik, B. (1970). Clinical Experience with Thiocarlide (Isoxyl). *Antibiotica et Chemotherapia*, vol. 16, pp.117-123, ISSN 0376-0227.

Velasco, M., Castilla, V., Sanz, J. et al. (2009). Effect of simultaneous use of highly active antiretroviral therapy on survival of HIV patients with tuberculosis. *Journal of Acquired Immune Deficiency Syndromes*, vol. 50, no. 2, pp. 148–152, ISSN 1525-4135.

Venkatachalam, T. K., Sudbeck, E.A., Mao, C. et al. (2000). Stereochemistry of halopyridyl and thiazolyl thiourea compounds is a major determinant of their potency as nonnucleoside inhibitors of HIV-1 reverse transcriptase. *Bioorganic & Medicinal Chemistry Letters*, vol.10, No.18, pp. 2071-2074, ISSN 0960-894X.

Venkatachalam, T. K., Sudbeck, E.A., Mao, C. et al. (2001). Anti-HIV activity of aromatic and heterocyclic thiazolyl thiourea compounds. *Bioorganic & Medicinal Chemistry Letters*, vol.11, No.4, pp. 523-528, ISSN 0960-894X.

Venkatachalam, Mao, C., Uckun, F.M. et al. (2004).Effect of stereochemistry on the anti-HIV activity of chiral thiourea compounds. *Bioorganic & Medicinal Chemistry*, vol.12, No.12, pp.4275–4284, ISSN 0968-0896.

Vig, R., Mao, C., Venkatachalam, T. K. et al. (1998). Rational design and synthesis of phenethyl-5-bromopyridyl thiourea derivatives as potent non-nucleoside inhibitors of HIV reverse transcriptase. *Bioorganic & Medicinal Chemistry*, vol.6, No.10, pp.1789-1797, ISSN 0968-0896.

Wang, C. & Hickey, A.J. (2010). Isoxyl particles for pulmonary delivery: In vitro cytotoxicity and potency. *International Journal of Pharmaceutics*, vol.396, No.1-2, pp. 99–104, ISSN 0378-5173.

World Health Organization. (2010a). *Global tuberculosis control: WHO Report 2010*, WHO press, ISBN 978 92 4 156406 9, Geneva, Switzerland.

World Health Organization. (2010b). *Treatment of tuberculosis: guidelines* (4th ed.), WHO Press, ISBN 978 92 4 154783 3, Geneva, Switzerland.

8

Quality of Life Assessment in People Living with HIV/AIDS: Clarifying the WHOQOL-HIV and WHOQOL-HIV-Bref Instruments

Bruno Pedroso, Gustavo Luis Gutierrez, Edison Duarte, Luiz Alberto Pilatti and Claudia Tania Picinin
Universidade Estadual de Campinas – UNICAMP
Brazil

1. Introduction

Assessing the quality of life (QoL) of people living with HIV/AIDS has become increasing. From 1995 to 2003, more than 300 papers on the subject were published. This fact encourages researchers to question the existence of suitable assessment instruments. Virtually all existing instruments until 2003 had been developed in the USA (Skevington & O'Connell, 2003).

To apply these instruments in countries in which English is not the vernacular language, the instruments were subjected to literal translations, without the worry of a cultural adaptation. In this wise, came the proposal to develop an instrument from sundry centers, located in different countries (Skevington & O'Connell, 2003).

The fact that there is no consensus on the QoL concept is a major problem in developing instruments to assess the QoL, while it is not possible to state clearly what elements these instruments are assessing (Fleck, 2008).

From this premise, the starting point to build the instrument for QoL assessment of the World Health Organization (WHO) was to conceptualize QoL. In the concept adopted, QoL is understood as "individuals' perceptions of their position in life in the context of the culture and value systems in which they live and in relation to their goals, expectations, standards and concerns" (The WHOQOL Group, 1998a, p. 25).

In face of this concept, WHO embarked on building the World Health Organization Quality of Life (WHOQOL) instruments, which assess QoL globally, e.g. WHOQOL-100 and WHOQOL-bref, and due to specific aspects, e.g. WHOQOL-HIV, WHOQOL-OLD, and WHOQOL-SRPB. One of these instruments, the WHOQOL-HIV, used to assess the QoL of HIV carriers, is the object of this study.

Starting from the fact that 95% of people infected with HIV did not live in the USA but in developing countries of Asia, Latin America, and sub-Saharan Africa, WHO has developed a tool to assess the QoL directed to such audience. The instrument was designed based on the premise that a multidisciplinary approach, involving centers in several countries, would allow for greater dissemination of the developed instrument (O'Connell, 2003).

The WHOQOL-HIV is a complementary module for WHOQOL-100 instrument, and was also translated into other languages and validated in sundry studies, among which are a part of Starace et al. (2002), Zimpel & Fleck (2007), Saddki et al. (2009), Canavarro et al. (2011) and Mweemba et al. (2011).

Notwithstanding the significant diffusion of the WHOQOL, questions concerning the calculation and analysis of the results of those instruments constitute a limitation for its use. In this context, we aimed here at clarifying the mechanism predetermined by the WHOQOL-HIV Group to calculate the WHOQOL-HIV and WHOQOL-HIV-bref instrument scores. Additionally, we proposed an alternative way to perform such calculations.

2. WHOQOL-100

The development of an instrument for evaluation of quality of life purposed by WHO was conducted in 15 centers simultaneously, based in 14 countries. After developing the project WHOQOL, new centers were built. Currently WHOQOL instruments are available in over 50 languages (WHO Field Center for Quality of Life of Bath, 2008).
The development methodology of WHOQOL was sectioned into four major stages: clarifying the concept of quality of life, qualitative pilot study, development of a pilot and finally, field implementation. For the integrated centers, after the completion of the instrument, a protocol was established which consisted in its translation, preparation of the test pilot, development of the response scales and administration of the pilot (The WHOQOL Group, 1998a).
All questions of WHOQOL-100 are closed. It was used a five-point Likert scale, ranging from 1 to 5. These extremes represent 0% and 100%, respectively. There are four different types of response scales, as can be seen in Table 1:

SCALE	0%	25%	50%	75%	100%
INTENSITY	Not at all	A little	A moderate amount	Very much	An extreme amount
	Not at all	Slightly	Moderately	Very	Extremely
EVALUATION	Very dissatisfied	Dissatisfied	Neither satisfied nor dissatisfied	Satisfied	Very satisfied
	Very poor	Poor	Neither poor nor good	Good	Very good
	Very unhappy	Unhappy	Neither happy nor unhappy	Happy	Very happy
CAPACITY	Not at all	A little	Moderately	Mostly	Completely
FREQUENCY	Never	Seldom	Quite often	Very often	Always

Source: Adapted from The WHOQOL Group (1998b)

Table 1. Response scale of WHOQOL-100

WHOQOL-100 aims at measuring the quality of life globally through six domains: Physical, Psychological, Level of independence, Social relationships, Environment e Spiritual/Religion/Personal beliefs. To obtain the results of WHOQOL instruments applications, the WHOQOL Group recommends the software Statistical Package for the Social Sciences (SPSS).

2.1 WHOQOL-100 scores calculation

The results of the WHOQOL-100 implementation are expressed through the scores of each facet and domain. The WHOQOL-100 scoring procedure presents the following logic:

- Verification of all those 100 questions completed with values between 1 and 5;
- Reversal of the 18 questions whose answer scale is inverted;
- Scores of facets calculation from the simple arithmetic average of questions that compose each facet, followed by a multiplication by four. The multiplication by four is used so that, in case of a question has not been answered, the score of a facet compensates the invalidation of the question through the product by the number of valid questions that the facet should have. It will be computed only those aspects that have at least three valid items;
- Scores of each domain are calculated through the simple arithmetic average of the facets scores that compose each area. In domains composed of up to five facets, this will be calculated only if the number of facets not calculated is not equal to or greater than two. In domains consisting of more than five facets, the domain will be calculated only if the number of facets not calculated is not equal to or greater than three. In the case of facets in reversed scale (all questions within the facet have reversed response scale), there will be an inversion of that facet to proceed the calculation;
- Scores of domains and facets are converted to a scale from 0 to 100;
- Total number of items answered by each respondent is counted. In the calculation are computed only those respondents who completed at least 80 items correctly (80% of the instrument items).

The WHOQOL-100 results are expressed in two scales, a variant scale between 4 and 20 points, due to the fact that the facets scores calculation is achieved by multiplying the average of questions that constitute each facet by four. Once each domain is calculated by the simple arithmetic average of facets that composes it. The results are expressed on the same scale of facets. The results are also expressed on a scale from 0 to 100.

2.2 Questions and facets response scale conversion

The conversion of questions is used in order to standardize all the answers of the instrument, so that the most positive response is 5. Therefore, the most negative response must be 1. Thus, all questions of each facet are converted to the same scale, where the gradual increase in response is equivalent in the same proportion to the increase in the result of the facet.

In cases where all four questions that constitute a facet are arranged in inverted scale, that same logic is used, but only in the domain calculation. That is, the result of these facets is expressed in the original scale: without inversion (the closer to 1, the more positive the result; the closer to 5, the more negative the result). However, when calculating the scores of areas where such facets are found, the score of the latter is converted.

For the conversion of the response scale of questions, the minimum value of the inverted scale question should be replaced by the maximum value of the normal scale question, and the maximum value of the inverted scale question should be replaced by a minimum value of the normal scale question. The same should occur with intermediate values, following this same logic. Thus, the only value that remains unchanged is the central value, which will remain the same in both normal and inverted scales.

It is necessary to be attentive to this fact, because when comparing the results between the facets, the score of a facet with inverted scale cannot be directly compared to the score of a facet with normal scale. The answers 1, 2, 3, 4 and 5 are to take the values 5, 4, 3, 2 and 1, respectively. The same procedure is used in the conversion of inverted facets, where the scores 4, 8, 12, 16 and 20 are to take the values 20, 16, 12, 8 and 4, respectively.

2.3 WHOQOL-100 questions, domains and facets

Composed by 100 questions, the WHOQOL-100 is sectioned into 24 groups of four questions each, receiving the name of "facets". The group of facets constitutes a "domain". Unlike the composition of facets, the six WHOQOL-100 domains are not constituted by the same number of facets, and may vary from one to eight.
The questions that compose WHOQOL-100 are not arranged in the questionnaire in a logical sequence by domain or facet. They are grouped by type of answer scale. The distribution of WHOQOL-100 facets and areas are listed in Table 2:

DOMAINS	FACETS
Domain I - Physical	1. Pain and discomfort
	2. Energy e fatigue
	3. Sleep and rest
Domain II - Psychological	4. Positive feelings
	5. Thinking, learning, memory and concentration
	6. Self-esteem
	7. Bodily image and appearance
	8. Negative feelings
Domain III - Level of Independence	9. Mobility
	10. Activities of daily living
	11. Dependence on medication or treatments
	12. Work capacity
Domain IV - Social Relationships	13. Personal relationships
	14. Social support
	15. Sexual activity
Domain V - Environment	16. Physical safety and security
	17. Home environment
	18. Financial resources
	19. Health and social care: accessibility and quality
	20. Opportunities for acquiring new information and skills
	21. Participation in and opportunities for recreation/ leisure activities
	22. Physical environment (pollution/noise/traffic/climate)
	23. Transport
Domain VI - Spiritual/Religion/Personal Beliefs	24. Spiritual/Religion/Personal Beliefs

Source: The WHOQOL Group (1998a)

Table 2. Domains and facets of WHOQOL-100

WHOQOL-100 has a facet that is not included in any domain, the facet Overall Quality of Life and General Health Perceptions (The WHOQOL Group, 1998b). This aspect deals with a self-assessment of quality of life, where the respondents express their point of view concerning their satisfaction with their lives, health and quality of life.

2.4 Short version of WHOQOL-100 (WHOQOL-bref)

Aiming at providing a tool that demand less time to its filling out, and with satisfactory psychometric characteristics, the WHOQOL Group developed the short version of WHOQOL-100, the WHOQOL-bref (The WHOQOL Group, 1996).

The WHOQOL-bref is composed of 26 questions - two questions on self-assessment of quality of life and 24 issues representing each facet of WHOQOL-100. To compound the questions of WHOQOL-bref, it was selected the question of each facet that present the highest correlation with the average score of all facets (The WHOQOL Group, 1998c).

After the selection of issues, an analysis was conducted to see if they, factually, represented the corresponding facets. In six facets, the question selected was replaced by another question of the corresponding facet, for, under the bias of experts, there was another question that could best define these six facets (The WHOQOL Group, 1998c). The facets belonging to the domain Level of Independence were incorporated into the Physical domain and the facet belonging to the domain Spiritual / Religion / Personal Beliefs was incorporated into the Psychological domain. Thus, the WHOQOL-bref is composed by four domains: Physical, Psychological, Social Relationships and Environment, completing the configuration expressed in Table 3:

DOMAINS	FACETS
Domain I - Physical	1. Pain and discomfort
	2. Energy e fatigue
	3. Sleep and rest
	4. Mobility
	5. Activities of daily living
	6. Dependence on medication or treatments
	7. Work capacity
Domain II - Psychological	8. Positive feelings
	9. Thinking, learning, memory and concentration
	10. Self-esteem
	11. Bodily image and appearance
	12. Negative feelings
	13. Spiritual/Religion/Personal Beliefs
Domain III - Social Relationships	14. Personal relationships
	15. Social support
	16. Sexual activity
Domain IV - Environment	17. Physical safety and security
	18. Home environment
	19. Financial resources
	20. Health and social care: accessibility and quality
	21. Opportunities for acquiring new information and skills
	22. Participation in and opportunities for recreation/ leisure activities
	23. Physical environment (pollution/noise/traffic/climate)
	24. Transport

Source: The WHOQOL Group (1998c)

Table 3. Domains and facets of WHOQOL-bref

The calculation of scores of WHOQOL-bref follows the same logic of WHOQOL-100, except for the calculation of scores of facets. In WHOQOL-bref each facet is represented by a single question, and therefore the scores of facets are not calculated (The WHOQOL Group, 1996).

3. WHOQOL-HIV

Aiming at creating a tool for assessing the quality of life directed to people living with HIV, researchers from the Joint United Nations Program on HIV / AIDS (UNAIDS) and WHO carried out studies in people with HIV in nine different countries. The result of this study was the instrument WHOQOL-HIV, an additional module specifically designed for people with HIV or AIDS (WHO Field Center for the Study of Quality of Life of Bath, 2008).

WHOQOL-HIV evaluates the quality of life from six domains and 29 facets. The domains and facets are the same as in WHOQOL-100, with the addition of five specific facets for people living with HIV/AIDS. The facet of WHOQOL-100 that evaluates the quality of life from the perspective of the assessed person, not included in any domain, remains in WHOQOL-HIV. The specific facets for people with HIV, as well as the facets from WHOQOL-100, are composed of four questions (O'Connell et al., 2004). The additional facets of WHOQOL-HIV are:

- Symptoms of PLWHA: physical problems that people living with HIV/AIDS (PLWHA) could present;
- Social Inclusion: individual's acceptance in society that he/she lives;
- Forgiveness and blame: feeling of blame that the individual has about his/her HIV infection;
- Concerns about the future: fear and worries concerning changes in individual's lifestyle after HIV infection;
- Death and dying: worries about dead, such as place, reason and suffering before dying.

The additional facets of WHOQOL-HIV are included in the domains already existent in WHOQOL-100, featuring the following configuration (Table 4):

DOMAINS	**FACETS**
Domain I - Physical	50. Symptoms of PLWHA
Domain IV - Social Relationships	51. Social Inclusion
Domain VI - Spiritual/Religion/Personal Beliefs	52. Forgiveness and Blame
	53. Concerns about the Future
	54. Death and Dying

Source: Adapted from O'Connell et al. (2004)

Table 4. Domains and facets exclusive of WHOQOL-HIV

Based on the previously mentioned configuration, questions which constitute additional facets of WHOQOL-HIV, with inverted questions written in italics, are:

FACETS	QUESTIONS
Symptoms of PLWHA	*How much are you bothered by any unpleasant physical problems related to your HIV infection?*
	To what extent do you fear possible future (physical) pain?
	To what extent do you feel any unpleasant physical problems prevent you from doing things that are important to you?
	To what extent are you bothered by fears of developing any physical problem?
Social Inclusion	To what extent do you feel accepted by the people you know?
	How often do you feel you are discriminated against because of your health condition?
	To what extent do you feel accepted by your community?
	How much do you feel alienated from those around you?
Forgiveness and Blame	*How much do you blame yourself for your HIV infection?*
	To what extent are you bothered by people blaming you for your HIV status?
	How guilty do you feel about being HIV positive?
	To what extent do you feel guilty when you need the help and care of others?
Concerns about the Future	*To what extent are you concerned about your HIV status breaking your family line and your future generations?*
	To what extent are you concerned about how people will remember you when you are dead?
	To what extent do any feelings that you are suffering from fate or destiny bother you?
	How much do you fear the future?
Death and Dying	*How much do you worry about death?*
	How bothered are you by the thought of not being able to die the way you would want to?
	How concerned are you about how and where you will die?
	How preoccupied are you about suffering before dying?

Source: Adapted from Zimpel & Fleck (2008)

Table 5. Additional questions of WHOQOL-HIV

The syntax for calculation of WHOQOL-HIV domain and facets' score, correcting the error reported by Pedroso et al. (2010), is the following:

STEPS	WHOQOL-HIV SYNTAX
Check all 120 items from assessment have a range of 1-5	RECODE F11 F12 F13 F14 F21 F22 F23 F24 F31 F32 F33 F34 F501 F502 F503 F504 F41 F42 F43 F44 F51 F52 F53 F54 F61 F62 F63 F64 F71 F72 F73 F74 F81 F82 F83 F84 F91 F92 F93 F94 F101 F102 F103 F104 F111 F112 F113 F114 F121 F122 F123 F124 F131 F132 F133 F134 F141 F142 F143 F144 F151 F152 F153 F154 F511 F512 F513 F514 F161 F162 F163 F164 F171 F172 F173 F174 F181 F182 F183 F184 F191 F192 F193 F194 F201 F202 F203 F204 F211 F212 F213 F214 F221 F222 F223 F224 F231 F232 F233 F234 F241 F242 F243 F244 F521 F522 F523 F524 F531 F532 F533 F534 F541 F542 F543 F544 G1 G2 G3 G4 (1=1) (2=2) (3=3) (4=4) (5=5) (ELSE=SYSMIS).
Reverse negatively phrased items	RECODE F11 F12 F13 F14 F22 F24 F32 F34 F72 F73 F81 F82 F83 F84 F93 F94 F102 F104 F111 F112 F113 F114 F131 F154 F163 F182 F184 F222 F232 F234 F501 F502 F503 F504 F514 F512 F521 F522 F523 F524 F531 F532 F533 F534 F541 F542 F544 F543 (1=5) (2=4) (3=3) (4=2) (5=1) (1=5) (2=4) (3=3) (4=2) (5=1).
Compute facet and domain scores	COMPUTE PAIN=(F11+F12+F13+F14)/4. COMPUTE ENERGY=(F21+F22+F23+F24)/4. COMPUTE SLEEP=(F31+F32+F33+F34)/4. COMPUTE SYMPTOM=(F501+F502+F503+F504)/4. COMPUTE PFEEL=(F41+F42+F43+F44)/4. COMPUTE COG=(F51+F52+F53+F54)/4. COMPUTE ESTEEM=(F61+F62+F63+F64)/4. COMPUTE BODY=(F71+F72+F73+F74)/4. COMPUTE NFEEL=(F81+F82+F83+F84)/4. COMPUTE MOBIL=(F91+F92+F93+F94)/4. COMPUTE ADL=(F101+F102+F103+F104)/4. COMPUTE DEPEND=(F111+F112+F113+F114)/4. COMPUTE WORK=(F121+F122+F123+F124)/4. COMPUTE RELATIO=(F131+F132+F133+F134)/4. COMPUTE SUPPORT=(F141+F142+F143+F144)/4. COMPUTE SEX=(F151+F152+F153+F154)/4. COMPUTE INCLUSI=(F511+F512+F513+F514)/4. COMPUTE SAFE=(F161+F162+F163+F164)/4. COMPUTE HOME=(F171+F172+F173+F174)/4. COMPUTE FINANCE=(F181+F182+F183+F184)/4. COMPUTE CARE=(F191+F192+F193+F194)/4. COMPUTE INFO=(F201+F202+F203+F204)/4. COMPUTE LEISURE=(F211+F212+F213+F214)/4. COMPUTE ENVIRO=(F221+F222+F223+F224)/4. COMPUTE TRANS=(F231+F232+F233+F234)/4. COMPUTE SRPB=(F241+F242+F243+F244)/4. COMPUTE FORGIVE=(F521+F522+F523+F524)/4. COMPUTE FUTURE=(F531+F532+F533+F534)/4.

STEPS	WHOQOL-HIV SYNTAX
	COMPUTE DEATH=(F541+F542+F543+F544)/4. COMPUTE GENERAL=(G1+G2+G3+G4)/4. COMPUTE DOMAIN1=(PAIN+ENERGY+SLEEP+SYMPTOM)/4*4. COMPUTE DOMAIN2=(PFEEL+COG+ESTEEM+BODY+NFEEL)/5*4. COMPUTE DOMAIN3=(MOBIL+ADL+DEPEND+WORK)/4*4. COMPUTE DOMAIN4=(RELATIO+SUPPORT+SEX+INCLUSI)/4*4. COMPUTE DOMAIN5=(SAFE+HOME+FINANCE+CARE+INFO+LEISURE+ ENVIRO+TRANS)/8*4. COMPUTE DOMAIN6=(FORGIVE+FUTURE+DEATH+SRPB)/4*4.

Source: Adapted from The WHOQOL-HIV Group (2002)

Table 6. WHOQOL-HIV syntax

The calculation of WHOQOL-HIV results is similar to the method used in WHOQOL-100. However, some criteria used in WHOQOL-100 were not inherited by WHOQOL-HIV. The results of the WHOQOL-HIV are presented as follows:

- Verification of all those 120 questions completed with values between 1 and 5;
- Reversal of all the questions whose answers scale is inverted. Concerning the facets in inverted scale, all the questions pertaining to these facets are individually inverted;
- Scores of facets are calculated from the sum of the four questions of each facet, followed by a division by four, being represented in a scale of 1 to 5;
- Scores of domains are calculated by the sum of the scores of "n" facets that compound each area, divided by the number of the domain facets. The result is multiplied by four, being represented in a scale of 4 to 20;

Contrarily to WHOQOL-100, the scores of domains and facets represent the mean of these variables only when all the belonging items to these are correctly punctuated. The score of facets is calculated since these presents one or more answered question, while the score of domains is calculated since these owns at least one facet that has been scored. The scores are not converted to a 0-100 scale. The exclusion criterion for individuals who answered incorrectly or doesn't answer more than 20% of total items from instrument does not exist on WHOQOL-HIV syntax.

4. WHOQOL-HIV-bref

Under the same reason for the development of WHOQOL-bref, the WHOQOL Group developed an abbreviated version of WHOQOL-HIV. The WHOQOL-HIV-bref is based on WHOQOL-bref, in a way each facet is represented by one single question.

The 26 questions of WHOQOL-bref are repeated in WHOQOL-HIV-bref, being added to these five questions that represent the additional facets of WHOQOL-HIV (The WHOQOL-HIV Group, 2002). Contrary to what occurs in WHOQOL-bref, the facets belonging to the domains Level of Independence and Spiritual/Religion/Personal Beliefs are not incorporated to the Physical and Psychological domains, having, therefore, the same configuration of the domains of WHOQOL-HIV, presenting the following configuration:

DOMAINS	QUESTIONS
Domain I - Physical	*To what extent do you feel that physical pain prevents you from doing what you need to do?*
	Do you have enough energy for everyday life?
	How satisfied are you with your sleep?
	How much are you bothered by any physical problems related to your HIV infection?
Domain II - Psychological	How much do you enjoy life?
	How well are you able to concentrate?
	Are you able to accept your bodily appearance?
	How satisfied are you with yourself?
	How often do you have negative feelings such as blue mood, despair, anxiety, depression?
Domain III – Level of Independence	*How much do you need any medical treatment to function in your daily life?*
	H ow well are you able to get around?
	How satisfied are you with your ability to perform your daily living activities?
	How satisfied are you with your capacity for work?
Domain IV – Social Relations	To what extent do you feel accepted by the people you know?
	How satisfied are you with your personal relationships?
	How satisfied are you with your sex life?
	How satisfied are you with the support you get from your friends?
Domain V - Environment	How safe do you feel in your daily life?
	How healthy is your physical environment?
	Have you enough money to meet your needs?
	How available to you is the information that you need in your day-to-day life?
	To what extent do you have the opportunity for leisure activities?
	How satisfied are you with the conditions of your living place?
	How satisfied are you with your access to health services?
	How satisfied are you with your transport?
Domain VI - Spiritual / Religion / Personal Beliefs	To what extent do you feel your life to be meaningful?
	To what extent are you bothered by people blaming you for your HIV status?
	How much do you fear the future?
	How much do you worry about death?
Overall Quality of Life and General Health Perceptions	How would you rate your quality of life?
	How satisfied are you with your health?

Source: Adapted from The WHOQOL-HIV Group (2002)

Table 7. Questions of WHOQOL-HIV-bref

The calculation of WHOQOL-HIV-bref's score then follows a different logic regarding WHOQOL-bref instrument, consisting of the following command lines:

STEPS	WHOQOL-HIV-BREF SYNTAX
Check all 31 items from assessment have a range of 1-5	RECODE Q1 Q2 Q3 Q4 Q5 Q6 Q7 Q8 Q9 Q10 Q11 Q12 Q13 Q14 Q15 Q16 Q17 Q18 Q19 Q20 Q21 Q22 Q23 Q24 Q25 Q26 Q27 Q28 Q29 Q30 Q31 (1=1) (2=2) (3=3) (4=4) (5=5) (ELSE=SYSMIS).
Reverse negatively phrased items	RECODE Q3 Q4 Q5 Q8 Q9 Q10 Q31 (1=5) (2=4) (3=3) (4=2) (5=1).
Compute domain scores	COMPUTE Domain 1 = (Q3 + Q4 + Q14 + Q21)/4 * 4 COMPUTE Domain 2 = (Q6 + Q11 + Q15 + Q24 + Q31)/5 *4 COMPUTE Domain 3 = (Q5 + Q22 + Q23 + Q20)/4 * 4 COMPUTE Domain 4 = (Q27 +Q26 + Q25 + Q17)/4*4 COMPUTE Domain 5 = (Q12 + Q13 + Q16 + Q18 + Q19 + Q28 + Q29 + Q30)/8 *4 COMPUTE Domain6 = (Q7 + Q8 + Q9+ Q10)/4 *4

Source: The WHOQOL-HIV Group (2002)

Table 8. WHOQOL-HIV-bref syntax

The WHOQOL-HIV-bref syntax's textual transcription presents the following configuration:
- Verification of all those 31 questions completed with values between 1 and 5;
- Reversal of all the questions whose answers scale is inverted;
- Scores of domains are calculated by the sum of the scores of "n" questions that compound each area, divided by the number of the domain questions. The result is multiplied by four, being represented in a scale of 4 to 20;

As can be realized, just as WHOQOL-HIV, the WHOQOL-HIV-bref's Syntax presents the same present fragility found in WHOQOL-HIV regarding the domains and facets score calculation, because it's not accomplished the arithmetic mean of domain items. There is not also the conversion of domains and facets score for a 0-100 scale. Lastly, and is not existing the criteria of exclusion of individuals who doesn't answer or answered incorrectly a number of questions higher than 20% from the total instrument items.

5. Tools for the calculation of scores and descriptive statistics of WHOQOL-HIV and WHOQOL-HIV-bref instruments

To obtain the results to apply the WHOQOL instruments, WHOQOL Group recommends the use of SPSS software, a statistical software program that requires specific expertise for its use and is not for free distribution.

Looking for the removal of such limitations, tools were built from the software Microsoft Excel, a software program for broad accessibility, to calculate scores and descriptive statistics for WHOQOL-HIV and for WHOQOL-HIV-bref. Such tools were made in the same manner as the tool developed by Pedroso et al. (2009) to calculate scores and descriptive statistics of WHOQOL-100.

The tools proposed on this study automatically perform all calculations in the incipient syntaxes provided by the WHOQOL-HIV Group. The researchers who use it need only to fill in the specified cells the answers given by respondents.
After data insertion, to use the results of theirs research, researcher may copy the individual scores for each respondent, results of descriptive statistics, and graphics; however, without changing such results. Is allowed to insert and edit values just in the area to tabulate the answers of respondents.
To validate such tools, simulations were performed with real data applications of each of the WHOQOL-HIV and WHOQOL-HIV-bref instrument, comparing the results by using the proposed tools with those from SPSS. The results from both software programs were exactly the same, thus ensuring the reliability of tools, which are object of this study.
The tools were tested on different versions of the Microsoft Office: 2000, XP, 2003, 2007 and 2010. It was found that they are compatible with all versions tested, without differences in the results. The tools are available for download in the website: http://www.brunopedroso.com.br/whoqol-hiv(en). html.

6. Conclusions

Although the WHOQOL-HIV and WHOQOL-HIV-bref instruments are respectively additional modules for WHOQOL-100 and WHOQOL-bref instruments, the syntax of these instruments are not entirely derivative from its precursor syntax. Despite the widespread distribution and use of the WHOQOL-HIV and WHOQOL-HIV-bref, the difficulty to interpret the instrument syntax limits in choosing to use such tools.
Additionally, the WHOQOL Group interposition in making the syntax to calculate the WHOQOL scores with SPSS (a relatively high cost software program and which requires specific expertise for use) encourages another imbroglio, restricting the use of WHOQOL instruments.
Facing this struggle, we here investigate the instruments in question to facilitate their interpretation and use. Looking for the removal of the previously described limitations, the syntaxes are transcribed textually, detailing all the steps used to obtain the results from WHOQOL-HIV and WHOQOL-HIV-bref instrument. Were also built tools from Microsoft Excel 2003 software to calculate the scores and descriptive statistics of such instruments, in which the researcher is responsible only for data tabulation. The calculation is carried out automatically.
The developed tools were tested and proved compatible in the versions 2000, XP, 2007 and 2010 of Microsoft Excel. The results returned by the tools were compared by using real application data of WHOQOL-HIV and WHOQOL-HIV-bref instruments, with the results returned by SPSS, following the parameters established by the WHOQOL-HIV Group. The results were identical to both instruments.
We conclude that, despite being globally disseminated instruments, developed under a rigorous methodology, the instruments produced by the WHOQOL-HIV Group show limitations. Expecting to facilitate its use, was made an approach with a focus on clarifying these instruments. In this wise, we aimed to enable greater accessibility of the results promoted by the instruments, object of study here, thus expanding the investigation involving QoL empirical reality of people living with HIV/AIDS.

7. References

Canavarro, M.C. et al. (2011). Quality of life assessment in HIV-infection: validation of the European Portuguese version of WHOQOL-HIV. *AIDS Care*, Vol. 23, No 2, (February 2011), pp. 187-194, ISSN 0954-0121

Fleck, M.P.A. (2008). Problemas conceituais em qualidade de vida. In: *A avaliação de qualidade de vida: guia para profissionais da saúde*, Fleck, M.P.A., et al. (Eds.), pp. 19-28. Artmed, ISBN 978-85-363-0947-7, Porto Alegre, Brazil

Mweemba, P. et al. (2011). Validation of the World Health Organization Quality of Life HIV instrument in a Zambian sample. *Journal of the Association of Nurses in AIDS Care*, Vol. 22, No 1, (February 2011), pp. 53-66, ISSN 1055-3290

O'Connell, K. et al. (2003). Preliminary development of the World Health Organization's Quality of Life HIV instrument (WHOQOL-HIV): analysis of the pilot version. *Social & Science Medicine*, Vol. 57, No 7, (October 2003), pp. 1259-1275, ISSN 0277-9536

O'Connell, K. et al. (2004). WHOQOL-HIV for quality of life assessment among people living with HIV and AIDS: results from a field test. *AIDS Care*, Vol 16, No 7, (October 2004), pp. 882-889, ISSN 0954-0121

Pedroso, B. et al. (2009). Cálculo dos escores e estatística descritiva do WHOQOL-100 utilizando o Microsoft Excel. *Revista Brasileira de Qualidade de Vida*, Vol 1, No 1, (July 2009), pp. 23-32, ISSN 2175-0858

Pedroso, B. et al. (2010). Quality of life assessment in people with HIV: analysis of the WHOQOL-HIV syntax. *AIDS Care*, Vol. 22, No 3, (March 2010), pp. 361,372, ISSN 0954-0121

Saddki, N. et al. (2009). Validity and reliability of the Malay version of WHOQOL-HIV BREF in patients with HIV infection. *AIDS Care*, Vol. 21, No 10, (October 2009), pp. 1271-1278, ISSN 0954-0121

Skevington, S.M. & O'Connell, K. A. (2003). Measuring Quality of Life in HIV and AIDS: A Review of the Recent Literature. *AIDS Care*, Vol. 18, No 3, (June 2003), pp. 331-350, ISSN 0954-0121

Starace, F. et al. (2002). Quality of life assessment in HIV-positive persons: application and validation of the WHOQOL-HIV, Italian version. *AIDS Care*, Vol. 14, No 3, (June 2002), pp. 405-415, ISSN 0954-0121

The WHOQOL Group. (1998a). The World Health Organization Quality of Life assessment (WHOQOL): development and general psychometric properties. *Social Science & Medicine*, Vol. 46, No 12, (December 1998), pp. 1569-1585, ISSN 0277-9536

The WHOQOL Group. (1998b). *WHOQOL User Manual*. Geneva

The WHOQOL Group. (1998c). Development of the World Health Organization WHOQOL-BREF Quality of Life Assessment. *Psychological Medicine*, Vol. 28, No 3, (May 1998), pp. 551-558, ISSN 0033-2917

The WHOQOL Group. (1996). *WHOQOL-bref: introduction, administration, scoring and generic version of assessment*. Geneva

The WHOQOL-HIV Group. (2002). *WHOQOL-HIV Instrument Users Manual*. Geneva

WHO Field Center for the Study of Quality of Life of Bath. (2008). About the WHO Field Center for the Study of Quality of Life. In: *University of Bath*. Retrieved on 20.09.2008 Available from http://www.bath.ac.uk/whoqol/about.cfm

Zimpel, R. & Fleck, M.P.A. (2007) Quality of life in HIV-positive Brazilians: application and validation of the WHOQOL-HIV, Brazilian version. *AIDS Care*, Vol. 19, No 7, (August 2007), pp. 923-930, ISSN 0954-0121

Zimpel, R & Fleck, M.P.A. (2008). WHOQOL-HIV: desenvolvimento, aplicação e validação. In: *A avaliação de qualidade de vida: guia para profissionais da saúde*, Fleck, M.P.A., et al. (Eds.), pp. 83-92. Artmed, ISBN 978-85-363-0947-7, Porto Alegre, Brazil